Teacher's Guide to ADHD

WHAT WORKS FOR SPECIAL-NEEDS LEARNERS
Karen R. Harris and Steve Graham
Editors

Strategy Instruction for Students with Learning Disabilities
Robert Reid and Torri Ortiz Lienemann

Teaching Mathematics to Middle School Students with Learning Difficulties
Marjorie Montague and Asha K. Jitendra, Editors

Teaching Word Recognition: Effective Strategies for Students
with Learning Difficulties
Rollanda E. O'Connor

Teaching Reading Comprehension to Students with Learning Difficulties
Janette K. Klingner, Sharon Vaughn, and Alison Boardman

Promoting Self-Determination in Students with Developmental Disabilities
*Michael L. Wehmeyer with Martin Agran, Carolyn Hughes, James E. Martin,
Dennis E. Mithaug, and Susan B. Palmer*

Instructional Practices for Students with Behavioral Disorders:
Strategies for Reading, Writing, and Math
J. Ron Nelson, Gregory J. Benner, and Paul Mooney

Working with Families of Young Children with Special Needs
R. A. McWilliam, Editor

Promoting Executive Function in the Classroom
Lynn Meltzer

Managing Challenging Behaviors in Schools:
Research-Based Strategies That Work
Kathleen Lynne Lane, Holly Mariah Menzies, Allison L. Bruhn, and Mary Crnobori

Explicit Instruction: Effective and Efficient Teaching
Anita L. Archer and Charles A. Hughes

Teacher's Guide to ADHD
Robert Reid and Joseph Johnson

Teacher's Guide to ADHD

Robert Reid
Joseph Johnson

THE GUILFORD PRESS
New York   London

Printed in the United States of America

This book is printed on acid-free paper.

Last digit is print number: 9   8   7   6   5   4   3   2   1

The authors have checked with sources believed to be reliable in their efforts to provide
information that is complete and generally in accord with the standards of practice that
are accepted at the time of publication. However, in view of the possibility of human error
or changes in behavioral, mental health, or medical sciences, neither the authors, nor
the editor and publisher, nor any other party who has been involved in the preparation
or publication of this work warrants that the information contained herein is in every
respect accurate or complete, and they are not responsible for any errors or omissions or
the results obtained from the use of such information. Readers are encouraged to confirm
the information contained in this book with other sources.

Library of Congress Cataloging-in-Publication Data

Reid, Robert.
  Teacher's guide to ADHD / Robert Reid, Joseph Johnson.
    p. cm. — (What works for special-needs learners)
  Includes bibliographical references and index.
  ISBN 978-1-60918-979-2 (pbk.) — ISBN 978-1-60918-980-8 (hardcover)
  1. Attention-deficit-disordered children— Education—United States.   2. Hyperactive
children—Education—United States.   I. Johnson, Joseph.   II. Title.
  LC4713.4.R386 2011
  371.94—dc23

                                                          2011030576

For those who helped along the way

About the Authors

Robert Reid, PhD, is Professor in the Department of Special Education and Communication Disorders at the University of Nebraska–Lincoln. He has done extensive work nationally and internationally on children with ADHD and on cognitive strategy instruction. He has also conducted research with youth in residential settings and in out-of-home care. Dr. Reid has published over 100 articles and book chapters and presented at national and international conferences. He is coauthor of the *ADHD Rating Scale–IV,* which is now used in seven countries, and *Strategy Instruction for Students with Learning Disabilities.* He received the Special Education Student Research Award from the American Educational Research Association in 1992 and the Jeannie P. Baliles Child Mental Health Research Award from the Virginia Treatment Center for Children in 1996. Dr. Reid currently serves on the editorial boards of five journals and actively reviews for a number of others.

Joseph Johnson, PhD, is Assistant Professor in the Department of Educational Studies at the University of Wisconsin–La Crosse. Prior to earning his doctorate in special education, he taught in public secondary schools for over 13 years, including 6 years as a special education teacher in both resource and cotaught classrooms. His interests include cognitive strategy instruction and academic interventions for adolescents with ADHD.

Preface

Children with attention-deficit/hyperactivity disorder (ADHD) constitute from 5 to 7% of the school-age population. Treatment for children with ADHD may also involve a number of different professional groups, including psychologists, medical practitioners, family therapists, and educators. Of these groups, educators will spend by far the most time with these children. Because of this fact, schools should play a central role in their treatment. Unfortunately, educators all too often are provided little if any background knowledge and training in ADHD and effective interventions for working with children with ADHD.

Ironically, if educators attempt to seek out information on ADHD they encounter another problem. There is an ocean of information on ADHD, from periodicals, books, and scholarly articles, to support groups, "how-to" books, and websites, to name a few. Want to find "the latest and greatest miracle cure for ADHD"? It's out there—and someone will be glad to sell it to you. New techniques, "miracle cures," and treatments pop up, disappear, and reappear like clockwork. Unfortunately, many lack any semblance of a theoretical base, and, even more important, are not empirically supported by research. To further confuse the situation, myths, misconceptions, and misinformation about ADHD are abundant. Teachers need a sound factual working knowledge of ADHD. Many parents will approach teachers for advice on treatment options or with basic questions about ADHD. Teachers should be in a position to provide accurate information and should be knowledgeable about effective accommodations and interventions that can help children with ADHD succeed in the schools.

The purpose of this book is to provide practical, immediately useful information for educators who work with students with ADHD. The focus is on the "big ideas." In each chapter we identify key concepts/information that teachers need to know and provide practical "how-to" knowledge and useful resources. Rather than discuss a topic at the abstract level we provide specific information. When discussing interventions or accommodations, we provide step-by-step instructions on how to implement them.

Chapters 1 and 2 provide background information on ADHD. Chapter 1 is intended to dispel some widespread myths and misperceptions about ADHD and students with ADHD. It provides an overview of the extent of the problems posed by ADHD along with a brief historical overview. We stress that ADHD is not a recent phenomenon, but has been documented for hundreds of years. In Chapter 2 we describe the features of ADHD and present and explain the diagnostic criteria. The common comorbid conditions (e.g., oppositional defiant disorder, conduct disorder, depression) are noted and their ramifications discussed. Major theories of ADHD are also introduced.

Chapter 3 deals with the ADHD assessment process. We note the steps entailed in the assessment process and how teachers are involved; discuss the types of assessment instruments and how they are used in the assessment process; and list instruments commonly used in the ADHD assessment process in schools. We also discuss major issues/concerns in the ADHD assessment process.

Chapters 4 and 5 cover how children with ADHD are served in the schools. In Chapter 4 we discuss how these children fit in the special education system, and how Section 504 relates to children with ADHD. In Chapter 5 we introduce the multimodal treatment model for ADHD: medication, behavioral interventions, classroom accommodations, and ancillary services (e.g., social skills training). Educators will be involved to some degree in all of these treatments. Important program planning considerations are noted. Finally, we provide an overview of questionable treatments for ADHD and give tips for spotting them.

Parents are a critical part of the ADHD treatment process. Chapter 6 provides tips on how to involve parents in the treatment of their children and also discusses why it may sometimes be difficult for some parents to help. We review some of the problems that parents of children with ADHD may face. We also provide information on supports for parents and a simple home–school intervention that has been demonstrated to be effective.

Medication is a recommended and widely used treatment for ADHD. However, many educators have misconceptions about the effects of medication and what they could/should expect. In Chapter 7 we review the major types of medications that are used with children with ADHD; provide information on what to expect and not to expect from medication; and discuss common side effects and the school's role in medication treatment.

One aspect of ADHD that is often overlooked is the fact that the environment can shape and maintain problem behaviors. Functional behavioral assessment (FBA) is a process that can help teachers to identify the environmental antecedents and the consequences that can maintain problem behaviors. This in turn can lead to effective interventions. In Chapter 8 we provide an overview of FBA and an explanation of its purpose; list the steps in the FBA process; and provide examples of the FBA process along with sources of additional information.

In Chapter 9 we provide an overview of behavioral interventions that are effective with children with ADHD. We present guidelines for using behavioral interventions with children with ADHD and detailed examples of how two of the interventions (token economies and response cost) could be implemented in the classroom. Academic problems are common among students with ADHD, and Chapter 10 discusses specific instructional approaches that can be effective.

Current theory now views ADHD as a disorder that results from a deficit in self-regulation. For this reason, interventions that can help students self-regulate their behavior may be very useful. In Chapter 11 we provide an overview of self-regulation interventions that are effective for children with ADHD and step-by-step examples of how the interventions can be used in the classroom. In the final chapter, Chapter 12, we discuss "survival skills"—the social and organizational skills that can be a lifesaver for children with ADHD. We review social skills training and common classroom survival skills, and provide examples of organizational supports.

Helping students with ADHD succeed in schools is a challenge. Students with ADHD pose complex problems, and effective treatment requires attention to the academic, behavioral, and social aspects of ADHD. Moreover, it requires a coordinated approach that, ideally, is integrated across home and school. It is our hope that this book will provide teachers with knowledge and practical ideas that can help them work more effectively with students with ADHD in the classroom.

Contents

CHAPTER 1

Introduction

The great enemy of the truth is very often not the lie—
deliberate, contrived and dishonest—but the myth—
persistent, persuasive and unrealistic.
—JOHN F. KENNEDY

Attention-deficit/hyperactivity disorder (ADHD) is a problem that affects millions of students. It is the most commonly diagnosed childhood disorder. It is likely the most thoroughly studied psychological disorder in history. A search of one online database found approximately 10,000 scientific papers written on ADHD, and this number is likely an underestimate. ADHD is also firmly embedded in popular culture, having received a tremendous amount of attention in the media. Cover stories on ADHD appear regularly in national news magazines, and stories on ADHD appear frequently in major newspapers. However, even this amount of attention pales in comparison to the sources available on the World Wide Web. Googling the term "ADHD" resulted in over 36 million hits. Truly, there is an ocean of information on ADHD.

There is, unfortunately, a downside to this ocean of information. Many of the accounts of ADHD in the popular media or on the web are sensationalized. These stories often focus on dramatic first-person stories of success or failure. They feature the uplifting but often atypical account of how a child overcame ADHD or conversely how the problems of ADHD led to other much more serious problems. Some stories present the latest "miracle cure" which—as regular as clockwork—will soon be replaced by the next "miracle cure." Other stories report on purported causes of ADHD. Often coverage focuses on controversies. There is now what amounts to a cottage industry of critics who focus on controversies—real or contrived—

surrounding ADHD and the uncertainties of scientific knowledge. As a result, there remains an air of mystery about ADHD, and many people are unaware of exactly what ADHD is and how it affects individuals and ultimately society. Perhaps for this reason there are numerous misconceptions about ADHD. Some of these misconceptions have attained mythic status, and are, as Kennedy noted, persistent, persuasive, and unrealistic. They also can affect how ADHD is perceived and how educators respond to ADHD.

The purpose of this chapter is to provide background information on ADHD and to address some of the more common and pervasive misconceptions pertaining to ADHD. First, we address the notion that ADHD isn't even a real disorder. Second, we address the notion that ADHD is not a serious problem. We discuss the extent, impact, and far-reaching effects of ADHD. Third, we address the idea that ADHD is a newly "invented" disorder that suddenly sprang up out of nowhere in the last 10–20 years. To address this issue we provide a history of ADHD. Fourth, we address a particularly pernicious misconception—the notion that children with ADHD "could do it if they really tried." Finally, we address *what does not cause* ADHD. By discussing these misconceptions, we provide a more solid knowledge base for teachers working with students with ADHD and their parents.

THERE'S NO SUCH THING AS "ADHD"

Despite its lengthy history and the substantial research done on ADHD, there are those who continue to question the validity of ADHD as a disorder. Some of the commonly expressed arguments verge on conspiracy theories. For example:

> Essentially, then, A.D.D. appears to exist largely because of a unique coming together of the interests of frustrated activist parents, a highly developed psychopharmacological technology, a new cognitive research paradigm, a growth industry in new educational products, and group of professionals (teachers, doctors, and psychologists) eager to introduce them to each other—all of this taking place under the beneficent influence of governmental approval. (Armstrong, 1995, p. 10)

The notion of a vast cabal of doctors, parents, teachers, and pharmaceutical executives creating a psychiatric disorder is far-fetched—to put it charitably. Some critics allege that parents seek out an ADHD diagnosis in order to get special treatment for their children. This charge is especially troubling since it purports that there are parents who are willing to have their child labeled with a disorder so he or she can receive "special treatment." This special treatment would consist, presumably, of accommodations and modifications offered in school in order for the child to be more academically successful. Leaving aside the fact that in the great majority of cases children with ADHD are legally entitled to special services and the school is legally required to provide them, we are aware of no evidence to support this claim. However, there is evidence to the contrary. Bussing, Gary, Mills, and Garvan (2007) conducted a study focused on parental health beliefs, knowledge, and information sources related to ADHD. They found that even among parents who were knowledgeable about ADHD, few were aware of special school services for children with ADHD. Thus the evidence suggests that most parents do not automatically link an ADHD diagnosis with some type of special services provided in schools. Moreover, the study also found that it was not always easy for parents to accept school accommodations based on an ADHD diagnosis, as there remains a stigma associated with being labeled as a special needs learner.

Other arguments do have a grain of truth, and for that reason should be discussed. In this section we discuss three arguments against the existence of ADHD: (1) that there is no medical test for a definitive diagnosis; (2) that ADHD remains poorly and subjectively described; and (3) that the behaviors associated with ADHD are displayed by all people to some degree at various points and times.

Argument 1: "There Isn't a Medical Test to Diagnose ADHD"

One argument against the reality of ADHD is the fact that there is no proven medical test to confirm or disconfirm the presence of ADHD. This statement is entirely true. There is no blood test or DNA test for ADHD. ADHD cannot be seen in an X ray. New imaging techniques such as positron emission tomography or magnetic resonance imaging—techniques that are so powerful that they actually allow scientists to view brain activation—cannot see ADHD. Neither can other techniques that measure brain electrical activity such as electroencephalograms or evoked potential. In sum, there is no "gold standard" for the diagnosis of ADHD. At this point in time we cannot say objectively and definitively that based on an objective medical test Stevie has ADHD while Karen does not.

At first glance this would seem to be a powerful argument. If we cannot say with any certainty that an individual does or doesn't have ADHD, how can we say that ADHD exists? After all, this gets at a basic principle of science: we must be able to test a hypothesis. If we can't show that a hypothesis is incorrect, then we can't test the hypothesis, and consequently from a scientific standpoint the hypothesis is useless. The problem with the argument is that it raises a nearly impossible standard. In practice the world is not nearly as black and white, especially in the case of psychiatric disorders. For example, if we demanded that there be an objective medical test before we accepted the reality of a disorder, then we would have to dismiss the reality of depression, autism, and learning disabilities, just to name a few disorders that are universally recognized. The problem here is that at present we must rely on the observation of behaviors and the effects of these behaviors to make a diagnosis. For this reason, an ADHD diagnosis is a subjective diagnosis. That is, the diagnosis is a judgment call. This leads to a criticism discussed in the next section.

A closely related argument is that because there is no proven cause for ADHD it is fair to question the existence of ADHD. Even though there is a strong presumption that there is a neurological basis for ADHD, research has yet to pinpoint the cause(s). For example, critics note that no consistent pattern of high activity or inattention has been seen in children with established brain injury (Hertzig, 1983; Rutter, 1983); no consistent structural, functional, or chemical neurological marker is found in children with the ADHD diagnosis (Peterson, 1995; Zametkin, Ernst, & Silver, 1998); and that today's evidence of a genetic basis for the current diagnosis of ADHD cannot be taken as proof of an underlying brain abnormality (Sherman, Iacono, & McGee, 1997). Critics contend that considering the amount of research completed in regards to the brain structure of individuals with ADHD, a neurological basis should have been found by this time. Once again the criticism sets a nearly impossible standard. It also has a logical flaw—the fact that we don't know what causes a disorder doesn't mean that the disorder doesn't really exist. For example, as yet we don't know the cause of autism, yet autism is a very real disorder.

Argument 2: "ADHD Is Very Subjectively Defined"

The next point of contention that skeptics of ADHD often point to is that it is often poorly and subjectively defined. For example:

> ADHD is diagnosed using a *checklist of behaviors*. Teachers and parents fill out questionnaires and their answers are limited to the following: 1. *Never* 2. *Rarely* 3. *Sometimes* 4. *Often* 5. *Always*. Herein lies the first problem in the reliability and validity of the ADHD diagnosis. What exactly is the operational definition of "rarely"? of "sometimes"? of "often"? It could be argued that these limited answers are highly subjective and vary tremendously from one rater to the next. (Stolzer, 2007, p. 111)

> In some ways, the *DSM-IV-TR* criteria lack the specificity necessary to function as a working guide for diagnosis.... This lack of specificity introduces a high level of subjectivity into the diagnosis process. Such a high level of subjectivity will necessarily affect rates of prevalence and cloud an accurate picture of the illness' scope. (Schlachter, 2008, p. 156)

> In summary, several brief questionnaires are currently used clinically to diagnose ADHD, but they are highly subjective and impressionistic and should be regarded as no more than the perceptions and discomforts of parents and teachers, which are not as reliable as clinical interviewing and observations and are insufficient for diagnosis of brain malfunction. (Carey, 2002, p. 3-10)

Further, critics suggest that these subjective judgments are often made by those with a deep, often subconscious, emotional investment in the outcome. Parents and teachers looking for answers as to why a child behaves in a negative fashion may not be the most objective observers of said child's behaviors (Armstrong, 1995).

There are two arguments in this criticism. The first is that the criteria for ADHD are poorly defined. The second is that because the criteria are subjective, a diagnosis made on the basis of these criteria is suspect. We discuss each in turn.

Poorly Defined ADHD Criteria

In part this argument is inevitable because, as we discussed earlier, there is no objective test for ADHD. Instead we must rely on observation of behaviors, and defining exactly what constitutes a behavior can be tricky. Critics are correct to say that we rely on a shared understanding of what constitutes behaviors such as "fidgets" and the frequency with which they occur (e.g., pretty much, very much; Reid & Maag, 1994) and that this is a subjective judgment. Still this problem is not unique to ADHD. For example, the criteria for depression include descriptors such as "indecisiveness," "loss of energy," and "sad," which are equally subjective. It's also important to understand that simply because the criteria are subjective does not mean that they are fanciful or unrealistic. In fact, the current diagnostic criteria outlined in DSM-IV-TR are some of the most rigorous and empirically derived guidelines ever available in the history of ADHD (Barkley, 2006).

The current diagnostic criteria were developed by a committee of the leading experts in the field. The committee thoroughly reviewed the research on ADHD symptoms. Based on this review, a pool of symptoms was developed and subsequently tested in a field trial with 380 children from a number of different sites in North America (Applegate et al., 1997; Lahey et al., 1994). Following this trial, results were analyzed and discussed by the committee before the final criteria were adopted. There have also been steady improvements in the ADHD criteria over time. For example, the DSM-IV-TR used a field trial to establish a cutoff point for the number of symptoms necessary to diagnose ADHD, included a requirement that ADHD symptoms must be exhibited across at least two different settings (e.g., school, home, work) and, perhaps most critically, added the requirement of significant impairment. As we discuss in the next section, impairment is one of the key factors in establishing the presence of a disorder.

Even these criteria will likely change to some extent in the future. By nature, diagnostic procedures require review and modification over time. This is because science is self-correcting. With continued research, our understanding of ADHD improves and changes. This in turn requires improvements to the criteria. Such improvements may include, for example, more attention being paid to the subtypes of ADHD and how certain individuals do or do not fit into them, whether or not significant inattention should be required to diagnose ADHD, how well the current diagnostic criteria apply to different age groups, the appropriateness for the symptoms for different developmental levels, and whether or not the criterion for age of onset should be abandoned or changed, to name a few (Barkley, 2006).

Subjective Equals Suspect

The second argument—that because ADHD criteria are subjective a diagnosis made on this basis is suspect—is seen frequently. The problem with subjective criteria, critics claim, is that one person could say that a child had ADHD and another could say the opposite. This would mean that the criteria could not be used to reliably assess ADHD, which would be a serious problem. For any test or set of diagnostic criteria to be useful it must measure what it is supposed to measure *consistently*. Imagine that you were dieting and wanted to monitor your weight. However, each time you stepped on your scale at home your weight fluctuated wildly. One time the scale read 120 pounds, and the next it read 201. The scale would not be of much use in determining whether you were losing weight because the scale is not reliable. Diagnostic criteria must also be reliable. If the criteria could not be used with reliability (i.e., to measure ADHD consistently), then they would be of no use. Once again, the claim is literally true. It is *possible* that two professionals could use the ADHD criteria and disagree about whether an ADHD diagnosis was indicated. But this is a *hypothetical* situation. The important question is "Can the criteria be used reliably in practice to diagnose children?" The answer to this question is yes. This has been researched thoroughly, and there are numerous studies showing that the ADHD diagnosis can be made reliably. Moreover, children with ADHD can be reliably distinguished from other groups with similar symptoms such as children with learning disabilities or children with oppositional defiant disorder.

Argument 3: "Everyone Could Be Considered ADHD at One Time or Another"

The third point critics of ADHD like to make is that at some point all people display the associated symptoms of inattention, impulsivity, and hyperactivity. Instead of representing a disorder, the critics contend that these behaviors are simply part of our biological makeup. The critics of ADHD also believe that there is a broad range of normal child behavior that is often at odds with adult-controlled environments. Once again this argument is literally true—there is overwhelming evidence that the symptoms that we call inattention, impulsivity, and hyperactivity exist along a continuum. That is, people have more or less capacity for attending to a task for a long period, are more or less inclined to be planful or organized, and have greater or lesser degrees of normal activity levels. Moreover, there can be distinct differences in the levels of inattention, impulsivity, and hyperactivity that are situational. For example, your attention might drift in the middle of a long boring lecture. Everyone has suffered from buyer's remorse after they have made an impulsive purchase or failed to complete an important task because they were distracted by a more appealing alternative. And our activity level and actions while attending a football game are not typical: we don't normally jump up and down and scream in public gatherings. Thus we can literally say that practically everyone exhibits symptoms of ADHD at one time or another.

So if everyone acts a little ADHD-like at one time or another, how can we say that one person has ADHD and another doesn't? Or, put another way, "How do we tell when an individual's behavior is disordered as opposed to merely annoying or inappropriate?" This can be a surprisingly difficult question to answer. There is no "bright line" between normal and disordered. If the degree to which each of us exhibits inattention, impulsivity, and hyperactivity exists along a continuum (i.e., is a matter of degree), where do we draw the line between "normal" and "disordered?" This is a question that has bothered researchers for as long as we have had psychiatric disorders. For some disorders it is easier to draw the line. For example, schizophrenics who hear voices are "not normal." But for disorders such as ADHD the problem is much more difficult. As we noted before, the behaviors that we think of as symptomatic of ADHD are also exhibited by "normal" people.

One widely accepted approach to defining what constitutes a disorder is Wakefield's (1992). Wakefield distinguished between behavior that is a disorder and behavior that is abnormal but not disordered based on the idea of *harmful dysfunction*. A disorder "is a harmful dysfunction, wherein harmful is a value term based on social norms, and dysfunction is a scientific term referring to the failure of a mental organism to perform a natural function for which it was designed by evolution" (Wakefield, 1992, p. 373). From this perspective, if a person's behavior does not violate social norms, is not harmful to the individual or society or is not maladaptive, and there is no problem performing natural functions (i.e., normal tasks of everyday living) then there is not a disorder. As we noted earlier in the chapter, the behaviors of children with ADHD lead to serious problems at home, school, and in society. In fact, for an individual to be diagnosed with ADHD *requires* a maladaptive deficit that cause problems in a variety of social contexts. This requirement for the behavior to result in severe problems functioning in society is literally a part of the definition of ADHD.

In closing we note that the debate over the reality of ADHD has lost steam, overall, in the past several years. There are still some very vocal critics, many of whom do not base their ideas on research and some of whom base their critique on their religious beliefs. But the simple fact is that ADHD is accepted as a real disorder by the vast majority of those in the medical and educational fields. It is true that there are gaps in our knowledge of ADHD. We still do not know what causes ADHD, nor is there an objective, fool-proof test for ADHD. However, this is true for a great many disorders (e.g., autism, learning disabilities). Some day we may find conclusive and definitive evidence on the causes and "reality" of ADHD, but until that day comes it is appropriate to focus on the current research and what it tells us about the realities of ADHD. It should also be noted that to those who deal with ADHD on a daily basis, those with ADHD, their parents, families, teachers, and friends, the debate about ADHD's existence isn't a concern. Instead, their focus is on the reality of coping and functioning with the problems of ADHD, problems that can be very serious, as we discuss in our next section.

ADHD? IT'S NO BIG DEAL

It's not hard to find statements in the popular press or the professional literature from those who minimize the impact of ADHD or suggest that the problems associated with ADHD are not really serious. This is represented by statements such as "we need to let boys be boys" or "they will outgrow it." Sometimes, ADHD is portrayed as a by-product of the stress of modern life as opposed to a disorder (Walker, 1999). Others claim that the behaviors characteristic of ADHD are due to boredom (DeGrandepre, 2000) or are the by-product of giftedness. Still others suggest that ADHD is a dumping ground that allows society to avoid the messy business of understanding children's difficulties and avoid responsibility for raising and nurturing well-behaved children (Timimi & Radcliffe, 2005). Missing in all of these accounts is a realistic appraisal of the actual impact of ADHD on the lives of children, their families, and society. In fact, there is an overwhelming body of evidence, collected over several decades, that ADHD is a widespread problem that may have serious deleterious effects on children's lives, that ADHD affects them at home, in school, and in the community, and that ADHD is not a problem that can be "outgrown."

To understand the impact of ADHD, let's examine the extent of ADHD. The U.S. Census Bureau estimated that 55 million students would be enrolling in kindergarten through 12th grade in the fall of 2006 (*www.census.gov*, accessed on August 25, 2008). Couple that with the estimated 3–7% prevalence rate for ADHD (American Psychiatric Association, 2000), and we find that between 1.65 million and 3.85 million of these students would have ADHD. This means that a conservative estimate suggests that there are 2 million students with ADHD. Another way of visualizing the extent of ADHD is that approximately one child in every 20 has ADHD. Translated into the normal school environment, this means that on average every classroom in America has a student with ADHD. Thus, as many teachers already realize, working with students with ADHD is a fact of life. What many teachers may not realize is how important it is that schools understand the problems of ADHD and provide effective treatment for students. ADHD is not a "bump in the road." Rather, it is a chronic (i.e., lifelong) disorder. The need for effective treatment is clear when the risks associated with ADHD are understood. The problems associated with ADHD often impact individual's lives in far-reaching and possibly damaging ways.

Students with ADHD commonly experience multiple academic difficulties. On average, the achievement of children with ADHD is significantly lower than that of their peers in reading, math, and spelling (Frazier, Youngstrom, Glutting, & Watkins, 2007), and they are more likely to be retained one or more grades (Weyandt, 2001). They often have difficulties with organization, including attending class unprepared, not writing down assignments, not bringing necessary materials home to complete assignments, and not turning in class assignments on time (Gureasko-Moore, DuPaul & White, 2007). Teachers have described students with ADHD as disorganized, distractible, spacey, and restless. These students often do not follow through on assignments and are inconsistent and careless in their schoolwork (Hinshaw, 2002).

Students diagnosed with ADHD are more likely to drop out of school, less likely to graduate from college, often underperform at work, and are more likely to use tobacco or illegal drugs than the general population. There are additional negative social effects for those with ADHD. Children growing up with ADHD are more likely to become pregnant as a teenager, contract a sexually transmitted disease, speed excessively, or be involved in multiple car accidents. Many adolescents with ADHD also have conduct disorders, oppositional defiant disorder, and/ or experience depression or other personality disorders. The negative impact of ADHD continues on into adulthood. Adults with ADHD had fewer years of education and had lower-ranking occupational positions compared to adults without ADHD (Mannuzza, Klein, Bessler, Malloy, & Hynes, 1997). They may also be relegated to lower-paying, less secure employment. One study found that the most common occupation of adults with ADHD was skilled labor, followed by physical labor. Other studies have found that adults with ADHD are more likely to be fired from their jobs. Clearly the impact of ADHD is not limited to school-age children and can have a profound impact throughout an individual's life. Note, however, that *ADHD ranges in severity*. In many of the studies noted the individuals were those who were severely involved and had been referred to specialized treatment facilities. Additionally, many of the individuals had other associated problems. *ADHD is not invariably associated with negative outcomes*.

As the above discussion would suggest, ADHD has potentially detrimental effects on an individual's academic, social, and family life. Moreover, these problems are not limited to childhood, but continue on into adolescence and adulthood. There are also direct economic costs associated with ADHD. For example, students diagnosed with ADHD incur medical costs, including prescriptions, often require additional educational services, and may incur other costs related to ADHD (e.g., court costs). When all of these costs are compiled, the estimates of the economic cost of ADHD are between *42.5 and 52.5 billion dollars per year* (Pelham, Foster, & Robb, 2007). Incredibly these are conservative estimates. If other factors were included, such as costs associated with lost work time by family members, the costs would be even higher. Thus by any measure, ADHD is a serious problem at both the individual and societal level.

WHERE HAS ADHD BEEN?

Critics claim ADHD is a recent "invention," that ADHD is a disorder that did not manifest itself until the 1990s. For example, Stolzer (2007) stated that in the 1950s ADHD did not exist in America, argued that ADHD is a recently "constructed" phenomenon, and wondered "Why has this disease not been recorded across time? Across cultures?" (p. 109). Critics also cite an ADHD "epidemic" or an ADHD "explosion" which is followed by the question "Where have these children been all these years?" The point of these criticisms, at least to the critics, is that ADHD is not "real" because it is a recent creation. In truth, the history of ADHD reaches back more than 100 years and has been recorded across cultures. For example, a parent in Australia gleefully related to the first author how O'Henry's classic story "Ransom of Red Chief," written in 1910, aptly describes the trials of parenting a child with ADHD. An even earlier and equally apt example is the nursery rhyme "Fidgety

Phil" written in 1863 by German physician Heinrich Hoffman. As Barkley (2006) pointed out, it contains one of the earliest recorded references to a child displaying symptoms of what we now call ADHD:

> "Phil, stop acting like a worm,
> The table is no place to squirm."
> Thus speaks the father to his son,
> severely says it, not in fun.
> Mother frowns and looks around
> although she doesn't make a sound.
> But Phillip will not take advice,
> he'll have his way at any price.
> He turns,
> and churns,
> he wiggles
> and jiggles
> Here and there on the chair,
> "Phil, these twists I cannot bear." (Silver, 1999)

Whether "Fidgety Phil" would meet the current standards for ADHD is debatable, but clearly Hoffman accurately recorded the behavior of a child who was displaying ADHD-like behavior.

While the charge that ADHD did not exist in 1950 is not literally true, it is true the term ADHD was coined in 1987 (the term "attention deficit disorder" or ADD, was coined in 1980; American Psychiatric Association, 1980, 1987). Thus no one could have written about ADHD in 1950. However, that is not the same as saying that there were no children who displayed behaviors characteristic of ADHD. In fact, children who exhibit ADHD-type behavior have been described in scientific and popular literature for over a century. They have also had many different labels over the years, and these changing labels have added to the confusion. Figure 1.1 shows many of the different labels attached to children we would today call ADHD. Note that originally many of these terms were used to describe a heterogenous group of children comprised of children with learning disabilities, emotional–behavioral disorders, and ADHD.

It is true that there has been a noticeable increase in the number of children diagnosed with ADHD. For example, between 1990 and 1995 the number of children and adolescents diagnosed with ADHD more than doubled, increasing from

• Defect in moral control	• Minimal brain dysfunction
• Postenchephalatic behavior disorder	• Hyperkinetic reaction of childhood
• Minimal brain damage	• Attention deficit disorder
• Brain-injured child	• Attention-deficit/hyperactivity disorder

FIGURE 1.1. "Alias ADHD."

950,000 to more than 2.3 million. By 1994 ADHD was the most commonly diagnosed psychiatric disorder of childhood in the United States (Neufeld & Foy, 2006). Why the numbers of children diagnosed with ADHD have increased so dramatically is open to debate. Clearly, continued research efforts have contributed to awareness among medical professionals, and the coverage in the popular media have increased the awareness of ADHD among parents. This would lead more parents to seek, and more doctors to provide, a diagnosis of ADHD. However, this is not an unusual occurrence. For example, both learning disabilities and more recently autism spectrum disorders have experienced dramatic increases in identification for much the same reasons. These increases have not been due to some plot, but to the increased recognition of the occurrence of the conditions.

History of ADHD

The history of ADHD reaches back to the turn of the 19th century. The first recognized description of what we now look at as ADHD is generally attributed to George Still (Barkley, 2006). In a series of three published lectures to the Royal College of Physicians in 1902, Still described children in his clinical practice with typical cognitive abilities who displayed serious problems with attention; who were also quite overactive, displaying signs of aggression, defiance, and resistance to discipline; and who were being overly emotional (Still, 1902). Still believed these behaviors resulted from a "defect in moral control." Moral control of behavior meant "the control of action in conformity with the idea of the good of all." Still believed these children lacked the capacity to control their behaviors in such a manner as to conform to society's expectations. These children's lack of control put them in direct conflict with society's notions of how children should behave.

Still (1902) also noted that the children he observed had reached a point where they could understand that their behaviors were in conflict with society, yet that understanding was not enough to keep them from acting in an inappropriate manner. He believed that our will or consciousness influences our behaviors, and that clearly a moral defect had to be in play in children with negative behaviors not accompanied by any intellectual delay. Still concluded that the defect in moral control could develop in relation to three distinctive impairments: "(1) defect of cognitive relation to the environment; (2) defect of moral consciousness; and (3) defect in inhibitory volition" (p. 1011). Still also suggested a biological predisposition to these behaviors that was probably hereditary (Barkley, 2006). This was a perceptive and remarkably accurate description of ADHD as we understand it today.

The history of interest in ADHD in North America can be traced to an outbreak of encephalitis in 1917–1918. Many children who survived this brain infection were left with numerous behavioral and cognitive impairments. Many of these children exhibited characteristics now associated with ADHD, including inattentiveness, impaired ability to regulate activity, and impulsivity. The children also were often socially disruptive. Symptoms of what we now call oppositional defiant disorder, conduct disorder, and delinquency were also observed. That so many of these children displayed these types of behaviors led to the widespread use of the term "postencephalatic behavior disorder," believed to be linked to brain damage. The link to brain damage associated with these behaviors led to the concept of brain damage syndrome, and researchers for the next few decades spent a great deal of time studying the links between brain damage and characteristics of what is now commonly called ADHD, as well as learning disabilities and other disorders (Barkley, 2006).

Though there was a widespread belief among many researchers that brain damage was a probable cause of children's behavioral deficits, there was no definitive proof. The medical technology available at the time could not link brain damage to the deficits exhibited by the children observed. Some researchers compared the children's behaviors with those of primates, the subjects of frontal lobe studies for more than 60 years before the encephalitis outbreak. Lesions observed on the frontal lobes were known to contribute to excess restlessness, aimless wandering, and poor ability to sustain interest in activities. The brain damage hypothesis would continue on into the 1940s and beyond, even in instances where no evidence of brain trauma existed in a child's medical history. The term *minimal brain damage*, or MBD, was first used in the 1940s and into the 1950s to describe children whose difficulties with learning were believed to be tied to nervous system problems. Some students identified as MBD displayed signs of hyperactivity and distractibility (Weyandt, 2001). During this era the concept of the "brain-injured child" was introduced (Strauss & Lehtinen, 1947), and was applied to children with hyperactivity and distractibility even in cases, as noted above, where no evidence of brain damage was present (Barkley, 2006). Once again note that these children could have just as easily been displaying signs of learning disabilities or other disorders.

After continued observations and testing throughout the 1950s revealed no evidence of brain damage in many of these children with MBD, researchers concluded that the nature of the problem lay in how the brain functioned, rather than how it was structured. Acknowledging that brain damage was not in evidence, the terminology shifted to *minimal brain dysfunction* (Silver, 1999). The concept of MBD would die a slow death throughout the 1960s, as researchers realized it lacked research support and had little practical use. While MBD was slowly fading into the background, researchers turned their attention to the behavioral symptom of hyperactivity that many believed most characterized the disorder that would become ADHD (Barkley, 2006).

The efforts of multiple researchers, particularly Stella Chess, contributed to the idea that hyperactivity was the defining characteristic of the disorder, that objective evidence of the symptom needed to be more strongly considered, and that blame for the children's symptoms did not lie with the parents. Chess described 36 children diagnosed with "physiological hyperactivity," noting that most were referred prior to age 6, that educational difficulties were common among the group, and that many of the children displayed oppositional defiant behavior and had poor peer relationships. Chess also noted that impulsive and aggressive behaviors, as well as a poor attention span, were common. The shift to a more modern view of what would ultimately become known as ADHD had begun (Barkley, 2006).

It was not until the late 1960s, however, that the first official term in the medical classification system for children displaying hyperactivity was established. In 1968, with the publication of the second edition of the *Diagnostic and Statistical Manual of Mental Disorders* (DSM-II; American Psychiatric Association, 1968), the term "hyperkinetic reaction of childhood" was introduced. It became the label given to a child who exhibited symptoms of hyperactivity: overactivity, restlessness, distractibility, and a short attention span. After over 60 years of research efforts, official medical recognition was finally given to the disorder we now know as ADHD (Barkley, 2006).

In the 1970s researchers began to emphasize problems with sustained attention and impulse control in addition to hyperactivity. In 1983 Virginia Douglas theorized that ADHD comprised four major deficits: (1) maintaining attention and effort; (2) the inability to inhibit impulsive behavior; (3) the ability to modulate arousal levels to meet situational demands; and (4) an unusually strong inclination to seek immediate reinforcement (Douglas, 1983). As a result there was yet another name change that took into account deficits in attention and impulsivity along with hyperactivity (Barkley, 2006). In 1980 the name of the disorder was changed to attention deficit disorder (ADD) in the new *DSM-III*. This also marked the creation of a much more specific symptoms list, specific guidelines for the age of onset and duration of symptoms, and the requirement that other childhood psychiatric conditions be excluded as a cause for the symptoms. Two subtypes of ADD were defined, based on the presence or absence of hyperactivity. The creation of those subsets was controversial, as little empirical research on the issue existed (Barkley, 2006).

In 1987 another DSM revision occurred. In DSM-III-R the official classification changed to attention deficit hyperactivity disorder. The new diagnostic criteria featured: (1) a single list of symptoms along with a single cutoff score; (2) the need to establish the symptoms as being developmentally inappropriate for the child's age; and (3) the acknowledgment that mood disorders could co-exist with ADHD. Another key change was that ADHD was now classified as a behavioral disorder (Barkley, 2006).

In 1994, with the publication of DSM-IV, the official classification changed once again. The term ADHD was still used; however, three types of ADHD were delineated: (1) individuals who were primarily inattentive were called predominantly inattentive type; (2) individuals who were primarily hyperactive and impulsive were called predominantly hyperactive–impulsive type; and (3) individuals who were inattentive, hyperactive, and impulsive were called combined type. The new DSM-IV changes reintroduced the purely inattentive form of ADHD, required pervasive evidence of the disorder across settings, and required the demonstration of impairment in at least two major domains of life functioning (home, school, or work; American Psychiatric Association, 1994; Barkley, 2006).

Heading in to the 21st century, research on ADHD continued. There has been more emphasis in recent research on heredity, molecular genetics, and neuroimaging, along with efforts to link these fields together, seeking to identify the cause (or causes) for ADHD. Some research has attempted to establish subtypes of ADHD, leading to a possible new subtype called "sluggish cognitive tempo," or SCT. The characteristics of SCT are found in 30–50% of the children diagnosed with the predominantly inattentive type of ADHD. Another key focus of recent research has helped establish that other disorders may coexist with ADHD without having a common cause. For example, learning disabilities are commonly associated with ADHD, but may stem from separate causes (Barkley, 2006).

ADHD is far from a new disorder. It did not spring into existence in the 1990s but instead it has a long and well-researched history. While widespread *awareness* of the disorder may be called relatively new in the past two decades, the notion that ADHD itself is newly invented does not stand up to critical analysis. As we have shown, what we now call ADHD has gone by many names over the years, which has no doubt helped to fuel the notion that ADHD is a new disorder. However, the characteristics of the disorder and the children who have it have remained virtually unchanged. Accepting that ADHD has been around for quite a long time is an important part of understanding the scope of the disorder.

"HE COULD DO IT IF HE REALLY WANTED TO"

The basis for this misconception of ADHD is that students with ADHD have problems that are willful. That is, if children with ADHD really put forth a good and concentrated effort they could get past the negative effects of the disorder. They could pay attention, complete assignments, and stay on-task. The reason for this misconception is that there are times when a child with ADHD can perform well. For whatever reason(s) there are times when the stars align and the student can attend to the lecture, finish the worksheet, ignore distractions, and not wander around the room. When teachers see the child perform successfully, they may—mistakenly—conclude that the child should be capable of this level of performance on a regular basis. After all, if he or she did it once can't he or she do it every time?

Unfortunately, this is based on a serious misconception about the fundamental nature of ADHD. Put very simply, one of the core problems of children with ADHD is that they are "consistently inconsistent." For children with ADHD, wide variability in performance is *the norm* not the exception. This variability or inconsistency is a part of the disorder. It's not realistic to expect a child with ADHD to achieve a "personal best" performance every day. That's like expecting a champion golfer to make a hole-in-one on every shot or a runner to break a world record in every race. The expectation that the child with ADHD can simply decide to perform at personal-best level every day "if he really wanted to" is equally unrealistic. What is even more disturbing about this misconception is that it implies that children should overcome the debilitating effects of ADHD independently. It's their responsibility to summon the will or the motivation to succeed. This is exactly the same as telling people with depression that they can just "cheer up" it if they really want to.

IT AIN'T NECESSARILY SO

In the final section of this introductory chapter we focus on some of the misconceptions regarding the causes of ADHD. Although evidence points to a neurological cause for ADHD, at present we simply don't know for sure what causes ADHD. This is true for many common disorders. For example, even after 50 years of research, we can't say with certainty what causes learning disabilities or behavioral disorders. There is a long list of proposed causes for ADHD (we discuss these further in Chapter 2), ranging from lead poisoning to fluorescent lights to flu shots to open classrooms. Most have been laid to rest by ongoing research efforts. Unfortunately, this does not eliminate the misconceptions. They have a way of persisting despite all evidence to the contrary. Ironically, for teachers, it may be more important to know what *doesn't* cause ADHD, because some of the misconceptions about the causes of ADHD can be hurtful or expensive. Thus, it's important for teachers to be able to provide accurate information to parents.

ADHD Is Caused by Poor Parenting

One potentially harmful misconception is that ADHD is caused by poor parenting. The reasoning is that children raised in a chaotic environment lacking in discipline, limits, rules, or consequences for breaking rules will not learn to follow directions from adults, obey rules, or control their behavior. As a result, when children come to school where they are expected to follow rules and obey the teacher, they will engage in problematic behaviors. It is easy to understand why some people might believe poor parenting would cause ADHD. Children raised in such a home would have problems in just about any environment. It is also easy to see why teachers would be sensitive to poor parenting; teachers must deal with the consequences of home-based problems every day. However, there is *no evidence that poor parenting causes ADHD*. It is easy to find instances where two children raised in the same family have different outcomes—one has ADHD, the other has no problems to speak of. In fact there is ample evidence that children with ADHD will have difficulties even with exemplary parenting (Barkley, 2006).

The belief that ADHD may be caused by poor parenting may be related to problems experienced by parents of children with ADHD. Studies of parent–child interactions do indicate that parents of children with ADHD use more coercive parenting styles and are more likely to consider their parenting skills as lacking. They tend to be more disapproving, provide more controlling directions, and be more demanding and critical than parents of children without ADHD (Hechtman, 1996; Johnston, 1996; Kaplan, Crawford, Fisher, & Dewey, 1998; Marsh & Johnston, 1990; Thomas &

Guskin, 2001). At one time it was thought that these problems could cause ADHD. However, we now know that the coercive parenting styles are a *reaction to* problem behavior (Barkley, 2006). Additionally, parent training in effective behavior management techniques can improve parenting practices (and children's behavior).

ADHD Is Caused by Diet

The notion that ADHD was caused by diet began in the 1970s. It was thought that adverse reactions to food additives (e.g., food dyes, preservatives) caused allergic reactions in children (Feingold, 1975). The problem behavior associated with ADHD resulted from this allergic reaction. Proponents of this theory claimed that over half of all ADHD cases were due to diet (Barkley, 2006). To avoid having ADHD children needed to have a diet free of these additives. This was a widely believed idea during the 1970s. The relationship between food additives and ADHD has been tested in a number of studies. The evidence strongly suggests that food additives have little or no effect on behavior. In the 1980s refined sugar was also suggested as a cause. This is consistent with the commonly accepted but incorrect notion of the "sugar high." However, research does not support any relationship between sugar consumption and ADHD (Wolraich, Wilson, & White, 1995).

ADHD Is Caused by Too Much Television

Blaming behavior problems on various types of media has been common for many years. For example, at one time it was suggested that there was a link between comic books and criminal behavior. The notion that behavior problems are linked to television has been put forth in the popular media for years. The idea is that because television programs typically switch between scenes very rapidly, children who watch too much television (how much is "too much" is never actually defined) won't be able to develop sustained attention. Very few studies have been conducted on the relationship between television viewing and ADHD (Christakis, Zimmerman, DiGuiseppe, & McCarthy, 2004; Geist & Gibson, 2000; Levine & Waite, 2000). One study found a correlation between television viewing and teacher ratings of attention and impulsivity difficulties; however, those ratings were not reflected by parents nor were they consistent with the study's laboratory-based measure of attention (Levine & Waite, 2000). Another study that was featured prominently on a national news network link reported a correlation between the hours of television watched between ages 1 and 3 and attention difficulties at age 7. These results were interpreted by the media as indicating that early television watching caused later problems with attention.

   The problem with these studies and their interpretation by the media is that the studies could only show that in some instances there was a *correlation* between television watching and attention problems. In fact, as Barkley (2006) noted, the media made a very common error: they equated correlation with causation. That is they assumed that because there was a relationship between television watching and attention problems that television caused the attention problems. In fact, as Barkley (2006), stated we could just as easily conclude that ADHD causes children to watch television. There is some research to support the idea that children with ADHD enjoy television more and therefore spend more time watching, and it is possible that excessive television viewing could exacerbate ADHD problems (Acevedo-Polakovich, Lorch, & Milich, 2007), but there simply is not sufficient research to link too much television viewing to ADHD.

SUMMING UP

In this chapter we've provided some background information on ADHD and dispelled many misconceptions. There are additional misconceptions associated with ADHD; in fact, there are too many to address in one chapter. Here is a list of the major points you should remember.

- ✓ There is indeed a great deal of misinformation in circulation about ADHD. Be skeptical, especially of the popular media!
- ✓ ADHD is a serious problem for millions of individuals. If anything the impact of ADHD is understated rather than overblown.
- ✓ ADHD is not an "American fad" disorder. In fact, ADHD has been studied in Australia, Brazil, India, the Ukraine, France, China, and Japan, just to name a few countries.
- ✓ ADHD is not a new disorder. In fact, ADHD has a long history in the field of medical and psychological research.
- ✓ Even though the ADHD diagnosis is subjective, ADHD can be accurately and reliably assessed.
- ✓ The inconsistent performance of children with ADHD is not willful. Rather it is a result of problems inherent to ADHD.
- ✓ At this point in time we don't know what causes ADHD, but we do know that parenting, diet, and television *don't* cause ADHD.

CHAPTER 2

What Is ADHD?

It was six men of Indostan
To learning much inclined,
Who went to see the Elephant
(Though all of them were blind)
—JOHN GODFREY SAXE

In the classic parable "The Blindmen and the Elephant," six blind men of Indostan were given the task of examining an elephant. Each of the six men examined the elephant. Because each examined a different part of the elephant, each came to a different conclusion about what kind of animal it was. One, who examined the trunk, said the elephant was like a snake; another who felt a leg, declared that elephants were like trees. Even though each individual's observation was correct, none of them individually captured the totality of an elephant. ADHD has much in common with the elephant in the famous parable. ADHD is a very complex disorder that presents itself in different ways. Children with ADHD are a highly heterogenous group who can differ markedly even thought they have the same diagnosis. Additionally, because different adults (e.g., parents, teachers) see a child in different environments that place different demands on the child, and where adults may have different expectations, they may differ on the nature of the child's problem.

The complexity of ADHD is heightened by the fact that in many instances other disorders co-occur with ADHD. For this reason, characterizing ADHD in any simple, direct way is a very difficult undertaking—there simply is no such thing as a "typical" case of ADHD. In this chapter we give an overview of the nature of ADHD. We start by covering the current diagnostic criteria for ADHD and the three types of ADHD currently recognized. Next we discuss common characteristics of children with ADHD and other disorders that commonly occur in conjunction with ADHD. We also briefly list some of the leading theories that have attempted to explain ADHD. Lastly, we discuss several of the proposed causes of ADHD. Note that we cannot cover any of these topics exhaustively. Rather, we hope that our overview will provide a basic, practical understanding of ADHD.

COMMON CHARACTERISTICS OF CHILDREN WITH ADHD

It is difficult to describe common characteristics of children with ADHD because they are so heterogenous. There are no medical tests that reliably distinguish children with ADHD; as of yet, there are no chemical or genetic markers that distinguish children with ADHD. And there are no overt physical characteristics that would allow us to identify a child with ADHD. Still, there are some broad characteristics of ADHD and some factors that are not related to ADHD:

- There is a pronounced gender disparity (Barkley, 2006). Boys are much more likely than girls to be diagnosed with ADHD. In research samples, which use very rigorous diagnostic criteria, the male-to-female ratio is around 3 to 1. In community samples it is typically much higher, at around 7 to 1. Why this occurs is a matter of some debate. It may be that boys are more likely to externalize (i.e., act out) than girls, or there may be a genetic link between ADHD and gender.
- There is a difference between ADHD groups and non-ADHD groups on measures of intelligence. On average children with ADHD score around one-half standard deviation (around 8 points on an IQ test) lower than the non-ADHD group (Frazier, Demaree, & Youngstrom, 2004). This data should be interpreted cautiously. The range of scores for ADHD groups *mirrors that of non-ADHD groups* (i.e., they range from below average to well above average). It is quite possible that the lower scores is a reflection of problems with maintaining attention and motivation during an intelligence test. It is also possible that this reflects a referral bias—students with lower intelligence may be more likely to experience school-related problems and thus be referred and diagnosed with ADHD.
- Children with ADHD are at high risk for academic failure. This may include failing courses, grade retention, dropping out of school, or referral for special education services (Barkley, 2006). Most children are diagnosed with ADHD between the ages of 5 and 9 that corresponds to early school years and increasing demands children face.
- ADHD is not limited to any ethnic group or race and occurs across groups of all socioeconomic status (SES; Barkley, 2006). Low SES is thought to be a risk factor for ADHD (Counts, Nigg, Stawicki, Rappley, & von Eye, 2005) because of increased family adversity and increased exposure to environmental stresses.

ADHD DIAGNOSTIC CRITERIA

The fourth edition (text revision) of the Diagnostic and Statistical Manual of Mental Disorders (DSM-IV-TR; American Psychiatric Association, 2000) is a publication of the American Psychiatric Association. It contains diagnostic criteria for all the psychiatric disorders that are recognized by the American Psychiatric Association, including ADHD. It is in essence a catalogue of psychiatric disorders intended for use by health professionals. The health professional would identify the problems that a child exhibits and compare them to the DSM-IV-TR diagnostic criteria for disorders. The disorder or disorders (a child can have multiple disorders) that fit the criteria would then be diagnosed. DSM-IV-TR is intended for use as a diagnostic tool by health professionals (e.g., physicians, pediatricians, psychiatrists, psychologists). It is not intended to be used by individuals without clinical training—this can lead to inappropriate application of its contents. The DSM-IV-TR criteria for a diagnosis of ADHD are shown in Figure 2.1. As Figure 2.1 shows, ADHD is characterized by three main symptoms: inattention, impulsivity, and hyperactivity. Together or separately, these symptoms are the hallmarks of ADHD.

Inattention

"Attention" typically refers to selectively concentrating on one aspect of the environment while screening out other aspects. For example, a child who listens to the teacher during a lesson would be paying attention. Problems with attention (i.e., inattention) are a hallmark symptom of ADHD. Figure 2.2 lists characteristics commonly associated with inattention. When considering inattention it is necessary to be cautious because (like the elephant in the poem) inattention in ADHD can present itself in multiple ways (Barkley, 1988, 1994; Hale & Lewis, 1979; Mirsky, 1996; Strauss, Thompson, Adams, Redline, & Burant, 2000). Attention can refer to:

- *Sustained attention*. This refers to keeping focused on a task through completion. Sustained attention is the type of inattention with which children with ADHD experience the most difficulty. That is, they often lack persistence in completing a task. This is seen most often in situations requiring children to sustain effort in completing dull and repetitive tasks (Barkley, DuPaul, & McMurray, 1990). For example, if a child with ADHD was given an assignment that was not particularly motivating, such as a long drill and practice activity, he or she might have trouble sustaining attention and thus have great difficulty successfully completing the assignment.

- *Alternating attention*. This refers to the ability to shift between tasks that have different cognitive requirements or make different demands on the individual. For example, in a science class a student might have to apply math skills, listening skills, and writing skills in the same activity. If the student has trouble shifting between the skills required for different parts of the activity, he or she will struggle with task completion. Tasks that require shifting attention can cause problems for students with ADHD.

A. Either (1) or (2):

   (1) six (or more) of the following symptoms of **inattention** have persisted for at least 6 months to a degree that is maladaptive and inconsistent with developmental level:

   Inattention

     (a) often fails to give close attention to details or makes careless mistakes in schoolwork, work, or other activities

     (b) often has difficulty sustaining attention in tasks or play activities

     (c) often does not seem to listen when spoken to directly

     (d) often does not follow through on instructions and fails to finish schoolwork, chores, or duties in the workplace (not due to oppositional behavior or failure to understand instructions)

     (e) often has difficulty organizing tasks and activities

     (f) often avoids, dislikes, or is reluctant to engage in tasks that require sustained mental effort (such as schoolwork or homework)

     (g) often loses things necessary for tasks or activities (e.g., toys, school assignments, pencils, books, or tools)

     (h) is often easily distracted by extraneous stimuli

     (i) is often forgetful in daily activities

   (2) six (or more) of the following symptoms of **hyperactivity–impulsivity** have persisted for at least 6 months to a degree that is maladaptive and inconsistent with developmental level:

   Hyperactivity

     (a) often fidgets with hands or feet or squirms in seat

     (b) often leaves seat in classroom or in other situations in which remaining seated is expected

     (c) often runs about or climbs excessively in situations in which it is inappropriate (in adolescents or adults, may be limited to subjective feelings of restlessness)

     (d) often has difficulty playing or engaging in leisure activities quietly

     (e) is often "on the go" or often acts as if "driven by a motor"

     (f) often talks excessively

   Impulsivity

     (g) often blurts out answers before questions have been completed

     (h) often has difficulty awaiting turn

     (i) often interrupts or intrudes on others (e.g., butts into conversations or games)

B. Some hyperactive–impulsive or inattentive symptoms that caused impairment were present before age 7 years.

C. Some impairment from the symptoms is present in two or more settings (e.g., at school [or work] and at home).

D. There must be clear evidence of clinically significant impairment in social, academic, or occupational functioning.

E. The symptoms do not occur exclusively during the course of a Pervasive Developmental Disorder, Schizophrenia, or other Psychotic Disorder and are not better accounted for by another mental disorder (e.g., Mood Disorder, Anxiety Disorder, Dissociative Disorders, or a Personality Disorder).

FIGURE 2.1. DSM-IV-TR criteria for ADHD. From American Psychiatric Association (2000). Copyright 2000 by the American Psychiatric Association. Reprinted by permission.

• Doesn't seem to listen.	• Can't work independently of supervision.
• Daydreams.	• Requires more redirection.
• Often loses things.	• Shifts from one uncompleted activity to another.
• Can't concentrate.	• Is confused or seems to be in a fog.
• Is easily distracted.	

FIGURE 2.2. Descriptions commonly associated with inattention. Based on Barkley et al. (1990) and Stewart, Pitts, Craig, and Dieruf (1966).

- *Focused attention.* This refers to the ability to focus on and respond to the important aspects of a task and/or choosing between different options to respond to a situation and applying those options appropriately. For example, at a four-way intersection with stop signs there is more than once choice for how to proceed through the intersection, but these choices are governed by basic driving rules depending on the location. Appropriate attention is needed to make the proper choice.

- *Selective attention.* This refers to the ability to maintain focus and screen out potential distractions. This is also called "freedom from distraction." Distractibility may be one of the most obvious forms of inattention. For example, if a student is supposed to be reading or writing or working on a math problem but instead spends most of the time looking out the window at another class at recess, the student has succumbed to distraction.

It's often difficult to determine if a student has a problem with sustained attention or with distractibility. Children with ADHD often spend much more time involved in off-task behaviors instead of attending to their assigned tasks (Sawyer, Taylor, & Chadwick, 2001). At first glance this might give the impression that the children are easily distracted, but the truth may be that they are having great difficulty sustaining their attention. Instead of being distracted they may just be unable to persist as well as others. This is a difficult distinction to make, but it is important to keep in mind that being easily distracted is actually different than having trouble sustaining appropriate attention (Hoza, Pelham, Waschburch, Kipp, & Owens, 2001). A student who appears more interested in what the rest of the class is doing may actually be experiencing great difficulty keeping focused on a math problem or a reading selection. How a competing activity is viewed may influence distractibility. If an alternate activity is viewed as reinforcing or offers immediate gratification, a child may gravitate to that activity away from the task that is more menial and much less rewarding (Barkley, 2006).

Impulsivity

"Impulsivity" means to be swayed by impulses. Children with ADHD often respond quickly, often without taking the time to assess what would be an appropriate response or to see if further guidance or directions might be forthcoming. This often leads to careless errors or failure to consider potentially negative or harmful consequences for the actions. Figure 2.3 lists some common impulsive behaviors of children with ADHD. First impressions of children displaying these behaviors often result in judgments that they have poor self-control, are overly talkative, immature, or "rude." As a result, these children often face more punishment and criticism from adults than do their peers without ADHD. The poor inhibition and regulation of activity associated with these symptoms may result in some of the attention problems displayed by these students. This means that inattention symptoms may actually be signs of impulsivity. It is possible that those attention problems may be secondary to a primary disorder of behavioral regulation that shows itself as impulsivity and hyperactivity (Barkley, 2006). The impulsivity associated with ADHD often involves deficits in executive functions (Scheres et al., 2004). Executive functions involve strategic planning, cognitive flexibility, self-regulation, and goal-directed behavior (Weyandt, 2005). Executive function deficits are well documented among individuals with ADHD. Poor executive functioning leads to undercontrolled behavior, inability to properly inhibit responses, and the quick responses and impulsive behaviors so commonly associated with ADHD.

Hyperactivity

"Hyperactivity" refers to excessive or developmentally inappropriate levels of activity, whether motor or vocal. Hyperactivity is often characterized by restlessness, fidgeting, or simply moving about much more than is necessary. These physical actions are problematic because they are often unrelated to the task at hand or inappropriate for the situation. Figure 2.4 includes some common descriptions of hyperactivity. There are numerous ways that hyperactivity presents itself in children with ADHD. Children with hyperactivity are clearly more active, restless, and fidgety throughout the day then their peers. These children often move about in classrooms without permission or play with objects not related to their academic task. This often occurs during activities requiring sustained attention. They may also make

---

- Often chooses to do work that offers an immediate reward over work that will lead to a long-term reward.
- Takes shortcuts in his or her work and puts forth minimal effort to complete it.
- Badgers someone to immediately fulfill a promise.
- Has difficulty awaiting his or her turn in a game or social play situation.
- Says things indiscreetly, without regard for the feelings of others.
- Blurts out answers.
- Interrupts the conversations of others.

FIGURE 2.3. Characteristics of impulsivity. Based on Barkley (2006).

- Is always up and on the go.
- Acts as if driven by a motor.
- Climbs excessively.
- Can't sit still.
- Talks excessively.
- Often hums or makes odd noises.
- Is squirmy.

FIGURE 2.4. Common behaviors associated with hyperactivity. Based on DuPaul, Power, Anastopoulos, and Reid (1998).

unnecessary sounds or have a tendency to provide a running commentary on activities taking place around them (Barkley, 2006).

Types of ADHD

There are three types of ADHD: ADHD predominantly inattentive type (ADHD-IA), ADHD predominantly hyperactive–impulsive type (ADHD-HI), and ADHD combined type (ADHD-C). The type of ADHD diagnosed depends on whether the child's problems relate to inattention, hyperactivity–impulsivity, or both. ADHD characterized primarily by inattention is diagnosed as ADHD-IA. ADHD characterized primarily by hyperactivity or impulsivity is diagnosed as ADHD-HI. Children who meet the criteria for both ADHD-IA and ADHD-HI are diagnosed with ADHD-C (American Psychiatric Association, 2000). ADHD-IA and ADHD-C are by far the most common types of ADHD. ADHD-HI is relatively uncommon, especially among school-age children.

Note that there are other criteria that must be met in addition to the symptoms listed in Figure 2.1. The additional criteria include:

- Individuals must have displayed the symptoms *for at least six months*. ADHD is not a temporary or an "on again off again" disorder. It is a life-long problem.
- Symptoms must occur to a degree that is *developmentally deviant*. The behaviors must be extreme for the age group. For example, an extremely high degree of motor activity is common in a 3-year-old, but not in a 12-year old.
- Symptoms appeared before 7 years of age. Behaviors associated with ADHD should be present from an early age. Most parents report that they noticed problems by age 3 or 4. Behaviors should *not* suddenly appear after age 7 or in adolescence.
- Impairment from the symptoms should be present in *two or more settings*. ADHD symptoms should not be situational (i.e., appear only at home or school). If problems occur in only one setting the problems are probably not due to ADHD.

- Clear evidence of *significant impairment*. ADHD should cause serious problems in social, academic, or occupational functioning. Remember that it is quite possible for a child to exhibit many of the symptoms of ADHD but still function effectively in school and socially.
- There are exclusionary factors. These factors should rule out an ADHD diagnosis (e.g., schizophrenia). Additionally the symptoms can't be better explained by another problem (e.g., a mood disorder). This is because other disorders can result in symptoms of inattention, impulsivity and/or hyperactivity.

Note that a new DSM version—the DSM-5—is currently in the works. The diagnostic criteria may change somewhat in the new version.

ADHD AND COMMONLY ASSOCIATED DISORDERS

When ADHD occurs with one or more additional disorders, it is termed "comorbidity." Children with ADHD have a high risk for comorbid disorders. For example, Wilens and colleagues found that 75% of the preschool children and 80% of the school-age children referred to a specialized psychiatric clinic had at least one other disorder besides ADHD (Wilens et al., 2002). There is currently no explanation for why comorbid disorders occur so often with ADHD. Teachers should be aware of the increased risk of a comorbid disorder for two reasons. First, they need to be aware that the symptoms of some disorders (e.g., depression, anxiety) closely resemble ADHD symptoms. It's possible that another disorder might better explain ADHD symptoms. Second, teachers need to understand that dealing with one disorder is difficult. When comorbid disorders are present it is even more challenging, especially for parents. Teachers need to be sensitive to this problem. Before we discuss comorbid disorders there is one note of caution. Many of the estimates of comorbidity will tend to be on the high side because they are based on children who were referred to psychiatric clinics or who are severely involved.

Oppositional Defiant Disorder

Oppositional defiant disorder (ODD) is by far the most common comorbid disorder. ODD is characterized by a continuing pattern of defiant, hostile, and disobedient behavior toward authority figures that presents consistently for at least 6 months. The behaviors associated with ODD are often aggressive in nature (e.g., losing one's temper, arguing with adults, actively refusing to comply with directions of adults, deliberately doing things that will annoy people). These behaviors must occur more frequently than normal for a comparative age or developmental level, and must lead to significant impairment in social, academic, or occupational settings in order to be diagnosed as a disorder (DSM-IV-TR; American Psychiatric Association, 2000). A child with ADHD is 10 times more likely to also have ODD than a child without

ADHD (Angold, Costello, & Erkanli, 1999). Between 45 and 85% of children with ADHD will meet full diagnostic criteria for either ODD alone, or ODD combined with conduct disorder (Barkley & Biederman, 1997; Barkley et al., 1990; Biederman, Farone, & Lapey, 1992; Cohen, Velez, Brook, & Smith, 1989; Faraone & Biederman, 1997; Fischer, Barkley, Edelbrock, & Smallish, 1990; Pfiffner et al., 1999; Wilens et al., 2002).

Conduct Disorder

Conduct disorder (CD) is defined by a continued pattern of behaviors that violate the basic rights of others or age-appropriate societal norms. There are four groups of behavior problems: (1) aggressive conduct that causes or threatens physical harm to other people or animals; (2) nonaggressive conduct that causes property loss or damage; (3) deceitfulness or theft; and (4) serious violations of rules. Figure 2.5 lists some specific behaviors associated with each of the four CD groupings. Three or more of these behaviors must be present for 12 months, with at least one being present for 6 months, and they must cause significant impairment in social, academic, or occupational functioning in order for CD to be diagnosed. Estimates of comorbidity of CD and ADHD vary widely, ranging from 15–56% of children and 44–50% of adolescents (Wilens et al., 2002).

Aggressive behaviors
- Bullying, threatening, or intimidating behaviors
- Initiating frequent physical fights
- Using a weapon that can cause serious physical harm
- Being physically cruel to people or animals
- Stealing while confronting a victim
- Forcing someone into a sexual behavior

Deliberate destruction of others' property
- Fire setting with the intention of causing serious damage
- Deliberately destroying others' property by smashing, puncturing, etc.

Acts of deceitfulness or theft
- Breaking into someone's house, building, or car
- Frequently lying or breaking promises to obtain goods or favors or to avoid debts or other obligations
- Stealing items of nontrivial value without confronting the victim (i.e., shoplifting)

Serious violations of rules
- Staying out late at night despite parental prohibitions
- Running away from home overnight
- Being truant from school

FIGURE 2.5. Some behaviors associated with the four CD groupings. Based on American Psychiatric Association (2000).

CD often occurs in conjunction with ODD. In fact, it is much more common to find someone diagnosed with both ODD and CD than simply CD. At first glance it seems that CD and ODD have much in common. One key difference between ODD and CD is that the disruptive behaviors associated with ODD are often less severe than those associated with CD. Individuals with ODD only typically do not display aggression toward people or animals, for example, nor do they engage in destruction of property or a pattern of theft or deceit. However, nearly all of the features of ODD are usually present in CD (DSM-IV-TR; American Psychiatric Association, 2000).

Depression

Depression may be present if there is a period of at least 2 weeks during which there is either a severely depressed mood or loss of interest or pleasure in nearly all activities. This mood may be more irritable than sad in children and adolescents. These episodes must also include at least four additional symptoms such as changes in appetite or weight, decreased energy, feelings of worthlessness or guilt, difficulty in thinking or concentrating, or recurrent thoughts of death or suicide (DSM-IV-TR; American Psychiatric Association, 2000). A child with ADHD is five times more likely to also have a depressive disorder than a child without ADHD (Angold et al., 1999).

Psychosocial risk factors (events related to both social and psychological development) may have contributed to comorbidity (Drabick, Gadow, & Sprafkin, 2006). Boys who displayed social problems were much more likely to have symptoms of depression, as were boys from family environments characterized by frequent conflict. These findings may suggest that in some cases the presence of one disorder creates an environment conducive to the development of a second disorder. An example might be where a child's ADHD creates significant family stress. In such a case the child's ADHD might lead to a great deal of tension and arguing among the family. If the child feels responsible for causing the family's problems, he or she might internalize a feeling of guilt that could lead to symptoms of depression.

Anxiety Disorders

Anxiety disorders include several specific disorders, such as panic disorder, social phobia, postraumatic stress disorder, and acute stress disorder. In each of these anxiety disorders a heightened sense of anxiety reaches a strong enough level to debilitate an individual (DSM-IV-TR; American Psychiatric Association, 2000). Angold et al. (1999) found that the presence of ADHD in a child made it three times more likely that the child would also have an anxiety disorder. It is estimated that 25–35% of children with ADHD experience anxiety disorders (Biederman, Newcorn, & Sprich, 1991; Tannock, 2000). Additionally, about 15–30% of children diagnosed clinically with anxiety disorders were likely to have ADHD (Tannock, 2000).

Obsessive–Compulsive Disorder

Obsessive–compulsive disorder (OCD) occurs when an individual experiences recurrent obsessions or compulsions that are severe enough to be extremely time-consuming, cause significant distress, or cause marked impairment. These obsessions and compulsions are not caused by any physiological effects from medication or drugs, and are not the result of a general medical condition, such as an illness or injury. As with all disorders, the severity of the symptoms culminating in impairment is paramount in recognizing the presence of the disorder (DSM-IV-TR; American Psychiatric Association, 2000). Very few studies have assessed comorbidity between ADHD and OCD. The general consensus is that 3–5% of children with ADHD also have OCD. Brown (2000) estimated that between 6 and 33% of children with OCD also had ADHD. More research needs to be done to understand the possible link between these two disorders, but there is sufficient data to link OCD to ADHD (Barkley, 2006).

Bipolar Disorder

Bipolar disorder (BPD; previously referred to as manic–depression) is a complex mental disorder. The most commonly occurring form of BPD has separate criteria sets depending on whether the disorder is marked by manic or depressive episodes (we previously covered the symptoms of a depressive episode), or a mixture of the two. A manic episode is characterized by an abnormally and continuously elevated, expansive, or irritable mood lasting at least a week. This mood can include such characteristics as inflated self-esteem, decreased need for sleep, flight of ideas, and distractibility. The disturbance associated with these symptoms must be severe enough to cause marked impairment in social or occupational functioning or to require hospitalization, or be associated with psychotic features (i.e., hallucinations, hearing voices). Individuals with BPD can go through rapidly shifting moods (euphoria, irritability, sadness) and display symptoms including agitation, insomnia, irregular appetite, psychotic features, and suicidal thinking (DSM-IV-TR; American Psychiatric Association, 2000).

Most studies report the comorbidity for BPD and ADHD at around 10 to 15% (e.g., Biederman, Farone, & Lapey, 1992; Milberger, Biederman, Faraone, Murphy, & Tsuang, 1995) though some have reported rates of nearly double these amounts (Wilens et al., 2002). With different studies producing different percentages concerning coexisting ADHD and BPD, it is difficult to state definitively just how frequently the overlap occurs. BPD among children is somewhat controversial because the number of children diagnosed with BPD has increased 40-fold over the last decade, particularly among children with ADHD (Blader & Carlson, 2007). This has led some researchers to suggest that some children are being inappropriately diagnosed as BPD. Some researchers believe that children who have extreme difficulty regulating their emotions exhibit may exhibit behaviors that resemble symptoms of BPD and may be inappropriately given the BPD diagnosis.

Final Thoughts on Comorbidity

Individuals with ADHD are at high risk for also having one or more additional disorders. Teachers should be aware that additional disorders may be present. It is very possible that some disorders will include symptoms that mirror the symptoms of ADHD. Hopefully, our brief coverage of some of the disorders often comorbid with ADHD will prove useful, especially if someone with ADHD is displaying additional symptoms. Coping with ADHD alone is a complex undertaking; when additional disorders are present, coping with the demands becomes even more difficult and stressful. *Remember this when dealing with parents or caregivers.*

THEORIES OF ADHD

At present there is no generally accepted theory or body of research that adequately explains ADHD. Figure 2.6. summarizes some of the more influential theories of ADHD. In terms of practical use for the classroom teacher the most important theory is Barkley's (1997a).

Barkley's Theory

In Barkley's theory, ADHD is due to a deficit in self-regulation. He views problems with behavioral inhibition as the primary cause of ADHD behavior. Children with ADHD may be unable to stop their initial reaction to a situation. This initial reaction comes so quickly and automatically that it overwhelms executive functions that would normally help to guide behavior. Children with ADHD fail to monitor situations, assess whether an action is appropriate to the situation, act planfully, or consider the consequences of their actions. This results in impulsive behavior. For example, during a lesson a child with ADHD might notice that his pencil is dull. His immediate reaction would be (quite reasonably) to jump up to sharpen it. However, he would not consider that this was not appropriate during a lesson, that the teacher could be angry, and he could even be punished. In the words of the famous cartoon character Dennis the Menace, "By the time I've thought about what I'm gonna do I've already done it." ADHD is *not* the result of a lack of skills or knowledge. As Barkley puts it, ADHD is not a problem with knowing what to do, rather it's a problem with doing what one knows (Barkley, 2006). This is one reason why teachers are often so frustrated with children with ADHD. Children with ADHD do things that they know (at least in retrospect) will cause problems. Teachers need to realize that this is normal for ADHD. This type of problem is at the core of ADHD.

Barkley's theory provides an explanation for many of the problems of behavioral inhibition. It focuses on four processes that are critical to self-regulation of behavior: (1) nonverbal working memory, which includes self-awareness, sense of time, retrospective function (hindsight), and prospective function (foresight); (2) internalization of speech, which includes self questioning and problem solving;

Inhibited BIS

Based on the belief that our brains have a behavioral inhibition system (BIS) and a behavioral activation system (BAS). In the Quay–Gray model, the BAS is activated by signals of reward or avoidance and escape, and the BIS is activated by signals of punishment or frustrated nonreward. Quay stated that the impulsivity commonly associated with ADHD possibly arose from diminished function in the brain's BIS, that those with ADHD did not respond appropriately to signals that they should inhibit a behavior (Quay, 1988a, 1988b).

The "race model"

Also associated with the inhibitory deficits of ADHD. It is based on the "race" model proposed by Logan in which environmental stimuli provide signals for both activation and inhibition responses in the brain. The belief is that a signal for activation to create a response toward the stimuli is in a "race to the brain" with a signal for inhibiting a response toward the stimuli, and that whichever signal arrives first is the winner. Those with ADHD have a slower inhibition response, and also a slower ability to adjust their responses when required to do so by an individual task (Schachar, Tannock, & Logan, 1993).

Delay aversion

The impulsivity characterizing ADHD stems from an aversion to delay or waiting. This theory proposes that children with ADHD act more quickly than their peers without ADHD to terminate delays and achieve gratification (Sonuga-Barke, 2002; Sonuga-Barke, Taylor, & Hepinstall, 1992).

Reward dysfunction

Theory states that ADHD involves difficulty in how behavior is regulated by rules and the motivational factors in the task. The fundamental difficulty in the disorder is a deficit in responding to behavioral consequences, that those with ADHD have a "reward dysfunction" problem in regulating their behavior (Haenlein & Caul, 1987).

Optimal stimulation

ADHD seen as based on a difficulty maintaining sufficient arousal. Those with ADHD engage in sensation-seeking behavior in low-stimulation tasks and settings. This behavior can result in hyperactivity, difficult in waiting/delaying a response, and a preference for novel situations that results in a failure to attend to tasks at hand (Zentall, 2006).

FIGURE 2.6. Theories of ADHD.

(3) self-regulation of affect/motivation/arousal which includes objectivity; and (4) reconstitution (planning), which include analysis of behavior and planning.

Nonverbal Working Memory

Nonverbal working memory refers to our ability to keep information in mind that can be used to control our response to various stimuli. It is our ability to make use of our memories or skills appropriately in a given situation. We are able to call up what we have learned from previous experience when we encounter a similar situation at a later time. Nonverbal working memory incorporates past experiences and uses our memory of those experiences to help us regulate our actions. For example, in the pencil sharpening example above, we would remember that it was not OK to jump up during a lesson. It gives us the ability to imitate complex sequences of behavior, or to learn a skill by observing it practiced by someone else. Nonverbal working memory also includes the concepts of hindsight, our ability to look back at an experience and reflect on it, and forethought, our ability to consider the future and what actions we should take to accomplish a particular goal, or consider the future consequences of our actions. Our ability to remember a sequence of events also gives us a sense of time, and allows us to manage our behavior relative to time (i.e., time management).

Internalization of Speech

Internalization of speech is the concept of "self-talk." It is the "little voice in your head" that tries to give you advice on how to handle situations or solve problems. Self-talk helps us deal with problems by literally talking ourselves through things. For the most part self-talk is internal (i.e., it's inside our head) though in some instances it becomes externalized and we actually speak aloud to ourselves. There are plenty of examples of times where people have literally had conversations with themselves when thinking about how to handle a situation. For example, while driving someone notices that a tire has gone flat. The following internal dialogue might ensue, "Oh, great, a flat tire. What do I need to do? First I need to get over off the road, as far as I can. I do have a spare tire in the back, don't I? Yes, I remember seeing it the other day. And the jack is there, too. So I've got what I need to handle this situation, especially since the jack handle also helps take the tire off the car." In a very short "self-talk," the situation has been appraised and a plan to deal with the situation has been made. This type of self-speech is considered description and reflection. That is, we describe whatever is happening and then briefly reflect on how to respond to the situation. There are other types, such as self-questioning ("What's the formula for solving this problem?"), rule-governed behavior ("I know the teacher doesn't allow chewing gum, so I need to get rid of mine"), and moral reasoning ("I'd feel bad if someone treated me that way, so I'm not going to treat my friend like that").

Self-Regulation of Emotion/Motivation/Arousal

The ability to self-regulate our emotions, motivation levels, and general arousal levels in response to the environment is very important. Being able to control our actions based on an emotional response is a very significant part of self-regulation. External events have the power to generate an emotional response that may create a physical response. Most of us have the ability to rein in those emotions and not overreact. For example, if our favorite team loses a close game, we may be upset, but we can control ourselves and not smash the television out of frustration. We also have the ability to self-regulate our motivation. Self-regulation of motivation helps us maintain our efforts so we can reach a goal. People have differing levels of self-motivation, but when most of us are given a job we know how to do we find a way to get it done. The last component, the self-regulation of arousal, is closely tied to motivation in that we must also keep ourselves alert, oriented, and focused on goal-directed actions. Arousal is closely tied to our ability to persist at a task. Both motivation and arousal are related to drive, willpower, determination, and "sticking to it," attributes that may be difficult for individuals with ADHD (Barkley, 2006).

Reconstitution

Reconstitution refers to our ability to analyze behaviors, either our own or others, and then synthesize those behaviors into new behaviors needed to handle different situations. Planning, strategic behavior, and flexible problem solving are key elements of reconstitution. For example, imagine the common situation of a teenage girl who is constantly rushing around in the morning before school trying to find her books, school ID, papers, and so on. As a result she is seldom ready to leave on time—which angers her mother. Rather than continue with this pattern, she decides to gather all her materials and put them on the table so she is ready to go in the morning. The girl has analyzed the problem, and planned and implemented a strategy. Reconstitution also involves the ability to mentally simulate what might result from a new combination of behaviors or to see yourself in a situation. In our example the girl might mentally compare her typical behavior (searching frantically for books while her mother does a slow burn) with how much simpler it would be to simply pick up her backpack from the table. Unfortunately, children with ADHD will seldom if ever engage in this type of analysis independently. In sum, reconstitution involves the planful ordering of our actions to reach a specific goal.

POSSIBLE CAUSES FOR ADHD

Despite intensive effort and decades of research, as yet no cause or causes for ADHD have been found. To put it simply, we don't know what causes ADHD or even if there is a single cause or multiple causes. Many times research does not result in "the answer," but instead raises new questions or points to new directions.

Research on ADHD is no exception. While it has not produced a final, definitive cause for the disorder, it has provided many tantalizing possibilities, and made it possible to infer some possible causes for ADHD. This final section focuses on a few of these possibilities.

Neurological Factors

The brain has been one of the dominant areas of study. The well-established relation between behavior problems and specific regions of the brain is the driving basis for the belief in a neurological cause for ADHD (Barkley, 2006). Research suggests ADHD is related, to some degree, to structural and or/functional abnormalities in the frontal lobes, basal ganglia, and cerebellum portions of the brain, which are located in the front of the brain. Executive function deficits, which are associated with the frontal–striatal–cerebellar region of the brain, are commonly associated with ADHD symptoms. These include an inability to control behavioral responses, difficulties with working memory and verbal fluency, and difficulties with planning. Also included are difficulties with motor coordination and sequencing. These are problem areas for many children with ADHD, and thus suggest a neurological basis for ADHD (Barkley, 2006).

Recent studies suggest that cortical development may be delayed in children with ADHD, generally by several years (Shaw et al., 2007). The delay was most prominent in prefrontal regions important for control of cognitive processes including attention and motor planning. However, although the research showed a delay, there were no abnormalities in the cortex's structure. Other research has focused on transmission fibers in the posterior region of the brain. Transmission fibers carry chemical messages to and from different parts of the brain. Children with ADHD were shown to have fewer transmission fibers, which resulted in less activation in the frontal part of the brain due to deficient communication. The posterior region of the brain is responsible for accessing information from previous situations, while the frontal brain applies that knowledge to the situation at hand. Knowing the difficulties children with ADHD have in these areas, it is possible that fewer transmission fibers may be linked with ADHD (Semrud-Clikeman & Pliszka, 2005). Inefficient connections may also be a problem. Inefficient connections would lead to inefficient communication that can result in a poorer level of functioning, though not a total loss of function (Goldman-Rakic, 1987; van Zomeren & Brouwer, 1994). Some research suggests that brain networks that are separated work together to carry out attentional functions. If connections between these networks are deficient, then it is possible an individual may exhibit difficulty in carrying out tasks that require attention to multiple and overlapping demands (Corbetta & Shulman, 2002).

Brain research has advanced at a prolific rate over the past few decades, especially with technology that allows closer examinations of brain structures and brain functions. With the amount of data already collected in regards to neurological processes and ADHD, it is easy to infer a neurological basis for the disorder. While a definitive neurological component in the cause of ADHD remains elusive, the evidence at hand strongly suggests something in the brain is responsible for the development of ADHD.

Genetic Factors

Strong evidence from multiple lines of research suggests a genetic basis for ADHD. Research shows that if a child has ADHD, between 10 and 35% of the immediate family members are also likely to have the disorder, with the risk to siblings of these children being approximately 30% (Biederman, Farone, Keenan, et al., 1992; Biederman, Keenan, & Faraone, 1990; Levy & Hay, 2001; Welner, Welner, Stewart, Palkes, & Wish, 1977). If a parent has ADHD, the risk to their offspring is over 50% (Biederman, Farone, et al., 1995). Identical twins are commonly used in genetic studies because they share an identical genetic makeup. Numerous studies have demonstrated that if one twin has ADHD it is highly likely the other does also. This is strong inferential evidence of a genetic basis for ADHD. Multiple studies have supported the idea that some specific genes can be tied to ADHD, but more work needs to be done in that area. Similar to the results of neurological research, there is sufficient evidence to infer a genetic basis for ADHD, though as in most research efforts, it is not yet possible to state ADHD has a genetic basis (Barkley, 2006). It's important to interpret "genetic basis" correctly. ADHD is not like inheriting brown eyes or blue eyes. It is much more complicated. It's more accurate to say that individuals can inherit a *predisposition* to ADHD-type behaviors. It is unlikely that ADHD results from a single gene. It is more likely that there is complex of genes involved in ADHD.

Other Possible Causes

Food additives/diet, environmental toxins, prenatal cigarette and alcohol exposure, maternal smoking during pregnancy, and low birthweight have all been suggested as possible causes of ADHD (Banerjee, Middleton, & Faraone, 2007). Psychosocial causes have also been suggested. In this section, we discuss these possible causes.

Environmental Toxins

Exposure to environmental toxins can result in problems that are similar to ADHD. Lead contamination can result in distractibility, hyperactivity, restlessness, and lower intellectual functioning. Those characteristics are very similar to the diagnostic criteria used for ADHD (Needleman, 1982). Manganese exposure can also result in behavioral characteristics similar to those found in ADHD (Collipp, Chen, & Maitinsky, 1983). However, few students diagnosed with ADHD have been shown to suffer from any type of lead contamination (Barkley, 2006). It's questionable whether exposure to toxins could account for a significant percentage of ADHD cases, and whether ADHD would be the appropriate diagnosis in those cases.

Prenatal Cigarette and Alcohol Exposure

The effects of fetal exposure to maternal smoking and alcohol consumption have been well documented. High levels of fetal exposure to alcohol can lead to the impairment of cognitive abilities including overall intellectual performance, learning and memory, language, attention, reaction time, and executive functioning (Huizink & Mulder, 2006). Maternal tobacco use during pregnancy can adversely affect cognitive development and behavior in children and adolescents (Wasserman et al., 1999). However, as with environmental toxins, it is not certain how many cases of ADHD could be the result of prenatal cigarette and alcohol exposure.

Psychosocial Factors

Several psychosocial factors have been associated with ADHD. Children who have been physically of sexually abused have significantly greater incidences of ADHD and oppositional disorders (Famularo, Kinscherff, & Fenton, 1992; McLeer, Callaghan, Henry, & Wallen, 1994). Marital distress, family dysfunction, and exposure to maternal psychopathology are also risk factors for ADHD (Biederman, Milberger, et al., 1995).

SUMMING UP

In this chapter we gave an overview of the nature of ADHD, and the theory and causes of ADHD. There is a great deal of information on the behaviors associated with ADHD, and teachers need to understand the core problems of ADHD (i.e., inattention, impulsivity, and hyperactivity). It's obvious that there are many gaps in our knowledge, but this must be put in perspective. It's useful for teachers to have a working knowledge of the theory and possible causes for ADHD, especially when working with parents. However, in classroom practice, teachers don't need to know what causes ADHD to work effectively with children with ADHD.

- ✓ ADHD is complex. There are many different problems and combinations of problems. Bottom line—there's no such thing as a "typical" kid with ADHD.
- ✓ Inattention, impulsivity, and hyperactivity are the central problems of ADHD.
- ✓ Impulsivity is likely the core deficit in ADHD.
- ✓ For a diagnosis of ADHD, there must be *significant impairment*, that has occurred for at least 6 months, across two or more settings.
- ✓ It's likely that students with ADHD will also have other problems such as ODD, CD, depression, or anxiety. Comorbid disorders makes dealing with

ADHD much more difficult for parents and teachers. *Be sensitive to this issue.*

✓ ADHD is likely the result of problems with self-regulation. This is the result of deficits in executive functions involved with regulation of behavior. This means that problems with planning and organization are common.

✓ ADHD is not a problem of knowing what to do, it's a problem of doing what one knows (Barkley, 2006). Don't confuse this problem with willful disobediance.

✓ We don't know what causes ADHD. In practice it may not matter for teachers.

CHAPTER 3

Assessment of ADHD

I have yet to see any problem, however complicated, which, when looked at
in the right way did not become still more complicated.
                                                    —POUL ANDERSON

Assessment for ADHD is not always a straightforward process, for several reasons. First, there is no single test(s) that can be used to objectively and definitively diagnose ADHD. An ADHD diagnosis is subjective and must be made on the basis of informed judgment. Second, there is not a single assessment path. The diagnosis of ADHD can and should be made on a unique and individual basis (Barkley & Edwards, 2006). For example, a child who is displaying significant levels of inattention may not be assessed in exactly the same manner as a child whose problems are due to impulsivity. Third, ADHD is a diagnosis that requires ruling out other possible causes for symptoms (e.g., depression, anxiety disorders). Finally, the assessment process should involve both parents and teachers, and information should be collected across multiple settings. The current recommended assessment model is the *multimethod* assessment of ADHD. The multimethod approach involves multiple sources of information (e.g., interviews, rating scales, observations) from multiple informants (e.g., teachers, parents, caregivers) who have experience with the child in different settings. This information provides details on the extent to which ADHD symptoms are present, their severity, and the degree of impairment. This allows health professionals or schools to determine if a child meets the DSM criteria for ADHD.

The multimethod approach to assessment of ADHD is intended to reduce the possibility of misdiagnosis. Misdiagnosis of ADHD is most likely to occur in situations where a single practitioner makes a diagnosis based on limited information from a single source and environment. Misdiagnosing a disorder can have serious consequences in terms of treatment and services. For example, a child might be prescribed medication that would be totally ineffective. Thus, the assessment process should be as thorough as possible, taking sufficient time to collect all pertinent information before any final decision is made. The more information collected, the more accurate the final diagnosis will be (Handler & DuPaul, 2005).

Teachers are critical informants in the assessment process because they regularly observe students' behaviors and monitor academic performance. Teachers can provide information on student behavior because they observe it on a daily basis. They can often point out behaviors that are symptomatic of ADHD. Additionally, teachers are familiar with students' normal behavior; therefore they are likely to know if a student is behaving in a manner that is developmentally inappropriate. They also know if a student is struggling academically and are familiar with the nature of the difficulty (e.g., has trouble completing assignments or performs poorly on tests). They also are in a position to assess whether a student's troubles are caused by problems that are symptomatic of ADHD such as inattention during instruction, difficulty following directions, or frequently being off task. Typically, the teachers' role will be limited to providing information. While teachers provide critical information for the assessment, they should *never* be responsible for interpreting results and making the decision on whether an ADHD diagnosis is warranted.

Our focus in this section is to describe how the multimethod assessment of ADHD works and the teacher's role in the process. Our description includes coverage of the most commonly used assessment tools available for diagnosing ADHD: interviews, rating scales, direct observation of the student, review of academic records, academic and achievement testing, and a medical examination. Note that diagnosing ADHD is only one part of an assessment. Other steps, which include developing a treatment plan, specifying treatment goals, and monitoring an individual's progress in dealing with ADHD are discussed in subsequent chapters (Pelham, Fabiano, & Massetti, 2005).

INTERVIEWS

The assessment process often begins with interviews. Interviews are a simple and effective way to gather basic information about a student. There are two different interview formats: structured and semistructured. Structured interviews require those administrating the interview to read the questions exactly as written and in the order presented. Informants mostly respond categorically—either yes or no. Semistructured interviews allow the interviewer more freedom to inquire about certain aspects of the student's behaviors and to ask follow-up questions. The semistructured interview also allows the interviewer to more closely examine the severity of the behaviors (e.g., how much of a disruption is caused by the student's off-task behaviors, do inattentive behaviors require the teacher to constantly repeat directions to the student). The main goal of either interview format is to formulate a list of the student's specific problem behaviors. This list will then be compared to the DSM criteria for ADHD (Anastopoulos & Shelton, 2001).

Parents or caregivers are often the first interviewed because some information crucial for an ADHD diagnosis can only be provided by parents or caregivers. For example, the age at which symptoms appeared is important because an ADHD diagnosis requires that symptoms were present before age 7. Parents will be asked to provide basic background information on the child. This background information can be used to determine if there were previous behavior problems indicative of ADHD, if there was anything in the child's developmental history that stood out as abnormal, if the child ever showed signs of an emotional disturbance, and if the child had trouble adjusting socially. Parents can answer questions about the child's medical history and whether previous assessments/evaluations have been conducted. They will be able to provide information on when problem behaviors first occurred. Age of onset is important information, as we discuss later. Parents can also provide a family history, which might indicate that others in the child's family have ADHD. If other family members had received an ADHD diagnosis it may support the ADHD diagnosis for the student.

Teacher interviews can provide critical assessment information. Teachers are often the first to notice symptoms that might be caused by ADHD because they are familiar with developmentally normal behavior, and can easily detect behavior that deviates substantially from the norm (Sax & Kautz, 2003). In the course of normal daily activities, teachers directly observe students' classroom behaviors that may indicate ADHD. The teacher interview will include questions to help specify whether behaviors fitting DSM ADHD criteria (e.g., inattention, impulsivity) are present. The teacher interview also should collect information on whether or not the student's problematic behavior is subject to environmental influences. Possible antecedents for problem behavior that may cause or maintain problem behaviors should be identified. For example, are the student's problem behaviors more evident during individual or group tasks? Does the student have particular problems during transitions from one activity to another? Do the problem behaviors appear to depend on how others in the class react to those behaviors? The teachers should also be asked if any particular class management techniques have been effective in dealing with the student's behaviors because this information will be useful in the later stages of assessment and in intervention planning (DuPaul & Stoner, 2003).

The teacher interview also addresses the student's academic performance and social adjustment. Information on academic performance is important because most students with ADHD exhibit academic skill deficits. Students with ADHD are more likely to have handwriting that is difficult to read, careless approaches to academic tasks, and poorly organized work materials. A teacher interview can verify if a student has these types of problems (Barkley, 2006). Teachers will also be asked about any other disorders that could cause the behavior problems being observed. For example, students with learning disabilities often exhibit problems paying attention. It's important to rule out other disorders that could better account for the symptoms or to identify the presence of a comorbid disorder. Finally, teachers will be asked about social functioning. Teacher observations of the student's social interactions and his or her acceptance by peers can help determine whether the student has social skills deficits. Social skills deficits are common among students with ADHD. For example, many students with ADHD engage in a controlling and aggressive interaction pattern with their peers that often results in social rejection (Stormont, 2001).

RATING SCALES

Behavior rating scales are commonly used in the ADHD assessment process. They are an efficient way to gather important behavioral data on a student from multiple sources. They are simple to use and can often be completed relatively quickly (e.g., in 15 minutes). Rating scales typically consist of a series of statements (e.g., Fails to complete work) followed by a numerical rating (e.g., 1 = rarely, 2 = sometimes, 3 = often, 4 = very often). Users are asked to rate the child on each statement based on his or her typical behavior over the last 6 months. Rating scales are valuable because they can directly assess the presence and severity of symptoms that may be the result of ADHD. Additionally, many rating scales have norms that allow comparison of a child with his or her peer group. A thorough assessment requires both teachers and parents to fill out rating scales (Anastopoulos & Shelton, 2001). The rating scales results are an important piece of evidence for diagnosing ADHD.

There are two types of behavior rating scales: broad range and narrow range. Broad-range scales assess a wide array of behaviors and symptoms; they are not limited to ADHD. They can be used to help diagnosis many different disorders (e.g., ADHD, ODD, CD). They are important because they can rule out the presence of other disorders as the cause of symptoms or suggest the possibility of a comorbid disorder. There are many broad-range rating scales. Different scales have different features that might make them a more suitable choice for a particular case. For example, some broad-range rating scales include computerized scoring, which enables a user to quickly see the results. Some include a feature that allows for interview-style questions to be asked to elaborate on any areas of concern indicated by the scale. Because broad-range scales are used to assess the possibility of a number of different disorders they are much longer than narrow-range scales. Broad-range scales can range from 80 items to as many as 122 items. Also, some broad-range scales include different formats for different ages (e.g., one meant for children ages 5–12 and one meant for teens ages 13–18; Anastopoulos & Shelton, 2001). Figure 3.1 includes a brief description of some commonly used broad-range rating scales.

Narrow-range rating scales differ from broad-range scales in that narrow-range ADHD rating scales address only the specific behaviors that are symptomatic of ADHD (e.g, inattention and hyperactivity/impulsivity). These scales cannot be used to identify other disorders. Some of these narrow-band scales do go beyond

CRS-R

The Conners' Rating Scales—Revised (CRS-R; Conners, 1997) was designed to evaluate problem behaviors, and is now commonly used in diagnosing ADHD. There are forms for parents, teachers, and child self-report, each with short and long versions. Both versions ask raters to rate the frequency of behaviors on a 4-point Likert scale. The short form for teachers includes 28 items; the long form includes 59 items. The time to complete any of the forms is estimated to be 10–20 minutes. Subscale scores are available for Oppositional, Cognitive Problems/Inattention, Hyperactivity, Anxious–Shy, Perfectionism, Social Problems, Psychosomatic, Global Index, ADHD Index, DSM-IV, and Symptom subscales. The standardization sample for the teacher short form included 3,870 students, the sample for the long form included 6,880 students.

BASC-2 TRS

The Behavior Assessment System for Children–2 Teacher Rating System (BASC-TRS; Reynolds & Kamphaus, 1992) is designed as a comprehensive evaluation of a student's functioning. It also includes a Student Observation System (SOS). Teachers are asked to rate a child's behavior on a 4-point scale. There are at least 100 items depending on the child's age. The time to complete the scale is estimated to be between 10 and 20 minutes. Five composite scores can be derived: Behavioral Symptoms, Externalizing Problems, Internalizing Problems, School Problems, and Adaptive Skills. Scores can also be derived for Adaptability, Aggression, Anxiety, Attention Problems, Atypicality, Conduct Problems, Depression, Hyperactivity, Leadership, Learning Problems, Social Skills, Somatization, Study Skills, and Withdrawal. The standardization sample for the TRS included 4,650 students (Gladman & Lancaster, 2003).

CBCL-TRF

The Child Behavior Checklist—Teacher Report Form (TRF; Achenbach & Rescorla, 2001) includes 118 items. Respondents rate each behavior on a 3-point scale: not true (0), somewhat or sometimes true (1), or very true or often true (2). The TRF provides scores for Withdrawn, Somatic Complaints, Anxious/Depressed, Social Problems, Thought Problems, Attention Problems, Delinquent Behavior, and Aggressive Behavior. The CBCL also contains items about activities, social relationships, academic performance, chores, and hobbies, which are summarized in three competence scales: Activities, Social, and School scales. The standardization sample for the CBCL included 2,368 children.

FIGURE 3.1. Broad-band behavior rating scales commonly used in assessing ADHD.

the specific ADHD symptom criteria to identify additional warning signs indicative of the disorder. For example, the Adolescent Behavior Checklist includes scores for such additional indicators as conduct problems, poor work habits, and social problems/competence (factors consistently identified as weak in students with ADHD) (Anastopoulos & Shelton, 2001). Figure 3.2 includes a brief description of some commonly used narrow-band rating sales.

Like the broad-range scales, the narrow-range scales have different features that may be desirable or useful. For example, some scales include versions for both parents and teachers. This is very useful when comparing teacher and parent ratings. It can also provide critical assessment information because for an ADHD diagnosis

ADHD Rating Scale–IV

The ADHD Rating Scale–IV (DuPaul, Power, Anastopoulos, & Reid, 1998) has parallel versions for both parents and teachers. Each version consists of 18 items, and should take about 10 minutes to complete. Each item is scored on a 4-point scale from *not at all* to *very often*, generating scores for both inattention and impulsivity/hyperactivity. A Total Score is derived from the inattention and impulsivity/hyperactivity subscores. The standardization sample for both the parent and teacher versions included 2,000 students.

ADDES-2

The Attention Deficit Disorders Evaluation Scales–2 (ADDES-2; McCarney, 1995) includes forms for both parents and teachers. The school version is intended for children ages 4–19. The home version includes 46 items; the school version includes 60 items. The estimated completion time is 15–20 minutes. Both versions consist of the same response format, with items rated on a 5-point scale, from (0) *does not engage in the behavior* to (4) *one to several times per hour*. Subscale scores are produced for Inattentive and Hyperactive/Impulsive Symptoms. The standardization sample for the home version included 2,415 children; the sample for the school version included 5,795 students (Angello et al., 2003).

SNAP–IV

The SNAP–IV (Swanson, 1992) is an updated version of the SNAP Questionnaire. It consists of nine inattentive and nine impulsive–hyperactive symptoms from the DSM-IV symptom list for ADHD. Teachers and parents use the same version. The SNAP-IV uses a 4-point scale (0 = *Not At All*, 1 = *Just A Little*, 2 = *Quite A Bit*, and 3 = *Very Much*) for rating each item. Cut scores for inattentive, hyperactive/impulsive, and combined type ADHD are included. The SNAP-IV is available at *www.myadhd.com/snap-iv-6160-18sampl.html*.

FIGURE 3.2. Narrow-band behavior rating scales.

symptoms must be present across multiple settings (e.g., home, school). Some scales provide separate scores for each ADHD symptom (i.e., inattention, impulsivity, and hyperactivity). Some scales have versions for different age groups (e.g., an elementary school teacher would fill out a different rating scale than would a middle or high school teacher). This can be helpful as both problem behaviors and environmental demands change over time. Some rating scales are very brief to administer, taking roughly 15 minutes to complete, while others are much more involved and may incorporate such additional features as direct observation data. One important feature is separate norms for different age groups.

Figure 3.3 shows an example of a commonly used narrow-range scale: the ADHD Rating Scale–IV: School Version (DuPaul, Power, et al., 1998). The scale presents the nine DSM-IV criteria for inattention and the nine DSM-IV criteria for impulsivity/hyperactivity in alternating fashion (inattention in odd-numbered positions and impulsive/hyperactive in even-numbered positions). To complete the scale, teachers read over the 18 items and circle the number (0 for Never or rarely, 1 for Sometimes, 2 for Often, and 3 for Very Often) they believe best describes the frequency of specific student behaviors. After the scale is filled out, the raw scores are tabulated by totaling the scores for the odd-numbered responses for an Inattention

	Never or rarely	Sometimes	Often	Very often
1. Fails to give close attention to details or makes careless mistakes in schoolwork.	0	1	2	3
2. Fidgets with hands or feet or squirms in seat.	0	1	2	3
3. Has difficulty sustaining attention in tasks or play activities.	0	1	2	3
4. Leaves seat in classroom or in other situations in which remaining seated is expected.	0	1	2	3
5. Does not seem to listen when spoken to directly.	0	1	2	3
6. Runs about or climbs excessively in situations in which it is inappropriate.	0	1	2	3
7. Does not follow through on instructions and fails to finish work.	0	1	2	3
8. Has difficulty playing or engaging in leisure activities quietly.	0	1	2	3
9. Has difficulty organizing tasks and activities.	0	1	2	3
10. Is "on the go" or acts as if "driven by a motor."	0	1	2	3
11. Avoids tasks (e.g., schoolwork, homework) that require sustained mental effort.	0	1	2	3
12. Talks excessively.	0	1	2	3
13. Loses things necessary for tasks or activities.	0	1	2	3
14. Blurts out answers before questions have been completed.	0	1	2	3
15. Is easily distracted.	0	1	2	3
16. Has difficulty awaiting turn.	0	1	2	3
17. Is forgetful in daily activities.	0	1	2	3
18. Interrupts or intrudes on others.	0	1	2	3

FIGURE 3.3. ADHD Rating Scale–IV: School Version. From DuPaul, Power, Anastopoulos, and Reid (1998). Copyright 1998 by the authors. Reprinted with permission from The Guilford Press.

subscale score, and the even-numbered responses for a Hyperactive–Impulsive sub-scale score. These scores can then be combined for a total score. The raw scores can also be converted into percentile scores. There are norms for boys and girls bro-ken down into four age groups: 5–7, 8–10, 11–13, and 14–18. For example, consider a 7-year-old boy who receives a maximum raw score of 27 on the hyperactivity/impulsivity subscale. A raw score of 27 equals a percentile score of 99. That means the boy scored in the top 1% for his age group and gender. This score would support a diagnosis of ADHD. Note that this would only *support* a diagnosis. No single score on a rating scale should be considered as diagnostic of ADHD in and of itself. The student would still have to meet other criteria noted in Chapter 2 (e.g., behaviors cause serious problem in functioning, symptoms appeared before age 7) and other sources for the problem (e.g., depression) would need to be ruled out. The ADHD Rating Scale–IV manual includes detailed information on cut scores. *Cut scores* are thresholds that are predictive of the presence or absence of ADHD. For example, if a student's percentile score for Inattention is greater than or equal to .90, research has shown that, if the rest of the diagnostic criteria were met, the child will very likely fit the diagnostic criteria for ADHD-IA. Conversely, a student who scores below the 90th percentile for Inattention will very likely not meet the criteria for an ADHD diagnosis. The same is true for scores for Hyperactivity–Impulsivity and for the combined type of ADHD (DuPaul et al., 1998).

In summary, teachers should remember that rating scales are not a "one size fits all" proposition (Anastopoulos & Shelton, 2001). Teachers should realize that—depending on the situation—they might be asked to fill out different scales for different students being assessed for ADHD. In some cases more than one form may be needed for the same student. In fact, in a thorough assessment, a teacher would likely be asked fill out both a broad-band and a narrow-band rating scale. The broad-band rating scale would be used to check for the presence of a comorbid disorder; the narrow-band scale would focus on ADHD. If a teacher were only to fill out a narrow-band scale specifically seeking ADHD, the presence of another disorder could be missed. The only situation where assessment would be limited to narrow-band scales would be if there was no reason to suspect that another comor-bid disorder was present (DuPaul & Stoner, 2003).

DIRECT OBSERVATION

Direct observation of the student in home and classroom situations is a valuable tool. Observations can provide immediate evidence of ADHD symptoms. Through direct observation it is easy to determine if students exhibit behaviors that are symptoms of ADHD such as high rates of off-task behavior, gross motor activity (fidgeting), or inappropriate vocalizations (e.g., speaking out of turn, interrupting others, animal noises). Several observations of the student performing independent academic work should be conducted. These observations can provide information on what symptoms of ADHD (inattention, impulsivity, and/or hyperactivity) relate to student's academic difficulty. Figure 3.4 lists some common observation tools available for use during an ADHD assessment (Anastopoulos & Shelton, 2001).

Although direct observation is considered part of the "best practice" of assessment, in practice it is not employed as often as it should be (Handler & DuPaul, 2005). Few doctors, psychologists, or psychiatrists make the time to leave their offices, go to a child's school or home, and observe a child's behavior. Instead many health professionals depend on the information obtained from interviews and the scores on rating scales to make the diagnosis. In essence, they consider the teachers and parents who are interviewed and complete the rating scales as observers. The parents and teachers become the health professionals' eyes and ears, so to speak, providing the kinds of information the doctor would find by conducting a direct observation (Handler & DuPaul, 2005). Direct observation is more commonly included in a school-based assessment, where the school psychologist would visit

---

DOF
The Direct Observation Form and Profile for Ages 5–14 (DOF; McConaughy & Achenbach, 2004) consists of 96 items developed from norms obtained from observing 287 children ages 5–14 in classroom settings. The system allows for tabulation of On-Task, Internalizing, Externalizing, and Total Problems scores, and once fully processed produces a computer-scored profile including six additional scales: Withdrawn–Attentive, Nervous–Obsessive, Depressed, Hyperactive, Attention-Demanding, and Aggressive. The DOF includes a section for the observer to write a more detailed description of student behavior.

BASC SOS
The BASC Student Observational System (SOS; Kamphaus & Reynolds, 1992) allows coding of directly observed adaptive and maladaptive classroom behaviors. After a 15-minute observation, the observer completes three sections. The first is a frequency checklist of 65 behaviors in 13 categories (four adaptive and nine maladaptive). The second section is a recording of behaviors during thirty 3-second observations spread across the 15 minutes. The third section is a place to note any additional observations, including the teacher's response to the behavior or teacher–child proximity during the behavior. The system allows the observer to note whether any particular behaviors disrupted the class. The SOS system is useful because it records the degree to which certain maladaptive behaviors may be disruptive, and it also proves useful in determining the effectiveness of any applied interventions.

AD/HD Behavior Coding System
The AD/HD Behavior Coding System (Barkley, 1990) requires observation of a child or adolescent completing an independent academic task. The child's behavior during the activity is then observed for 15 minutes and is coded in five categories: off-task, fidgeting, leaving the seat, vocalizing, and playing with toys and objects. The observer checks for any of those five behaviors every 30 seconds, and the percentage of each behavior and total occurrence for all behaviors is calculated. The number of problems completed and completed correctly is also calculated.

FIGURE 3.4. Direct observation tools available for use during an ADHD assessment.

the child's classroom and conduct the observation. The school psychologist would then combine the observation data with rating scale scores and interview information to assist the diagnostic process.

RECORDS REVIEW

Another important part of a multimethod assessment is a review of the student's school records. This review is to determine whether or not there were any earlier problems that may be indicative of ADHD. These signs include a history of academic difficulties such as grade retention, problems with work completion, and consistent low marks. Records should also be examined for evidence of prior behavioral problems. For example, disciplinary actions such as suspensions or office referrals may suggest ADHD-related problems. There may have been referrals for screening made earlier in the student's school history. In many schools teachers grade the quality of a student's work habits and behaviors and include those grades on report cards. These reports can provide information on student's' work habits. Additionally, teachers often include comments about why a student received low marks for work effort and behavior, and those comments may provide additional evidence for when a student began to display ADHD symptoms (DuPaul & Stoner, 2003).

A records search can be as simple as examining a child's file and writing down relevant information. Unfortunately, this unstructured approach risks overlooking important information. There are structured approaches to records review such as the School Archival Records Search (SARS; Walker, Block-Pedego, Todis, & Severson, 1998) that offer several advantages. The SARS uses a standardized format to collect information concerning 11 categories, such as number of schools attended, number of days absent, grades retained, and academic/behavior referrals. This reduces the risk of omitting important information. The data obtained for each of the 11 variables is used to create scores for three areas: Disruption, Needs Assistance, and Low Achievement. There are standardized cut scores that point to potential problems in any of those three areas. This allows for comparisons to the norm group. Students with ADHD, or other behavior disorders, often receive scores indicative of problems with Disruption and Low Achievement. Structured approaches such as the SARS can be helpful in the ADHD assessment process because they provides a standardized method of gathering information pertinent to an ADHD diagnosis (DuPaul & Stoner, 2003).

ACADEMIC TESTING

Academic testing is an important part of the assessment process because ADHD will usually have an impact on classroom performance. There is some debate over what type of information—standardized tests or curriculum-based measures—is most useful and should be collected. Standardized tests do provide valuable information concerning a student's cognitive and academic strengths and weaknesses. They also allow comparison to norm groups. Additionally, they may prove useful in determining whether a student has a disability other than or in conjunction with ADHD (e.g., a learning disability). In many cases this information may already be available because of the normal achievement testing process. The drawback to standardized tests is that they provide very general information. An achievement test may tell us that a student is low in reading, but won't provide information on student's specific problems or on day-to-day performance. Some researchers believe it is more useful to directly assess a student's day-to-day performance on academic tasks. They believe that examining completion and accuracy rates on in-class assignments and homework, acquisition of skills being taught in the curriculum, and organizational skills can provide more useful information for intervention. Students with ADHD often experience difficulties in these areas so gauging a student's performance in these areas should be included in the assessment process (DuPaul & Stoner, 2003). We would agree that this is useful information. Moreover, it is simple to collect. Completion rates for assigned tasks can be obtained by comparing the amount of work completed by the student with the amount of work expected or the amount of work completed relative to classmates. Task accuracy can be determined by computing the number of items completed correctly. Curriculum-based measurement (CBM; Shinn, 1998) can be used to gauge a student's acquisition of skills taught in the curriculum. A student's organizational skills can be assessed by observation (e.g., how organized desk and materials are in comparison to the rest of the class). We believe that day-to-day performance information can provide important data. However, there is a potential concern about this information. There is a possibility that preconceptions could influence assessment. For example, if there was a strong belief that a child had ADHD, a record search might focus on information that suggested ADHD and ignore contradictory information, or a single lost assignment might be seen as indicative of a serious organizational problem. It's important that this information be interpreted as objectively as possible. Once again note that this information should be used in conjunction with other sources mentioned previously.

MEDICAL EXAMINATION

A medical examination may or may not be included in assessment. If a medical examination is done it would be to rule out other potential causes for symptoms that seem to indicate ADHD (Barkley, 2006). A number of medical conditions can cause ADHD-like symptoms such as sleep disturbances, thyroid dysfunction, head trauma, central nervous system infections, allergies, anemia, and vision and hearing impairments (Barkley, 2006; Hoban, 2008; Leo, Khin, & Cohen, 1996; Monastra, 2008). In addition, adverse reactions to medication for asthma or seizure disorders may be associated with problems with inattention and impulsivity. To rule out these types of problems, some doctors will include a physical examination as part of their assessment for ADHD.

ASSESSMENT "RED FLAGS"

Some aspects of ADHD assessment are as yet poorly understood. In this section we address four factors—gender, ethnicity, age of onset, and "halo" effects—that can affect assessment. Teachers should be aware that these factors might affect whether students are correctly diagnosed or referred for an ADHD diagnosis.

Gender

As we noted in Chapter 2, there is a pronounced gender disparity among children diagnosed with ADHD. The ratio between males to females ranges from 4:1 to 9:1, depending on whether a community-based or clinic-based sample is used (Barkley, 2006). This gender disparity has remained relatively unchanged over the last 40 years. Exactly why this disparity occurs is not well understood. One possible explanation is that males are more prone to ADHD-type behaviors. Interestingly, the behaviors used to define ADHD symptoms in the DSM-IV were created from a sample made up primarily of males (Frick et al., 1994; Lahey et al., 1994). Another explanation is that boys are more prone to disruptive behaviors and comorbid ODD or CD that upset teachers and parents. For example, boys with ADHD are more likely than girls to be expelled or suspended from school (Bauermeister et al., 2007) and girls are rated lower on ADHD hyperactivity and impulsivity symptoms (Gaub & Carlson, 1997; Gershon, 2002). It is also possible that girls with ADHD are more likely to have the predominantly inattentive subtype and that girls are more prone to comorbid depression or anxiety disorders (Barkley, 2006; Gaub & Carlson, 1997; Gershon, 2002). Thus girls may not be noticed because they don't exhibit behaviors that disrupt the classroom. Unfortunately, gender differences among children with ADHD are not well studied and there are conflicting results. Some recent research that has focused on differences between boys and girls with ADHD suggest that there are few if any differences in how the disorder presents, risk factors associated with ADHD, comorbid disorders, and school and family functioning (Bauermeister et al., 2007; Biederman et al., 2005; Silverthorn, Frick, Kuper, & Ott, 1996).

Another well-documented gender difference is that girls typically are rated lower than boys on behavior rating scales (e.g., Reid et al., 2000). The concern here is that if norms are based on averages that combine both boys' and girls' results, then boys may tend to be overidentified and girls may tend to be underidentified. One study found a subset of girls with elevated rating scale scores compared to other girls (Waschbusch & King, 2006). The girls with elevated rating scale scores also had significantly more problems with inattention, hyperactivity, and oppositional behavior than the girls in the average range; however, the girls with elevated scores did not meet DSM-IV-TR criteria for ADHD. Overall, the research suggests that there are girls with ADHD who may not be identified. This means teachers need to pay close attention for ADHD-like behaviors in girls who experience difficulties in the classroom. The girls most likely to be overlooked are not the ones who act out, but those who may appear to be more withdrawn, inattentive, or disorganized.

Cultural Diversity

The assessment of culturally different students with special needs is an ongoing problem. Minorities consistently have been disproportionately represented in categories of disability (Dunn, 1968; Mercer, 1973). For example, African American and Hispanic students are diagnosed and placed into special education (Coutinho & Oswald, 2000; Oswald, Coutinho, Best, & Singh, 1999) at higher than expected rates. The effect of cultural diversity in the ADHD assessment process is still not well understood. However, it is a significant concern because the number of children from minority groups has increased dramatically over the last decades—soon the combined minority groups will become the majority. Thus, teachers need to be aware of the possible effects of culture on ADHD assessments. The major area of concern is the use of rating scales with students from different cultural backgrounds. Teachers' ratings of students consistently differ across Caucasian and African American groups, with African American students receiving significantly higher ratings. Ratings of Caucasian and Hispanic groups show inconsistent results. Some studies have reported differences and some have not. This is important because of the potential for rater bias (i.e., teacher ratings inflated because of ethnic status) that could lead to overidentification of ADHD in certain ethnic groups.

There are several possible explanations for the differences across groups. One possibility is that some teachers may be less tolerant of behaviors not in line with their own cultural expectations (Gerber & Semmel, 1984; Lambert, Puig, Lyubansky, Rowan, & Winfrey, 2001). Some evidence suggests that Caucasian teachers may have lower thresholds of tolerance for problem behaviors exhibited by African American students (Puig et al., 1999). Another possibility is that differences in ratings may reflect an underidentification of Caucasian students (Hosterman, DuPaul, & Jitendra, 2008). Still another possibility is that there are real differences in behavior across groups. There is some evidence to support this notion. Epstein et al. (2005) compared African American and Caucasian students with ADHD. They found distinct differences in the amount of classroom activity levels between the groups. However, differences could also be due to different classroom environments across groups. On the whole, the classrooms with African American students with ADHD tended to have more activity and less on-task behavior than the classrooms with the Caucasian students with ADHD. When the average activity level of a classroom was controlled, the differences across groups were not significant. In other words, the activity level of the African American children did not stand out nearly as much in the context of the overall activity level in the classroom. To further complicate matters the researchers found that there were differences in SES across the groups. When SES was controlled there were no differences across the groups.

More research needs to be done on this topic, but as stated earlier, rating scale scores for ethnically diverse students should be evaluated carefully (Hosterman et al., 2008). Additional data should be gathered and examined to confirm the results obtained from the rating scales. For example, schools might want to compare the activity level or inattention of students suspected of having ADHD to his or her peers. Additionally, schools should consider the extent to which the behaviors of concern are maladaptive. Teachers should remember that rating scales alone should not be the sole evidence used to diagnose ADHD in any student, and *especially not in a minority student* (Reid et al., 1998).

Age of Onset

If a student meets all other diagnostic criteria for ADHD, obvious symptoms that cause significant impairment in multiple settings, but there is no evidence that those symptoms were present prior to age 7, does that mean the student definitively does not have ADHD? DSM-IV-TR requires that for ADHD to be diagnosed, "Some hyperactive–impulsive or inattentive symptoms that caused impairment were present before age 7 years" (American Psychiatric Association, 2000). The reason the age-of-onset requirement was initially included was that there were believed to be distinct differences between individuals who displayed symptoms prior to age 7 and those who did not. Many individuals in the field trials for the DSM-IV-TR criteria who displayed ADHD symptoms at age 6 or earlier had more severe and consistent problems when compared to those who had later onset. Further studies showed that these difficulties were matters of degree and not type. That is, even though onset of symptoms before age 7 might lead to more serious problems with the disorder, the same problems were still evident in those who did not display symptoms until after age 7. Thus, no clear qualitative distinctions emerged between those who exhibit ADHD symptoms before age 7 and those who exhibit them after age 7 (Barkley, 2006). There is also evidence to suggest that up to 10% of children with ADHD do not demonstrate onset before age 7 (Todd, Huang, & Henderson, 2008). The age of onset requirement may be changed in the next revision to the DSM.

The "Halo Effect"

The term "halo effect" (Guilford, 1954) refers to how perceptions of one set of behaviors can influence the perception of another set of different, unrelated behaviors. Put simply, we see one behavior and as a result believe we see other behaviors that actually are not present. Halo effects are a concern because they could potentially influence the results of behavior rating scales. The concern is that oppositional behaviors (e.g., noncompliance, defiance) could cause teachers to endorse the presence of behaviors symptomatic of ADHD (e.g., inattention, impulsivity) and result in an inaccurate diagnosis. Additionally, there is evidence that factors such as ethnicity and low SES can produce halo effects and result in ratings that are inflated (Stevens, 1980). The impact of halo effects on the assessment of ADHD has not received a great deal of research attention. However, there is evidence that halo effects can significantly influence teachers' ratings of ADHD symptoms. When elementary school teachers viewed videos of a student displaying behaviors associated with ADHD and ODD, teachers were accurate in their assessments of inattention and hyperactivity (i.e., ADHD symptoms); however, when students exhibited behaviors associated with ODD (e.g., opposition, noncompliance) *but not ADHD*, teachers would endorse behaviors associated with ADHD even when they were not present (Abikoff, Courtney, Pelham, & Koplewicz, 1993; Jackson & King, 2004; Stevens, Quittner, & Abikoff, 1998). That means that the teachers mistakenly rated the child exhibiting only oppositional behaviors as also displaying ADHD symptoms. Gender can also result in halo effects. Jackson and King (2004) found that when boys and girls display the same amount of ODD symptoms, teachers tended to rate the boys as displaying more ADHD symptoms. However, the reverse is true for ADHD symptoms: girls who display ADHD symptoms are rated higher on ODD symptoms than boys.

It is difficult to gauge the impact of halo effects on the assessment process because it may not be possible to say, "Well, clearly this is a case of halo effects." The only way to make such a distinction is through observation by someone adequately trained to distinguish differences. This emphasizes the need for multiple types of assessments in the ADHD assessment process. However, knowing that factors such as gender and oppositional behavior can produce halo effects may help to lessen their potential impact. Unfortunately, it is highly unlikely that halo effects can be totally removed from the assessment process. Note that halo effects don't equate to discrimination—teachers are not trying to see behaviors that are not actually present. A better analogy would be an optical illusion. Just as an optical illusion fools the eye, the presence of oppositional or ADHD behaviors can sometimes distort teacher's perceptions. This should also underscore the importance of multimethod ADHD assessments.

SUMMING UP

In this chapter we provided an overview of the ADHD assessment process and the teacher's role in it. By now it should be obvious that making an ADHD diagnosis isn't as simple as looking at an X-ray or the results of a blood test. It's a judgment call. The presence of comorbid disorders can complicate the process. Teachers should never be called on to make an actual diagnosis. This is the province of a health professional (e.g., physician, pediatrician, psychiatrist, clinical psychologist). Few school psychologists, who are typically trained at the master's level, would have the training to make an ADHD diagnosis, and in survey, only 23% of school psychologists reported using best practice in ADHD assessment (Handler & DuPaul, 2005). However, teachers and school psychologists are a source of critical information on school functioning.

✓ There are no *objective* measures for diagnosing ADHD. There *is no single test or information source* that can be used in isolation for an ADHD diagnosis.

✓ Teachers are critical components in the assessment process. They may be asked to be the health professional's eyes and ears.

✓ Teachers and parents may be asked to supply different types of information on students such as rating scales, interviews, and possibly observations.

✓ Direct observations and records reviews should be included in the assessment process.

✓ Assessments may also address comorbid disorders if they are suspected.

✓ The DSM age-of-onset criterion for ADHD may be raised or eliminated in the next revision of the DSM.

✓ Academics should be a part of the ADHD assessment process. This might include examining achievement test scores and curriculum-based measures.

✓ Girls with ADHD may be overlooked, especially if they don't act out.

✓ Be careful when dealing with students from different cultural groups. There could be a potential for misdiagnosis.

✓ Be careful when dealing with students who have oppositional behaviors. There is a possibility for halo effects. An experienced professional is needed to differentiate between ADHD and ODD.

CHAPTER 4

ADHD in the Schools

School and education should not be confused;
it is only school that can be made easy.
—ANONYMOUS

Schools have a tremendous responsibility. They are expected to educate millions of students who have a vast array of individual skills, talents, and needs. The school is responsible for the gifted student who needs advanced calculus, the student with developmental disabilities who needs functional living skills, and all those in between. Schools are also responsible for students with ADHD. Students with ADHD can pose problems for schools because they often combine chronic behavior problems, academic difficulties, and other problems (e.g., social difficulties). Schools must have programs in place to help these students. Schools must also be aware of the legal rights of students with ADHD and the services they are entitled to under federal law. In the case of students with ADHD this can be confusing because ADHD straddles the fields of medicine and education. ADHD is a *medical diagnosis* not an *educational category*. However, the great majority of students with ADHD qualify for services and legal protections under *education* law. As we noted in Chapter 2, academic difficulties are common among students with ADHD, and a problem functioning effectively in the school environment is expressly mentioned in the diagnostic criteria. While every student with ADHD does not experience school-related problems, these cases *are the exception* rather than the rule. It is important for teachers to have a working knowledge of the legal rights of students with ADHD and the services and protections they are entitled to, both for the good of the student and good of the school. In this chapter we discuss the two federal laws that directly impact services for ADHD students, their legal rights and safeguards, and the service provision options available to them.

FEDERAL LAWS THAT IMPACT STUDENTS WITH ADHD: THE INDIVIDUALS WITH DISABILITIES EDUCATION ACT AND SECTION 504

Individuals with Disabilities Education Act

The Individuals with Disabilities Education Act (IDEA) is the modern version of Public Law 94-142, the Education for All Handicapped Children Act, passed by Congress in August 1975 to protect the educational rights of children with disabilities. IDEA covers students from birth to age 21. It defines 13 categories of disability and provides the criteria for each of the categories of disability. To receive services under IDEA, a student must meet the requirements for at least one category of disability. IDEA provides federal funding to state and local education agencies to allow them to provide services to any student identified as having a disability. The intent of IDEA is to ensure that local school districts are able to provide an appropriate education to all students with special needs. IDEA contains three key components that impact special needs students, including students with ADHD: (1) free and appropriate public education (FAPE), (2) placement in a least restrictive environment (LRE), and (3) an individualized education plan (IEP) for these students.

FAPE goes to the heart of IDEA. The intent is to provide students with special needs the opportunity to benefit from education. It mandates that all students with disabilities are provided with *appropriate* educational services and that these services must be provided at public expense. Parents *are not responsible* for the costs of appropriate services associated with their child's education. Furthermore, IDEA states that special education services are to be provided under public supervision and direction, and must include an appropriate preschool, elementary school, or secondary school education. FAPE also includes the right to appropriate assessment and identification. This means that FAPE ensures students with ADHD can receive a proper school-based assessment, which in turn will help guide the creation and implementation of school-based interventions (U.S. Department of Education, 2006a). In the case of students with ADHD, this means that the school is obligated to provide appropriate accommodations and services (discussed in Chapters 5 and 6).

The concept of the LRE grew out of concerns that children with special needs might be placed in school environments that effectively isolated them from their peers. The intent of LRE is that a student be educated in a situation that is as close to "normal" as possible, given individual circumstances. To the maximum extent possible, schools must educate special needs students with their peer group. If a student with ADHD demonstrates the capacity to succeed in all regular classes with various accommodations provided, then regular classes would be considered that student's LRE. Conversely, if a student with ADHD clearly demonstrates that he or she requires more intensive and direct interventions in some subjects, then a resource setting for one or more classes may be justified as the LRE. Both *least* and *restrictive* in the term LRE are open to serious interpretation on a case-by-case basis which adds some complexity to placement discussions (U.S. Department of Education, 2006b). Where students are placed is discussed in more detail later in the chapter.

A third part of IDEA relevant for students with ADHD is the requirement for an IEP. IDEA requires schools to develop and implement an IEP for all special education students, to ensure that these students are receiving the accommodations and services needed to profit from an education. An IEP is a critical document for students with disabilities. An IEP includes (1) a written statement of the student's present level of educational performance; (2) measurable annual goals and short-term objectives related to meeting the child's needs that result from the disability; (3) special education, related services, supplementary aids/services, and program modifications to be provided for the student; (4) any modifications needed for the student to participate in state or local assessments (and, if the student will not participate in such assessments, why not and how they will be assessed differently); (5) date services are to begin and their expected duration; (6) explanation to what extent, if any, the student will not participate in regular classes; (7) beginning at age 14, transition service needs focusing on the child's course of study; and (8) how the student's progress toward annual goals will be measured. The IEP contains a great deal of information that should, on a daily basis, directly affect students with ADHD and how they are served in school (U.S. Department of Education, 2006a).

To ensure that school districts are providing the appropriate services and accommodations to students with special needs, IDEA includes legal protections termed *due process procedures* for parents and guardians to follow if they have any concerns about their child's education. The rights guaranteed by IDEA are enforced by the U.S. Office of Special Education, the federal agency that works with state departments of education, which in turn are responsible for monitoring local school districts for IDEA compliance. Figure 4.1 summarizes some of the key provisions of IDEA.

Section 504

Students with ADHD may also be served under Section 504 of the Rehabilitation Act of 1973. Section 504 is not an education law per se; rather, it is a civil rights law intended to prevent discrimination. It prohibits any institution that receives federal funds from discriminating on the basis of disability. A student would qualify for services under Section 504 is he or she has "a physical or mental impairment that substantially limits one or more major 'life activities' (including: walking, breathing, speaking and/or hearing, seeing, learning, performing manual tasks, and caring for oneself)." Because these major life activities include learning many students with ADHD would qualify. Further, Section 504 states that students can be considered as having a disability if they have a history of impairment or are regarded as having such an impairment. Section 504 impacts schools because most public schools in the United States receive some funds from the federal government. However, in contrast to IDEA, schools do not receive money to pay for services provided under Section 504. Section 504 is important to students with ADHD because, if a student does not meet IDEA criteria for services, he or she may qualify for services under Section 504 (U.S. Department of Education, 2006a). There are no formal guidelines

- IDEA guarantees all individuals with disabilities from birth to age 21 the right to a free and appropriate public education. This includes special education and related services, at no cost to the parents.

- If a student is suspected of having a disability, he or she may be referred for a full evaluation. This formal evaluation will determine whether or not a student has a disability and if the student requires special education or related services. If it is determined that the student has a disability, an individualized education plan (IEP) will be created for the student by the IEP team.

- The IEP team will always include the student's parents, teachers, special educators, related service providers, and a representative of the local school district knowledgeable about IDEA requirements. When appropriate, the student will also participate directly in the creation, implementation, and annual review of the IEP.

- An IEP includes (1) a written statement of the student's present level of educational performance (PLOP); (2) measurable annual goals and short-term objectives related to meeting the child's needs that result from the disability; (3) special education, related services, supplementary aids/services, and program modifications to be provided for the student; (4) any modifications needed for the student to participate in state or local assessments (and, if the student will not participate in such assessments, an explanation of why not and how he or she will be assessed differently); (5) date services are to begin and their expected duration; (6) explanation to what extent, if any, the student will not participate in regular classes; (7) beginning at age 14, transition service needs focusing on the child's course of study; and (8) how the student's progress toward annual goals will be measured.

- The IEP is reviewed annually, and a new IEP is written to reflect any changes in the student's ability or needs.

- Students should be fully reevaluated every 3 years to determine whether they still meet the criteria for a disability and to obtain up-to-date information on the student's ability level and needs.

- ADHD is not a specific handicapping condition under IDEA. However, students with ADHD may qualify for services under one of IDEA's other categories of disability. Most commonly, students with ADHD receive services under IDEA with the label of other health impaired (OHI), specific learning disability (SLD), or emotional disturbance (ED).

FIGURE 4.1. Key provisions of the Individuals with Disabilities Education Act (IDEA). From U.S. Department of Education (2006a).

for determining whether a student should be referred for services under Section 504. Smith and Patton (1998) suggested that Section 504 referral might be considered if a student:

- Is suspended or expelled.
- Has ongoing behavior problems.
- Is believed to have ADHD.
- Was evaluated for IDEA but did not meet criteria.
- Was referred for IDEA but was not evaluated.

Figure 4.2 lists some of the key provisions of Section 504, including more examples of what the law includes as major life activities. Because the major life activities are not explicitly defined, Section 504 is more open to interpretation than IDEA. That is, there is some leeway in who would be classified as having a disability. Like IDEA, Section 504 requires local school districts to provide a free and appropriate public education to any student identified as having a disability. Schools must provide an assessment for any student suspected of having a disability. However, the assessment process schools must follow is not explicitly described. If a student meets Section 504 criteria for additional educational assistance or services, a 504 plan is developed to establish what will be done to accommodate the student's disability. Note that providing services is the responsibility of general education, not special education. A 504 plan is very similar to an IEP, but while IDEA requires the development and monitoring of an IEP, an IEP is not formally required by Section 504

- Section 504 of the Rehabilitation Act (P.L. 93-112) is a federal civil rights law that prohibits discrimination against people with disabilities. Section 504 is enforced by the Office of Civil Rights (OCR).

- There is no federal funding attached to Section 504, but the OCR has the power to withhold federal funds otherwise provided to school districts that do not comply with the law.

- The definition of "handicapped person" in Section 504 is "anyone with a physical or mental impairment that substantially limits one or more major 'life activities' (including: walking, breathing, speaking and/or hearing, seeing, learning, performing manual tasks, and caring for oneself)."

- Based on the definition of a handicapped person listed above, many students with ADHD who do not qualify for services under IDEA may qualify for services under Section 504.

- Section 504 requires a student to be evaluated by a team, generally referred to as the student assistance team or student study team, consisting of teachers, administrators, and any other educational practitioners with knowledge of the evaluation process. Such an evaluation may be requested by a student's parents.

- If, after the evaluation, a student is deemed eligible for services under Section 504, a 504 plan is created to assist the student. Unlike the IEP required by IDEA, a 504 plan is simpler, and is the responsibility of general education, not special education.

- A 504 plan includes the interventions and accommodations the evaluation team agrees are necessary for the student to have the opportunity for academic success. It is the responsibility of the student's teachers to appropriately implement these interventions and accommodations.

- Section 504 states that a student with a disability should be provided an education in a regular classroom unless it is proven that such an education in a regular environment with supplementary aides and services cannot be achieved.

- Students who qualify for services under IDEA are also protected by Section 504.

FIGURE 4.2. Key provisions of Section 504 of the Rehabilitation Act of 1973. From U.S. Department of Justice (2000).

(U.S. Department of Education, 2006a). If the results of a school-based assessment suggest that a student does not have a disability, Section 504 provides guidelines for parents to follow if they disagree with the district's decision. IDEA and Section 504 have many commonalities, but there are also significant differences. Figure 4.3 compares IDEA and Section 504. In our next section, we focus more directly on how students with ADHD are served in schools.

IDEA CLASSIFICATION

Before we discus IDEA, it's important to note the categories under IDEA are derived from the *educational system*. ADHD, in contrast, is a medical diagnosis. The two systems are separate and distinct, as are the diagnostic categories. For example, a student could have ADHD, but not have a learning disability (and vice versa). Around half of the students with ADI ID will receive special education services under IDEA because they meet the criteria for one of the categories of disability (Reid, Maag, & Vasa, 1994), and around 60% of students who receive special services under IDEA also have ADHD (Schnoes, Reid, Wagner, & Marder, 2006). Note that a diagnosis of ADHD *does not* automatically qualify a child for services under IDEA. ADHD is not a category of disability under IDEA. To qualify for services under IDEA, students must meet the criteria for one or more of the categories of disability as they are defined in the law. There are different criteria for each category of disability. However, one critical component of the criteria for any disability category is that there must be a documented *problem with achievement*. A student with no achievement problems would not be eligible for services under IDEA. The school's involvement in identifying students for services can vary. A medical diagnosis might be needed in some instances, while in others a school-based assessment would be sufficient.

The great majority of students with ADHD qualify for services based on a co-occurring diagnoses of learning disabilities (LD), emotional–behavioral disorders (EBD), other health impaired (OHI), and speech–language impairment (SLI) categories. Students with ADHD make up a sizable proportion of students in special education. According to a recent national study, the percentage of students with ADHD in those categories is 20% for LD, 57% for EBD, 65% for OHI, and 5% for SLI (Schnoes et al., 2006). Note that these are the categories in which students with ADHD are most commonly served. There are almost certainly students with ADHD in many of the other categories of disability. For example, it is perfectly possible for a child to be hearing-impaired or vision-impaired and also have ADHD. In this section we provide an overview of four categories of disability—LD, EBD, OHI, and SLI—and how they relate to ADHD.

Learning Disability

Under IDEA, LD is defined as a disorder in the basic psychological processes involved in understanding or using language, either spoken or written, that

	IDEA	Section 504
Purpose	• Supports states' efforts to provide services for students with disabilities. • Ensures the rights of children and their parents.	• Broad civil rights law. • Protects rights of individuals in federally funded programs or activities. • No funding is provided for school's expense.
Who qualifies	• Children ages 3–21 identified in specific categories in one of 13 categories. Children with ADHD typically qualify under other health impairment, emotional disturbance, specific learning disabilities, or speech language impairments.	• Children who have, have had, or are regarded as having a disability that substantially limits one or more of life's major activities (e.g., learning).
Eligibility based on	• A comprehensive evaluation is required after informed consent. Reevaluation is required at least once every 3 years unless parent and district agree it is unnecessary. • Multidisciplinary team determines specific disability eligibility. • An independent evaluation at school's expense may be required if parents disagree with school evaluation data.	• A formal individual assessment is not required. • Parental consent is not required, only notice. • Evaluation team members must be knowledgeable about student, evaluation data, etc., and agree on a plan of services and accommodations. • Reevaluations are required only for changes in placement.
Services	• Requires a written IEP. • Requires the provision of related services and a continuum of placements, including general education. • IEP changes allowed without reevaluation.	• Requires a plan but not necessarily a written document. • Requires reasonable accommodations, such as tutoring or altered testing.
Legal rights	• Requires written notice and parent or guardian consent before conducting evaluation, identification, or placement. • Requires an individualized education plan (IEP) outlining services to be provided and their duration. • Requires consent for services noted on IEP.	• Requires notice to parent or guardian only in the case of significant placement changes.

FIGURE 4.3. Comparing and contrasting IDEA and Section 504. From U.S. Department of Education (2006a) and U.S. Department of Justice (2000).

manifests itself in impairments in the ability to listen, think, speak, read, write, spell, or do mathematical calculations (U.S. Department of Education, 2006a). LDs are generally broken down into three groups: Reading, Written Expression, and Mathematics Calculations (Fletcher et al., 2002; Fletcher, Morris, & Lyon, 2003; Lyon, Fletcher, & Barnes, 2003). Because different researchers may apply different criteria to what constitutes a LD, there is a wide degree of variability in the estimates of how many students with ADHD also have LD. If a rigorous approach to identifying LD is used, approximately 8–39% of students with ADHD are estimated to also have a reading disability, 12–30% a math disability, and 12–27% a spelling disability. Note that ADHD and LD are *not synonymous*. They are separate and distinct conditions. There are children who have only ADHD, there are children who have only LD, and there are children who have both ADHD and LD.

ADHD and LD appear to have a strong link because of the problems students with ADHD often demonstrate in academic performance and achievement. Students with LD who are diagnosed with ADHD have poor performance in school as a common trait. In part this may be due to the diagnostic criteria that specifically list school as an environment where there must be problems. The number of students with co-occurring ADHD and LD is likely one of the underlying reasons why serious problems with academics are common among student with ADHD. Students with ADHD often score below their classmates by 10–30 standard score points on standardized achievement tests in reading, spelling, math, and reading comprehension (Barkley et al., 1990; Brock & Knapp, 1996; Cantwell & Satterfield, 1978; Casey, Rourke, & Del Otto, 1996; Dykman & Ackerman, 1992; Fischer et al., 1990; Semrud-Clikeman et al., 1992). However, it's important to distinguish between problems caused by ADHD-related difficulties (e.g., forgetting to hand in assignments, losing schoolwork) and those related to learning disabilities (e.g., problems with phonological processing, number concepts). For teachers, it probably is best to consider ADHD and LD as comorbid conditions where the presence of LD *adds significantly* to the problem of ADHD and vice versa.

Emotional–Behavioral Disorder

EBD is diagnosed when a child exhibits one or more of the following five characteristics: (1) an inability to learn that cannot be explained by intellectual, sensory, or health factors; (2) an inability to create and maintain appropriate interpersonal relationships with peers and/or teachers; (3) inappropriate types of behavior or feelings under normal circumstances; (4) a general and pervasive mood of unhappiness and depression, and (5) a tendency to develop physical symptoms or fears associated with personal or school problems (U.S. Department of Education, 2006a). These problems must occur over a long period of time, to a marked degree, and must adversely affect a student's educational performance. Once again note that ADHD and EBD are separate and distinct conditions. Research suggests that the majority of students receiving special education services in the EBD category have been diagnosed with ADHD (Schnoes et al., 2006). This high incidence of students with ADHD receiving an EBD label may be due to the fact that EBD characteristics (e.g., aggressive behaviors and noncompliance) are reflective of disorders that commonly co-occur with ADHD (e.g., ODD and CD). Thus a high degree of overlap between ADHD and EBD should not be too surprising.

Other Health Impaired

Students in the OHI category are those with limited strength, vitality, or alertness that results in limited alertness in regards to the educational environment. It also includes students with a heightened alertness to environmental stimuli. This limited alertness is due to chronic health problems, and must adversely affect a student's educational performance. The IDEA definition includes ADHD as one of the chronic health problems that may qualify a student for an OHI diagnosis (U.S. Department of Education, 2006a). The inclusion of ADHD in the federal definition of OHI followed a change to the law in 1991, when the concept of "limited alertness" was added (Davila, Williams, & McDonald, 1991). This revision allowed many students with ADHD to qualify for special education under the OHI category. Between 1998 and 2002, 68% of students newly classified as OHI had a diagnosis of ADHD (Forness & Kavale, 2002). At present the majority of students with OHI have ADHD (Schnoes et al., 2006). If the trend continues, OHI may become synonymous with ADHD.

IDEA does not specifically state how local school districts and states should verify that a student has a chronic health problem. The majority of states require a medical diagnosis to confirm that a student has a chronic health problem. If a school requires a medical diagnosis, it must be provided at no cost to the parents (Grice, 2002). When such a diagnosis is provided, students *must also meet the OHI criteria of academic impairment*. IDEA does not include explicit guidelines for establishing how a student's academic performance is negatively impacted by a health problem. To prove a student's health problem is causing academic difficulties, states require various forms of documentation (e.g., the results of achievement tests, IQ tests, or curriculum-based measurements showing significant underachievement) as evidence. In situations where the documentation shows academic difficulties, but not a medical diagnosis of a chronic health problem, the student will not qualify as OHI. In such a case, the student may be able to qualify for services in a different special education category.

Speech–Language Impairment

SLI is defined as a communication disorder, including a language or voice impairment, adversely affecting a child's educational performance (U.S. Department of Education, 2006a). In the case of students with ADHD, the language-based problems are the most serious. The SLI category contains the smallest percentage of students with ADHD. For example, Reid, Vasa, Maag, and Wright (1994) found that 7.8% of students with ADHD were served in the SLI category, and Schnoes et al.

(2006) found that 4.5% of students with SLI also had ADHD. Problems with speech and language are well-documented among children with ADHD. ADHD has been associated with an increased risk for delayed speech development (Hartsough & Lambert, 1985; Szatmari, Offord, & Boyle, 1989) and problems with expressive language (Barkley et al., 1990; Munir, Biederman, & Knee, 1987). Up to 64% of children with SLI are likely to have a comorbid disorder. ADHD is the most common of these comorbid disorders, found in 16–46% of children with SLI (Baker & Cantwell, 1987; Cohen et al., 1998).

When some students with ADHD face tasks requiring them to organize and generate speech, they tend to talk less, be more dysfluent (e.g., using many pauses, fillers such as "um," and misarticulations), and be less competent in organizing their speech (Hamlett, Pelligrini, & Conners, 1987; Purvis & Tannock, 1997; Zentall, 1985). Many of these speech problems are commonly associated with SLI. Teachers need to be especially aware of the possibility of language-related problems. Problems with expressive or receptive language can directly affect school performance. For example, students might have difficulty completing assignments that involve written expression because of problems formulating their thoughts. Students might have difficulty following directions because they had difficulty processing oral language. Note that these problems could appear to be due to ADHD-related problems (e.g., poor organization, inattention) when in reality they would be due to language-based problems. Once again this underscores the difficulty and complexity of an ADHD diagnosis.

PLACEMENT

Where students with ADHD are served—referred to as "placement"—depends to some extent on whether they qualify for service under Section 504 or IDEA. For students served under Section 504 placement is straightforward: these students spend 100% of their time in the general education classroom. For students served under IDEA placement is more complicated. The great majority of these students are placed in one of three educational environments:

- *General education classroom.* The student is served in the general education classroom. The teacher typically is provided with supports (e.g., paraeducator, consultation with a specialist) and necessary academic and behavioral accommodations are provided.
- *Resource.* The resource setting is a class that is aimed at providing specialized instruction in a small-group or one-to-one setting. It is typically centered on academics, though there are also behaviorally centered resource rooms. Students with a resource placement will leave the general education class to attend a resource setting for a part of the school day. However, they will generally spend most of the day in the general education classroom.
- *Self-contained.* The self-contained setting is a special classroom where students

can receive intensive instruction. Typically there are a small number of students that allows for increased attention and teacher time for each student. Students may spend all or the majority of their time in the self-contained classroom. However, students typically spend at least some portion of the day in the general education classroom.

These are the most common placements. However, there are other placements for students with ADHD. A much smaller number of students who are severely involved (e.g., extremely disruptive or aggressive) may be served in special schools or in residential settings. A sizable proportion of students in special schools or residential settings have ADHD (Casey et al., 2008). There is not a great amount of research on the educational placements for students with ADHD. Table 4.1 shows data from a national survey comparing special education students with ADHD to special education students without ADHD on the time spent in the general education classroom. As the table indicates, the majority of ADHD special education students spent a majority of their school day in general education classrooms. This should emphasize the fact that ADHD is *not only a special education problem*. General education teachers should be aware they often will be primarily responsible for students with ADHD.

Deciding the most appropriate placement for a student is based on the principle of the *least restrictive environment* (LRE). LRE means that a student should be educated in an environment that is as close as feasible to their peers as possible, given individual circumstances. If a student with ADHD demonstrates the capacity to succeed in all regular classes with various accommodations provided, then regular classes would be considered that student's LRE. Conversely, if a student with special needs clearly demonstrates that he or she requires more intensive services, then a resource setting for one or more classes may be justified as the LRE.

TABLE 4.1. Percentage of Time Spent in General Education Classrooms by Special Education Students with and without ADHD

Time in general education classroom	With ADHD ($N = 467$)	Without ADHD ($N = 952$)
Mean percentage of time spent in general education classroom	63.1%*	69.4%
Percent of students' time in general education classrooms		
More than 80%	28.33%**	44.1%
61% to 80%	33.9%*	24.5%
21% to 60%	30.8%	22.3%
1% to 20%	2.9%	4.5%
None	4.2%	4.7%

Note. Data from Schnoes, Reid, Wagner, and Marder (2006).
*$p < .05$; **$p < .001$.

The most appropriate placement for a student with ADHD depends on a number of factors. Perhaps the most important factor is how severely the student is affected by ADHD, that is, the extent and severity of the ADHD symptoms the student exhibits. Another factor is the presence of comorbid conditions (e.g., ODD or CD). Other factors include the student's overall academic ability (Is the student on grade level with basic skills or in need of intensive remediation?), the student's ability to function in classes containing large numbers of students (Will the student be better served in the smaller class sizes commonly associated with resource or self-contained settings?), and just how much direct assistance the student with ADHD requires in order to succeed academically and socially in a school environment. Students with ADHD often experience great difficulties with task completion and organization skills, two additional areas of concern that should be considered when making placement decisions. The main point is that placement decisions for students with ADHD are not simple matters, and require a great deal of careful consideration.

School Services

Schools may be called on to provide a wide range of services for students with ADHD. Table 4.2 lists the percentage of students with ADHD receiving many of the various nonacademic and academic services that schools provide. Around 90% of students with ADHD receive some type of academic services (see Chapter 5 for more detailed discussion on academic services). Around two-thirds of special education students with ADHD receive at least one type of nonacademic service through schools, such as a behavior management program, mental health service, or occupational therapy. Note also that social services or family counseling/training may also be provided. The emotional and social needs of these children *may be just as important* to address as their behavioral or academic problems. These numbers

TABLE 4.2. Services to Special Education Students with and without ADHD

Services provided	With ADHD ($N = 464$)	Without ADHD ($N = 932$)
Academic services	91.0%**	80.3%
Behavior management program	37.1%***	10.1%
Mental health services	21.2%***	3.1%
Behavior interventions	16.7%***	1.8%
Social work services	12.7%**	2.5%
Family counseling/training	8.3%*	1.4%
Speech–language therapy	23.0%***	5.3%
Occupational therapy	10.8%	9.4%
Self-advocacy training	5.5%	4.4%

Note. Data from Schnoes, Reid, Wagner, and Marder (2006).
*$p < .05$; **$p < .01$; ***$p < .001$.

suggest that students with ADHD who are served under IDEA often are more likely to receive special services than their non-ADHD counterparts.

SUMMING UP

In this chapter we provided an overview of federal laws that effect service provision for students with ADHD, legal rights and safeguards, and the service provision options available to them.

- ✓ Most students with ADHD should qualify for services under Section 504 or IDEA.
- ✓ Teachers should be aware of the provisions of both Section 504 and IDEA as they apply to students with ADHD. These are *federal law*; they are not some minor bureaucratic concern. Failure to comply can result in unpleasant consequences for a school and/or teacher.
- ✓ Remember that ADHD is not just a special education problem or a general education problem. Both general education and special education teachers will be involved with students with ADHD.
- ✓ There may be students with ADHD who do not qualify or have not yet been identified under Section 504 or IDEA. Teachers *don't need to wait* for a formal identification to help a student. As we discuss in Chapter 5 there are many simple, "commonsense" accommodations teachers can use with students with ADHD.
- ✓ Schools may be called on to provide a wide range of services that extend beyond the classroom.

School-Based Treatment for ADHD

School is hell.
—MATT GROENING

Imagine playing a game. It's a very important game, a high-stakes game. It's a game that you really want to do well at, but one that you absolutely hate. The game makes you feel awkward. You struggle even on a good day, and you frequently experience frustration and failure. It's a game filled with irritation—like taking a long hike with a stone in your shoe. You really try your best, but no matter how hard you try you seem to screw up regularly. It's a game that has rules, but for some reason you don't seem to quite understand them, and even worse, the rules seem to change for no apparent reason. You make a lot of mistakes in the game; often you're not even sure what you did that was wrong. It would be a lot more fun if you had a friend who could play too, somebody who might help you perhaps, but nobody seems to want to play with you. It's also a looooooonnnngggg game. It lasts 6 whole hours. Now imagine that the game occurs regularly Monday through Friday for 9 months. It's something you think about every day. Sometimes you even dread it. Now let's add the icing to the cake. The game is compulsory. There is no choice—you must play the game for 12 whole years. Does this sound like a lot of fun?

For many children with ADHD, school is a lot like our fictional game. You could not design a situation that would be more difficult and frustrating for children with ADHD than the school environment. It's *not intentional*, no one decided to make schools aversive for kids with ADHD; it's just that typical school activities and the expectations that come with them can be major obstacles for students with ADHD. Kids with high activity levels are expected to sit still, often for long periods of time.

Kids with problems focusing and maintaining attention must try to attend. Kids with problems maintaining effort, especially on tasks that are not particularly motivating (e.g., repetitive but necessary tasks such as drill and practice activities) are expected to perform these tasks. Discipline issues also occur, sometimes because of ADHD-related problems (e.g., losing recess for failure to finish their seatwork), and sometimes because of failure to read social cues (e.g., when the teacher is giving directions it's not a good time to suddenly talk about your new bicycle). Socially related problems are also common. Students with ADHD may have few (or no) friends. Now add on to this the possibility of a comorbid disorder such as depression and anxiety that can exacerbate these problems. This could be the reality of school for students with ADHD.

When teachers consider school from the point of view of the student with ADHD, it's a bit easier to put in perspective the challenges posed by ADHD. It is absolutely true that it is also tough for teachers to work with students with ADHD and balance their needs with those of other students. It is helpful, however, to remember that school is no bed of roses for students with ADHD. ADHD in the schools is a challenge. A student with ADHD will have difficulties even when provided with optimal treatment. There are no magic cures for the problems of ADHD, it is a chronic condition that will continue throughout a student's entire schooling (and lifetime). However, given a well-conceived, coordinated, and aggressive treatment plan, *the odds of successful outcomes are much greater*. In contrast, if ADHD is left untreated, the chances of successful outcomes are much lower.

Effective school-based treatment is critical in any treatment plan for ADHD. All of the school personnel involved with students with ADHD play a critical role in treatment. (Note that parents also are critical in treatment. They are discussed in Chapter 6.) The school is often the setting where many ADHD-related problems occur and where the problems may be most serious. The school is where children will spend much of their time. Consider this fact: many of the professionals involved in treatment of students with ADHD will spend very little time with a student with ADHD. A physician might have 2–4 contact hours per year. A psychologist, meeting weekly, might have 50 contact hours per year. In contrast, children with ADHD will have *over 1,000 contact hours* with school-based professionals—most notably classroom teachers—over the course of a single school year. Over the course of a child's educational career this amounts to over 12,000 contact hours. This comparison speaks volumes. Left untreated, ADHD-related problems can severely affect students' educational attainment, with serious ramifications for their future. Lack of treatment can also affect social functioning and can exacerbate comorbid conditions (e.g., anxiety, depression).

In this chapter we introduce the school-based multimodal model for ADHD treatment. We then provide an overview of each of the components in the multimodal treatment model and guidelines for implementing the model; each component is discussed in detail in subsequent chapters. Next, we present examples of schoolwide intervention programs for children with ADHD. Finally we provide an overview of interventions that are questionable or unsupported by research.

THE MULTIMODAL TREATMENT MODEL

ADHD is a disorder that typically affects cognitive, behavioral, and emotional functioning. Thus, an *optimal* treatment plan should address all these areas. Figure 5.1 shows the areas addressed by the multimodal treatment model. The model shown is based on the approach to school-based ADHD treatment proposed by Pfiffner, Barkley, and DuPaul (2006). The model includes four primary areas: medical management, behavior management, instructional accommodations, and psychological support (both for child and parent). The model is not new. Researchers have known for decades that this combination of treatments can be effective in positively altering outcomes for children with ADHD (e.g., Satterfield, Satterfield, & Cantwell, 1980, 1981). Research continues to support the need for integrated treatment plans that encompass the areas of medical management, behavior management, instructional accommodations, and psychological support. Approaches that combine these areas are more effective and more acceptable to both parents and schools than those that are limited to any single area (Conners et al., 2001; Pisecco, Huzinec, & Curtis, 2001; Power, Hess, & Bennett, 1995; Swanson et al., 2001).

There are two major considerations that must be addressed to implement the model. The first and most obvious consideration is how school-based treatment will be implemented. That is, what are the actual interventions (e.g., daily report cards, self-regulation) that will be used? These are discussed in subsequent chapters. Involving parents is also critical. There will also likely be a need to monitor response to medication (if prescribed). The second and often overlooked consideration is that to implement the model, the professional in charge of a treatment plan must be able to *manage the logistics* of multimodal treatment. For example, the professional in charge must consider whether there are staff training needs, define responsibilities, and allocate resources. Setting up and maintaining effective lines of communications is also a concern because treatment of ADHD cuts across the home, school, medical, and social settings. Time is also a factor. Implementing the

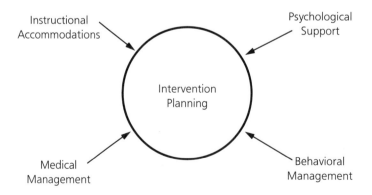

FIGURE 5.1. The multimodal intervention model.

multimodal model requires a serious, *long-term commitment* of time and effort on the part of all parties. We recognize that given real-world constraints on resources and expertise, it may not be possible or feasible for a school to fully implement all components of the model. However, the more components implemented, the more likely it is that the efforts of teachers and other school professionals can produce a positive, lasting change in behaviors. The payoff can be dramatic.

Implementing Multimodal Treatment

In the multimodal model (1) students are systematically evaluated from multiple viewpoints (i.e., multiple informants and settings), (2) a treatment plan is formulated to meet the needs of the student, (3) the plan is implemented within the school setting, and (4) progress is monitored on an ongoing basis. Figure 5.2 shows some of the steps involved in implementing multimodal treatment.

Professional Development

Training teachers and other school personnel in interventions and accommodations and helping them gain more knowledge of ADHD are critical in the implementation of multimodal treatment. Teachers who do not understand the nature of ADHD and grasp the need for treatment are less likely to effectively implement interventions (Pfiffner et al., 2006). Teachers have consistently expressed a desire for training in effective interventions for students with ADHD and lack of training is perceived as a significant barrier to working effectively with students with ADHD (Arcia, Frank, Sánchez-LaCay, & Fernández, 2000; Reid, Vasa, Maag, & Wright, 1994). Lack of training is a particularly serious problem among general education teachers. General education teachers will typically have a child with ADHD for most of the school day, yet often they have not received systematic instruction in skills critical to working with students with ADHD, such as behavior management techniques, in the course of their teacher training programs. They may also lack knowledge of medication management, effective accommodations, working with parents, and psychological support. Need for training is critical because there is evidence that insufficiently trained teachers may implement interventions incorrectly or in a manner that renders the intervention ineffective (Arcia et al., 2000; Fabiano & Pelham, 2003). General education teachers may also be more resistant to implement some interventions, especially those that involve altering instruction (Zentall & Stormont-Spurgin, 1995).

Implementation Considerations

Because students with ADHD are highly heterogenous, the specific interventions used will vary across students. However, there are overall aspects of the program that are consistent.

	Intervention	**Assess/monitor**	**Education**
Medical	• Ensure that medication is dispensed as prescribed and on consistent basis.	• Establish baseline rates (behavioral observations or behavior rating scales). • Establish lines of communication with physician(s). • Create mechanism for monitoring of administration, consumption, and resupply. • Assess medication response on ongoing basis across times and activities. • Monitor for side effects.	• Determine potential side effects and their symptoms. • Ensure **all involved staff** are knowledgeable about medication, medication effects, and possible side effects. • Teach staff behavior observation techniques and behavior ratings use. Stress need for ongoing monitoring.
Behavioral	• Utilize a functional approach that centers on problem behaviors and their possible causes. • Appoint a case manager. • Identify staff with intervention expertise. **or** • Create intervention "menus."	• Define target behavior(s). Collect baseline information on problem behaviors. • Use assessment information to select intervention. • Monitor intervention integrity. • Collect data—evaluate effectiveness.	• Stress functional approach. • Instruct staff in correct implementation of intervention(s) and data collection.
Academic	• Utilize a functional approach that centers on problem areas and their possible causes. • Define target behavior(s). • Develop interventions. **or** • Create intervention "menus" that address accommodations through alteration of (1) environment, (2) materials, (3) instruction.	• Collect baseline information on problem behavior. • Use assessment information to select intervention. • Collect data—evaluate effectiveness.	• Provide teachers with information on behavior of children with ADHD. • Provide teachers with information on appropriate accommodations and provide **support** for their implementation.

(cont.)

FIGURE 5.2. Steps in implementing school-based treatment.

	Intervention	Assess/monitor	Education
Psychological (family)	• Enlist involvement in home–school intervention(s) if feasible. • Provide training in effective behavior management techniques. • Provide information on support groups. • Provide information on respite care.	• Establish home–school communication. • Monitor home behavior change.	• Provide information on ADHD causes, treatments, and outcomes.
Psychological (child)	• Arrange for counseling services if indicated. • Provide instruction in social skills if indicated. • Structure environment to enable social engagement.	• Monitor school, home, and social functioning. • Monitor for affective problems, depression, and anxiety.	• Provide information on ADHD.

FIGURE 5.2. *(cont.)*

• First, planning is highly individualized and the focus is on the *specific behaviors* that cause the most difficulty in terms of functioning effectively in the classroom. The priority is on changing behaviors that would have the greatest impact on effective functioning in the classroom. It would be marvelous if there were a single intervention or accommodation that would work for *all* the problem behaviors for *all* students with ADHD. Unfortunately, there simply aren't any universal treatments for ADHD—*not even medication.* For children with ADHD, both the problems experienced and the most efficacious treatment vary widely. This requires collecting and analyzing information from a number of sources (e.g., parents, teachers, counselors) and a number of settings (e.g., home, school, playground). Note that a plan should include input from *both professionals and parents* if at all possible; the home setting can be a critical factor in success or failure of treatment.

• Second, the treatment regimen is *intensive and long-term*. As we noted in Chapter 2, problems associated with ADHD are lifelong, thus multimodal treatment is not something that you do for 6 weeks and you're done. Treatment typically must continue for years. Additionally treatment often will need to be changed as the student progresses through school because the nature of problems associated with ADHD will change as the student matures to adolescence (Robin, 2006). This means that schools must be able to maintain treatment regimens across school years and across school transitions.

• Third, the treatment includes regular assessment of treatment fidelity and student progress. Treatment fidelity is another way of asking "Has the intervention been implemented in the manner in which it was intended?" That is, are the interventions used being implemented correctly and consistently? This is a commonsense consideration—if an intervention isn't being implemented correctly or consistently, it's unlikely to produce desired results. Research clearly shows that interventions that are implemented correctly and consistently are more effective (Borrelli et al., 2005). Treatment fidelity is critical in the case of students with ADHD (Fabiano & Pelham, 2003).

• Fourth, the treatment planning and implementation must be *coordinated and integrated*. Remember that there are numerous professionals involved in treatment (e.g., classroom teacher, special education teacher, school psychologist, health professionals). Information from the family and professionals involved with the child should be utilized for intervention decisions. Based on this information, the parents and professionals can evaluate treatment results, make decisions on progress made, and determine what future course(s) of action should be considered. Remember also that the parents should be involved to the *maximum extent possible,* and that treatment often includes the school, the home, and other environments. Treatment teams must meet regularly to evaluate interventions and share information. It is critical that team members be aware of both their own individual responsibilities and the overall treatment program. This prevents individuals from working at cross-purposes or duplication of effort. It also helps in problem solving because a change in one aspect of treatment could affect other aspects of a child's treatment. Note also that communication among different professional groups (e.g., teachers, psychologists, physicians) and between professionals and parents is a serious concern. Learning the terminology of other groups and paying attention to situations where miscommunication might occur is also important.

• Fifth, teachers should be supported. It's all too common for teachers to be given "one more thing" to do. It may not be a large task, but unfortunately this is seldom followed up with "and here's what you can drop" or "and here are extra resources to do it with." Working with children with ADHD will require extra time and effort on the part of the instructor over and above what must be done in the course of normal duties (e.g., monitoring, record keeping, interventions). This can be especially difficult in the case of the general education teacher who may have 30 students in his or her class. Support from administration is needed to address the "one more thing" problem. Pfiffner et al. (2006) recommended that for general education teachers (1) educators should be provided with a behavior paraeducator when possible (even if it is for only part of the day); (2) there should be a source of support (e.g., school psychologist, behavior specialist) to help plan and troubleshoot interventions; and (3) teachers should be recognized for their efforts—this might include verbal recognition, letters of commendation, extra time for planning and professional development, or money for materials and books.

• Sixth, individual differences across teachers should be considered in selecting interventions. Some interventions tend to be more acceptable to teachers than others. For example, teachers tend to prefer interventions with positive consequences (e.g., the child receives a reward for positive behavior) more than those with negative consequences (e.g., the child receives punishment for inappropriate behavior; Piseco et al., 2001). The time and/or expertise required to implement the intervention should also be considered. Teachers may resist interventions that are perceived as time-consuming or cumbersome in the classroom. Forcing a teacher to use an intervention that he or she doesn't wish to use should be avoided to the extent possible. Remember that for an intervention to be effective it must be implemented correctly and consistently. One way to avoid this potential problem is to allow teachers to choose from among three or four acceptable interventions that have been identified as simple and effective. Note that acceptance of new interventions can be developed through professional development and team processes that support the use of new interventions

• Finally, there must be a clear delegation of responsibility for treatment—there should be a clearly identified person who is in charge of the overall treatment program. Individuals responsible for different components of treatment should also be clearly identified. This person in charge of the treatment program should have the authority to make final treatment decisions, should serve as an informational "clearinghouse," and should be notified if changes appear necessary or if problems occur. Although the model stresses a team approach to treatment, be aware that there should also be someone who has overall responsibility to serve as a case manager. Possible case managers could include special education teachers, SAT team leaders, school psychologists, or school counselors. The best person to be the case manager may vary for any number of reasons (e.g., whether the child is being served under Section 504 or IDEA; availability of personnel with necessary expertise; the setting where the child is being served).

IMPLEMENTATION MODELS

In the previous sections we outlined the multimodal treatment model, tasks that the school should accomplish, and considerations for implementing the model. Note that this was a *treatment model* not an *implementation model*. That is, a treatment model describes *what to do*; an implementation model describes *how to accomplish* the tasks detailed in the treatment model. There are no generally accepted implementation models for multimodal treatment, and there is no "best" implementation model. There are, however, several school-based implementation models that are research-supported. These implementation models are typically implemented schoolwide. They are useful not just for students with ADHD, but also for any students with academic or behavior problems.

Collaborative Consultation

School-based training in ADHD is well-meaning, but often ineffective (Pfiffner et al., 2006). A typical 1- or 2-day training session can provide teachers with useful information on ADHD and can expose teachers to effective interventions.

Unfortunately, such brief training sessions are unlikely to raise teachers' knowledge and skill level to the point where they can *effectively and independently* apply the knowledge and use the interventions in the classroom. To attain this level almost always requires additional support. Collaborative consultation approaches such as those developed by Shapiro and colleagues (Shapiro, DuPaul, Bradley, & Bailey, 1996) address this concern by first providing teacher training and then providing a 60-day intensive follow-up support period. After initial training, teachers meet with a consultant who is a professional with expertise and experience in ADHD and effective interventions. Together the teacher and consultant discuss the student's problem and work together to develop an appropriate intervention and progress-monitoring procedures. Student progress is evaluated on an ongoing basis and any necessary modifications to the intervention are made. Consultants may also help establish procedures to identify students with ADHD and in communicating with physicians.

ABC Program

The ABC Program (Pelham et al., 2005) is a schoolwide program intended to address problem behavior in the school. It is based on procedures used in a validated treatment program for students with ADHD developed by Pelham and Hoza (1996). The ABC Program begins with staff training and consultant support in the beginning stages to ensure that the program is *implemented correctly and consistently*. The program includes the following components, intended to be used universally by all school personnel: (1) school personnel are taught how to effectively use social reinforcement, give commands, and verbal reprimands; (2) schoolwide rules are systematically taught, student compliance is monitored, students are rewarded for following rules and consequences are administered for rule breaking; (3) students who follow the rules earn a daily positive note; (4) timeouts are enforced for serious rule violations; (5) students who earn a specified number of positive daily notes are eligible for enrichment activities (e.g., games, sports) on Friday afternoons; and (6) homework assignment sheets are used to inform parents of assignments, parents sign the sheet each night to indicate that homework was completed, and student receive rewards for returning signed assignment sheets. If a student is not responding to the universal components, an individualized plan may be developed. Additionally, social skills training may be included. When programs like ABC are used schoolwide and implemented correctly, they can dramatically decrease problem behavior (e.g., office referrals, hyperactive/impulsive behaviors), improve ratings of student–teacher relationships, and decrease teacher-rated academic impairment (Waschbusch, Pelham, & Massetti, 2005).

Key Opinion Leader Model

As previously noted, getting teachers to implement effective intervention in the classroom is a well-known problem. Schools often use outside experts or consultants to help train and support teachers, and this approach can be successful. Unfortunately, there can also be problems with this approach. There may be problems with communication difficulties, there may be resistance because experts are viewed as "outsiders," and typically experts are only available for a limited period of time after which teachers are left without support. The Key Opinion Leader (KOL) model is designed to help overcome this obstacle (Atkins, Graczyk, Frazier, & Abdul-Adil, 2003). In the KOL approach, all teachers in a school are asked to identify a colleague (the KOL) who they regard as knowledgeable and who they would go to for advice or assistance to help with a student's problem. The KOLs agree to serve as consultants for their colleagues. Next the KOLs are provided with intensive training in effective interventions for students with ADHD (e.g., positive reinforcement, response cost, home–school notes). Teachers in schools with KOL support were more likely to use effective intervention (Atkins et al., 2003). An advantage of the KOL approach is that it uses existing resources and is sustainable because it does not require additional resources (Atkins et al., 2003).

ALTERNATIVE TREATMENTS

There are many treatments for students with ADHD that have been proven to be effective. There are also alternative treatments (also referred to as complementary and alternative medicine) that are not well studied, not well supported, controversial, or simply ineffective. Fads, scams, and miracle cures literally have been around for centuries. This is an unfortunate fact of life in education. There is no educational equivalent of the U.S. Food and Drug Administration that requires that before a new treatment can be marketed it must be shown to be safe and effective. As a result, anyone can develop and market treatments without shouldering the burden of proving their effectiveness. The proponents of alternative treatments run the gamut from sincere professionals who genuinely want to help children with ADHD to those who are simply out to make a fast buck. What is consistent is that the alternative treatments are too often portrayed as "miracle cures" that promise immediate results with little or no effort (Silver, 1987).

Parents of children with disabilities—such as ADHD—are particularly vulnerable to the lure of the "miracle cure" for two reasons (Silver, 1987). First, it is completely understandable that parents would want to investigate a potential solution to the problem of ADHD. What parents wouldn't want to help their child? The promise of the "quick fix" often with little or no effort only adds to the allure. Second, alternative treatments are advertised in the popular press on the Internet, and on the websites of national ADHD organizations (Chan, Rappaport, & Kemper, 2003), which makes them readily available to parents. To illustrate, an Internet search for "alternative ADHD treatment" returned over 2 million listings. Many promised immediate cures if only you bought their product. In contrast to research-supported methods, such as those in the multimodal treatment model, which take a year of painstaking study and appear in research journals, "miracle cures" can literally pop up overnight on the Internet or popular press. Unfortunately, most parents don't read research journals. They will often ask educators (e.g., teachers, school psychologists) for information on alternative treatments. Thus teachers need a working knowledge of alternative treatments. Because the "miracle cures" pop up so rapidly, it is nearly impossible to investigate all of them. For this reason, teachers also need a means of examining the claims made so they can identify the "red flags" that are indicative of questionable treatments.

Overview of Alternative Treatments

Figure 5.3 lists some of the most common popular alternative treatments for ADHD. This is *not* a comprehensive list; any such list would be outdated by the time it appeared in print. For additional information on the treatments in Figure 5.3 and other alternative treatments see Arnold (2002) and Rojas and Chan (2005). It would be wrong to dismiss alternative treatments as a fringe issue. Alternative treatments are used by a significant number of parents. Estimates suggest that from 9 to 46% of parents have tried alternative treatments (Bussing, Zima, Gary, & Garvan, 2002), and the use of alternative approaches may be increasing (Chan et al., 2003). Additionally, religious or faith-based approaches are also commonly reported; 5% of parents reported using faith-based approaches to ADHD treatment (Bussing et al., 2002). Not surprisingly, parents who are regular Internet users are more likely to adopt alternative approaches (Bussing et al., 2002).

Dietary Treatments and Vitamins

Dietary treatments such as the Feingold diet have been suggested since the 1970s. These approaches are based on the premise that ADHD is caused by an adverse reaction to substance(s) in the diet. They involve reducing or eliminating additives or certain foods from the child's diet. The Feingold diet, which involves eliminating artificial colors and preservatives, has been studied extensively. There is solid evidence that this approach can have benefits. However, the benefits are limited to a small subset of children with ADHD and the effects are likely to be small (Schab & Trinh, 2004). Oligoallerginic and oligoantigenic diets are based on the idea that ADHD results from food allergies or sensitivities. These involve eliminating or reducing sugars, dairy products, wheat, corn, soy, and several other foods. These diets have not been thoroughly studied, but have some support (Rojas & Chan, 2005). Vitamin therapy, which involves providing the recommended daily allowance of vitamins, has been supported by one study, but benefits may be limited to children with poor diets (Arnold, 2002). There is no support for eliminating refined sugar from the diet. Hopefully all children with ADHD receive a balanced diet with sufficient vitamins and minerals, and reducing refined sugar might be beneficial in some instances. Megavitamins are not effective for ADHD (Arnold, 2002). Note that very large doses of vitamins can be toxic; this should not be tried without consulting with a physician.

Treatment	Theoretical basis	Evidence

• Restriction diets
  Feingold diet,
  Oligoallerginic/
  oligoantigenic diet
	ADHD caused by reactions to food additives (e.g., artificial colorings, flavorings, MSG) or sensitivity to certain foods. Treatment involves elimination of additives, "few foods" diet, or elimination of sugar.	Limited evidence that a small group of children with ADHD may respond to elimination of food additives or "few foods" diet. However, effects are small. No support for sugar elimination.

• Vitamins
  Recommended daily
  allowance (RDA),
  megavitamin,
  megadoses
	ADHD results in an increased requirement for vitamins. Three approaches used: RDA provides recommended vitamin levels; megavitamin provides high doses of needed vitamins; megadoses uses extremely high doses of a specific vitamin.	RDA may be useful for children with poor diets. No scientific support for megavitamins or megadoses. Extremely high doses of vitamins can actually be toxic.

• Nutritional
  Supplements
  Amino acids, fatty
  acids
	ADHD caused by imbalance in brain chemistry due to deficits in amino acids or fatty acids.	Some evidence that children with ADHD have lower levels than controls. No scientific support for benefits of amino acids supplements. Some support for fatty acids but research is not clear.

• Mineral Supplements
  Iron, zinc,
  magnesium
	Deficits in minerals needed for neural metabolism result in ADHD.	No definitive links between mineral deficiencies and ADHD. Some evidence children with ADHD have lower levels of iron, zinc, and magnesium than controls. Zinc deficiency may negatively affect medication response.

• Homeopathic or herbal medicine	The body can be helped to defend itself from diseases or disorders through use of herbal or other natural substances.	No effects for homeopathic treatments. Little research on herbal approaches.
• Biofeedback	Children can be taught to increase the types of brainwave associated with sustained attention and decrease the type associated with daydreaming/distractibility.	Numerous studies have claimed support, but studies did not adequately control for other sources of change. Treatment is time-consuming and expensive.
• Yoga	Yoga training can improve a child's focus and concentration.	One study reported promising results, but more rigorous studies needed. Might be useful adjunct to conventional treatments.
• Massage/relaxation	Helping children to relax can ease muscle tension and reduce ADHD-related problems.	Two studies found positive results, but more studies needed due to problems with the original studies.
• Green settings	Exposure to natural settings improves children's focus and task performance.	One study reported promising results, but the study has been heavily criticized.

FIGURE 5.3. Controversial treatments for ADHD.

Supplements

Diet supplements are a common alternative treatment. These treatments are based on the notion that ADHD is the result of an imbalance in brain chemistry caused by deficiency in materials needed for neural metabolism. Fatty acids and amino acids are essential elements for creation of the neurotransmitters necessary for brain functions. Several studies have reported some benefits for fatty acids; however, others found no differences, so the effects (if any) are not clear cut (Rojas & Chan, 2005). Deficiencies in iron, zinc, and magnesium have been suggested as possible factors in ADHD. Although one study reported that children with ADHD had lower levels of all these minerals, there is no strong evidence that suggest adding these minerals to the diet has any positive effect on ADHD symptoms. Note that excessive iron levels can be toxic. Zinc has received the most attention and two studies reported benefits of zinc supplements (Arnold & DiSilvestro, 2005), but as yet there is no conclusive evidence of effectiveness.

Homeopathic or Herbal Approaches

Homeopathic or herbal approaches attempt to help to stimulate the body's defense mechanisms to fight disease or disorders (Rojas & Chan, 2005). Because of the "bio-energy" of the molecules used in remedies, the remedies are extremely diluted. Homeopathic approaches are unlikely to cause harm; however, their effectiveness is questionable. A recent clinical trial found no effects for the homeopathic approach (Jacobs, Williams, Girard, Njike, & Katz, 2005). Herbal treatments are also used for ADHD. Estimates of the extent of herbal treatments vary widely, but one large study found that 17% of parents or caregivers of children with ADHD reported using herbal treatments (Cala, Crisomon, & Baumgartner, 2003). The most commonly used treatments were ginko biloba, echinacea, and St. John's wort. Herbal treatments are not well studied and the effectiveness of ginka biloba and echinacea for ADHD has not been scientifically demonstrated. St. John's wort appears to be ineffective (Weber et al., 2008). Note that herbal treatments are not regulated by the Food and Drug Administration. They can have serious side effects and can interact with other medications (Cala et al., 2003). Parents who wish to use herbal treatments should *consult their physician before starting any treatment.*

Biofeedback

Biofeedback treatment for ADHD has a long history. There are documented, but not yet well understood, differences in brain activity between children with ADHD and controls (Loo & Barkley, 2005). Proponents of biofeedback approaches suggest that changing children's brain waves can in turn affect behaviors. Biofeedback is one of the most controversial and contentious alternative treatments. Numerous studies have reported positive effects for biofeedback training. However, many of the studies were not well conducted. For example, many biofeedback studies were case studies that reported on one participant. However, the researchers used participants who had already completed training sessions. Thus the researchers already knew that a child had responded to biofeedback training before they wrote up their study. This is analogous to betting on a horse race after it is over—it's pretty easy to pick a winner under these circumstances. Had the student not responded, there likely would have been no study written. It's possible that only the successes are reported. Another concern is that it's not possible to determine whether the biofeedback training was what actually produced changes, because other treatments (e.g., reinforcement, therapist attention) are also used in conjunction with biofeedback. Additionally, the time (20–50 sessions) and expense required is a concern.

Yoga/Massage/Green Settings

Yoga training can affect body functions (e.g., heart rate). Proponents suggest that yoga training can increase focus and concentration in children with ADHD. Though not well studied, there is some support for the effectiveness of yoga (Rojas & Chan, 2005). Massage or relaxation therapy is based on the idea that massage or relaxation therapy can reduce muscle tension and help children with ADHD relax (Rojas & Chan, 2005). Again these approaches are not well studied, but there is some support (Arnold, 2002). The green settings approach (e.g., taking students outside into a park with grass and trees) is based on the idea that children with ADHD will do better on tasks conducted in the natural environment. One study reported positive effects for green settings; however, the results of the study have been questioned (Rojas & Chan, 2005). How useful this approach would be for school-based treatment is also questionable.

In summary, there are many alternative treatments for ADHD. Unfortunately very few are supported by research and some are demonstrably ineffective. The key point about alternative treatments is that *they should never be the main or only treatment* for a child with ADHD. They should only be used in conjunction with treatments that are known to be effective. They should never be done without consulting a physician, and hopefully they should be monitored by a physician.

Evaluating Alternative Treatments

As noted previously, new alternative ADHD treatments pop up with alarming regularity. What should teachers do if asked by a parent about an ADHD "cure" or a brand-new treatment? How do you tell a quack treatment from a potentially beneficial treatment? Park (2003), a noted author on pseudoscientific claims, offers some excellent guidelines for detecting quack treatments. Any of the following are major "red flags" suggesting questionable claims:

- *Consider the source.* Real scientific claims are reported in scientific journals not solely in the popular press or on the Internet. Scientific journals maintain high standards to ensure that what they report is credible. To appear in scientific journals, research must go through a rigorous review process in which every aspect of the research is scrutinized by a group of experts who systematically try to poke holes in it. *Beware of claims that only appear in the popular press or in advertisements.* Also beware of "reports" from impressive sounding "institutes." The reports may be baseless and the institutes may be little more than a post office box.

- *Suppressed knowledge.* It's very common to claim that the scientific establishment is trying to suppress some new knowledge or treatment. It's true that scientists by training are a skeptical lot who have little patience for wild, unsubstantiated claims. However, it's also true that scientists delight in reporting new knowledge. Far from wanting to suppress new findings, scientists want to shout about them from the rooftops.

- *Success stories/testimonials.* Testimonials or anecdotal evidence are compelling because they have a powerful emotional appeal. We all love a success story. For parents of a child with ADHD who desperately want to do something, testimonials may be very persuasive. Unfortunately, testimonials are unreliable because it is usually impossible to verify claims.

- *Ancient remedies.* The claim that the treatment has been used for centuries and that modern science can't explain it is common. However, longevity doesn't equal effectiveness. And, as Park (2003) put it, "Who would you trust more, ancient folk wisdom or modern science?"

- *The lone genius.* This claim features a lone genius who slaves in isolation for years, only to emerge with a tremendous, earthshaking, (fill in more superlatives), discovery. This is remotely possible, but in practice most advances or breakthroughs come from scientific teams who work for years right out in the open and advance knowledge slowly but surely. A related caution is to be leery of the "true believer." Proponents of alternative approaches often believe passionately in their effectiveness. Unfortunately this passion may lead them to "see" effects that don't really exist or that are due to other factors.

- *New laws of nature.* Some treatments propose totally new physical or neurological mechanisms to explain the effects claimed. Be very skeptical of claims such as these.

What to Look For

Real science has a distinct disadvantage in some sense because scientific findings are reported in scientific journals which, let's face it, are a bit on the dull side and are not always accessible to teachers and parents. Many teachers and parents rely on the media to some extent. So what should teachers look for? Here are a few tips that indicate the information is reliable.

• *Does the report mention that it is based on a study that appeared in a reputable scientific journal or was conducted at a research university?* Most news reports or trustworthy Internet sites will give this information (e.g., A recent study in *The New England Journal of Medicine* … " or "Researchers at Vanderbilt University reported the findings of a new study … " This is a good sign that the information is reliable. Even here it's a good idea to take new findings with a grain of salt. Sometimes preliminary findings don't pan out.

• *Was the study based on a randomized clinical trial?* The randomized clinical trial is the "gold standard" for evaluating the effects of treatments. This type of study involves rigorous controls to ensure that any differences that are found could only be attributed to the treatment, and uses participants that are randomly assigned to a treatment or control condition. Random assignment is critical to avoid situations where the participants in one group differ from another. For example, imagine a study that compared a group who volunteered for a treatment against a control group who was paid to participate. In a situation like this it's quite possible that there could be differences that were the result of group difference and not a treatment.

• *Was the study blinded or double-blinded?* Simply being in a research study can alter behavior. For example, a mom who knows that her daughter is receiving an experimental medication for ADHD might report improvements when in reality there is no change because she wants to see improvement. Similarly, a researcher collecting data on a participant who she knows is in a treatment condition might be unwittingly biased. For this reason, the most rigorous studies use a "double-blind" procedure. In the double-blind procedure neither the participant nor the researcher knows who is getting the real treatment and who is in a control condition (i.e., is not receiving the experimental treatment). For example, in medication studies participants would receive a pill to take. Neither the participant who takes the pill nor the researcher who monitors the effects of the pill know whether the pill was the actual medication being studied or a placebo (i.e., an inert substance that would have no effect). This eliminates any possibility of bias. When a double-blind study is not possible, a single-blind study, where the participants don't know whether they are in a treatment or control condition, may be used. Note that for behavioral interventions a double-blind or single-blind study often isn't possible. The next section discusses how this can be controlled for.

• *Did the study use a placebo condition?* Sometimes real behavior changes can occur even when no actual treatment is used. This is called a "placebo effect." It's a fairly common phenomenon in medication studies for participants to report changes when in actuality the pill they received was inert (e.g., a sugar pill). Researchers are aware of this and compare the results of the experimental medication with a placebo. To be judged effective, the experimental medication must be more effective than the placebo. Surprisingly, all too often the placebo has equal or larger effects. The same approach is also used in behavioral treatments. Because children in an experimental behavioral condition will receive increased attention and will have their routine altered, it's possible that any changes would be due to these factors. Good researchers try to equalize these factors. For example, children in the control condition might receive a benign treatment (e.g., playing a game, engaging in an activity) to ensure that factors such as increased attention or praise weren't responsible for differences.

SUMMING UP

In this chapter we've provided an overview of the multimodal model for school-based ADHD treatment. We also summarized tasks that schools need to consider when implanting multimodal treatment and provided examples of how the model could be implemented. Here is a list of the major points you should remember.

- ✓ School-based treatment for ADHD should be multimodal and must address medication, academic, behavior management, and psychological functioning.
- ✓ ADHD affects both school and home. Treatment should address both settings when possible.
- ✓ Multimodal treatment is individualized, intensive, and long term.
- ✓ Professional development is a critical factor. Teachers need to be taught to implement interventions effectively.
- ✓ Multimodal treatment should be coordinated.
- ✓ Teachers working with students with ADHD should be supported.
- ✓ There are different ways to implement multimodal treatment. There's no "best" way.
- ✓ Educators should be knowledgeable of alternative treatments. Alternative treatment should never be the main or only treatment. Teachers should stress that alternative treatments should only be used under the supervision of a physician.
- ✓ Educators need to be able to identify potential quack treatments.

CHAPTER 6

Working with Parents

Bringing up a child with ADHD may be the hardest thing
you ever have to do.
                                          —RUSSELL A. BARKLEY

Should teachers try to help parents be actively involved in their children's education? That's a pretty silly question, isn't it? It's like asking if you are in favor of world
peace, motherhood, or apple pie. Of course teachers should try to help parents be
involved in their children's education. Parents have an absolute right to be involved.
Parent involvement helps create a sense of community. It creates a shared commitment to maximizing student learning. Parent involvement is linked to higher teacher
ratings of student's academic competence, higher grades, and higher achievement
test scores; it's also correlated with lower dropout rates and higher high school graduation rates. Moreover, parent involvement can increase adaptive school behaviors
(e.g., attention to task) and improve engagement in schoolwork (Hoover-Dempsey
et al., 2005). It's clear that parent involvement is something teachers should want to
encourage, but getting parents involved isn't always easy.

One barrier is stress. It's becoming more and more difficult to be a parent. Parents and families are experiencing more stress today than at any other time in history (Knopf & Swick, 2008). Raising a child is hard work. It's difficult under the
best of circumstances, and it takes considerable time and effort. Factors such as
economic uncertainty, societal changes, the lack of extended family support networks, and more diverse family arrangements (e.g., blended families) can add to
parental stress and can reduce parent involvement in the schools (Knopf & Swick,

2008). The demands of parenting can result in parents who are mentally and physically exhausted; for these parents, finding time, energy, and motivation to become involved with the school can be a problem. Now add to this the problems faced by parents of children with ADHD. In this family, even the simplest activities, such as a trip to the mall, can be difficult because the parent must constantly be on watch for impulsive actions, and compliance with directions can't be assumed. Bedtime can result in arguments or temper tantrums. Chores can be an ordeal. Parents may be confused and frustrated because parenting practices that work with other kids don't seem to work with their kid. They wonder if they are doing something wrong and the problems are somehow their fault. Thus these parents may be even more stressed.

There's another potential problem in getting parents involved. Sometimes parents feel as though they aren't wanted. Consider the following statements from parents of a child with ADHD:

"The last time we had a school meeting there were six people there—his teacher, a psychologist, a social worker, someone called an LD specialist, his counselor, and the principal. I couldn't understand most of what they said. What can I do next time to avoid feeling intimidated and make sure my son gets the help he needs?" (in Barkley, 2000, p. 11)

"I get the feeling a lot of times that I'm being patronized. They really don't believe there is anything wrong with my son." (in Reid, Hertzog, & Snyder, 1996, p. 77)

Unfortunately, this is not an uncommon experience. Barkley (2000) noted that parents of children with ADHD often felt humiliated after meeting with educators. They described themselves as feeling lost or misunderstood. They believed that their views and opinions on how to address their children's problems often were dismissed out of hand. They felt that the school professionals' goal was simply to reach a quick conclusion, and to do what was most expedient for the school regardless of whether it was best for the child. As a result, parents experienced "disillusionment, dissatisfaction, and distrust in the parent–school relationship as well as a sense of loss of control over a child's fate" (Barkley, 2000, p. 11). Research suggests that parents of children with ADHD feel less able to help their child, feel less welcome at their child's school, and feel they have less time and energy to be involved in their child's education; however, they also receive more requests for involvement from the school (Rogers, Wiener, Marton, & Tannock, 2009).

We are *not* suggesting that teachers intentionally mistreat parents, nor are we suggesting schools don't want parents of ADHD to be involved in their child's education. There are many instances of parents and teachers working together effectively (e.g., Reid et al., 1996). Moreover, research has shown that teachers can be a significant source of support for parents (Bussing, Gary, Mills, & Garvan, 2003). However, for some parents the message being received is that their input and involvement is not valued or desired. Rather than getting support, these parents feel blamed or simply dismissed. In this chapter we provide information on how teachers can work more effectively with parents of children with ADHD. First, we discuss psychological and family stresses experienced by many parents that can affect parent–teacher relationships, child rearing, and involvement with home–school treatment. Second, we discuss resources for parents of children with ADHD. Note that these resources are also useful for teachers. Third, we discuss how teachers can increase the likelihood of parent involvement. Finally, we provide an example of an effective home–school intervention that can increase parent–teacher communication and improve a child's behavior and provide guidelines for helping parents and teachers deal with homework problems.

FAMILY STRESSORS

Parents of children with ADHD are more likely to experience psychological distress and high levels of family conflict. Compared to control groups, parents of children with ADHD are more likely to have ADHD themselves. From 12 to 20% of mothers and up to 50% of fathers reported symptoms of ADHD (Barkley, 2006). Mood disorders are more common among parents of children with ADHD (Johnston & Mash, 2001). Mothers of children with ADHD appear to be particularly vulnerable to depression, and there is considerable overlap between symptoms of depression and ADHD in mothers—mothers with ADHD were more likely to experience symptoms of depression (Chronis-Tuscano et al., 2008; Johnston & Mash, 2001). Up to 43% of mothers have reported symptoms of mood disorders, particularly depression. If the child has comorbid ODD or CD, mothers are five times more likely to experience depression than control group parents. Additionally, both mothers (15–17%) and fathers (13–31%) of children with ADHD have reported a childhood history of ODD or CD (Chronis et al., 2003). Interestingly, mothers with ADHD may actually respond more positively and affectionately to challenging behaviors compared to mothers without ADHD (Psychogiou, Daley, Thompson, & Sonuga-Barke, 2008). Note that teachers *should not assume* that parents of children with ADHD have psychological problems. "More likely" does not mean that all or even most parents experience psychological distress. It only means that they are at *increased risk compared to other parents*. The key point is that teachers should be *sensitive to the possibility* that parents of children with ADHD may experience psychological distress.

Stress is also a problem. Parents of children with ADHD report significantly higher levels of stress (Barkley, 2006) that begin in early childhood (DuPaul, McGoey, Eckert, & VanBrakle, 2001), and that is chronic (i.e., long lasting; Treacy, Tripp, & Bird, 2005). Higher stress levels are both global (e.g., dealing with everyday problems) and parenting-related (e.g., low opinion of parenting skills; Podolski & Nigg, 2001). Family conflicts are often a problem. Parents of children with ADHD report lower levels of marital satisfaction, fight more often, and experience higher divorce rates (Wymbs et al., 2008). A parent with ADHD increases the likelihood of family conflict (Biederman, Faraone, & Monteaux, 2002). Stress levels are usually higher if the child also has ODD or CD or is male (Barkley, 2006; Bussing et al., 2003). The difficulties associated with parenting a child with ADHD is thought to cause high stress levels (Barkley, 2006). Elevated stress levels are a problem because high stress levels are associated with ineffective, coercive, or maladaptive parenting styles; parenting problems can also contribute to stress (Johnston & Mash, 2001). In some families, there is a negative interactions cycle that results in continued family conflict that is stressful to the parent and child. The negative interaction cycles result from noncompliance by the child that then results in a reprimand or other negative reaction from the parent that in turn results in increased noncompliance. This negative interaction cycle increases a child's future risk for CD (Chronis-Tuscano et al., 2008).

Problems with parenting practices occur in some families (Chronis-Tuscano et al., 2008; Weiss, Hechtman, & Weiss, 2000). Some commonly reported parenting problems are:

- Less monitoring or knowledge of children's activities.
- Less responsive to requests for attention from the child.
- More negative, critical, or reprimanding interactions.
- Use of overly harsh or physical punishment.
- Problems maintaining consistent rules.
- Not using consequences or rewards for behaviors.
- Using inappropriate or inconsistent consequences.
- Not reacting to misbehavior.

These problems are serious because they can exacerbate problem behavior and increase parent stress levels. They can also interfere with home–school treatment. Problems with treatment compliance (e.g., remembering to reward a child for good behavior) are especially problematic if one or more parents have ADHD. Teachers should consider this when planning treatments with parents. Teachers should try to get a sense of how parents perceive their parenting skills and relationship with their child. Parents who report that problems seem intractable or that they can't seem to manage the child's behavior might benefit from additional resources described in the following section.

RESOURCES FOR PARENTS

One way that teachers can help parents deal more effectively with their children is to provide them with information on ADHD and with sources of support. This is especially important when parents suspect that their child may have ADHD or immediately after the child has been diagnosed. During this time parents are coming to grips with their child's diagnosis and trying to find ways to better deal with problem behavior. Note that parents of older children may already be aware of resources and support networks. Teacher can help provide three main resources:

information on ADHD, information on parent education programs, and information on parent support groups.

Information on ADHD

There are a number of excellent books on ADHD that are aimed at helping parents understand the nature of ADHD and what they can do to help their child succeed. There are also books designed to help children understand how ADHD affects them. Better understanding the nature of ADHD and how it affects their child can help parents can actually reduce parent stress. It can also help with feelings of guilt (i.e., that they are somehow to blame for the problem with ADHD; Harborne, Wolpert, & Clarke, 2004). Figure 6.1 provides examples of books that are useful resources for parents (and teachers). There are also many excellent resources on the Internet. Figure 6.2 shows some sites hosted by professional organizations or universities that provide reliable information on ADHD. Note that there is a great deal of misinformation on ADHD on the Internet. Some sites have impressive-sounding names designed to give the impression that the site is affiliated with a reputable professional organization when in reality the site is dedicated to hawking a product. Teachers should warn parents about this situation and encourage them to focus on sites sponsored by professional organization or universities. It's important for parents to be informed consumers (Barkley, 2000). Otherwise there is a risk of parents adopting ineffective treatments rather than effective treatments.

Information on Parent Education Programs

Some parents may feel the need for more than informational support. For these parents, parent-education programs could be useful. Parent education programs for parents of children with ADHD commonly provide (Anastopoulos, Hennis Rhoads, & Farley, 2006): (1) basic information on ADHD (e.g., symptoms, how ADHD is diagnosed, common treatments, comorbid conditions); (2) effective behavior management for children with ADHD (e.g., strategies for managing behaviors such as praise, use of a token economy, response cost), and (3) techniques to improve parent–child interactions (e.g., focusing on positive communication, while avoiding negative communication, attending to appropriate behaviors and ignoring inappropriate behaviors). Figure 6.3 shows topics commonly included in parent education programs. Programs typically involve from six to 12 training sessions that last 1 to 2 hours. Parent education programs can reduce problem behavior (e.g., oppositional behavior) and parent–child conflict; they can also lower parent stress levels and increase parents' confidence in their ability to cope with problem behavior (Anastopoulos et al., 2006). Parent education programs are often available through medical centers and health professionals who specialize in ADHD. There are also web-based resources for locating parent education resources. For example, the CHADD website (see below) provides a locator service, and the U.S. Center for Mental Health Services provides an online database of mental health providers (*store.samhsa.gov/mhlocator*).

Taking Charge of ADHD: The Complete, Authoritative Guide for Parents (rev. ed.) by Russell A. Barkley(Guilford Press, 2000). Written by a leader in the field of ADHD, this book is an excellent resource for parents (and teachers). The book covers the causes of ADHD, psychosocial aspects of the disorder, practical parenting issues (e.g., when a child should be evaluated for ADHD), effective behavior management techniques, problem-solving approaches, and pharmacological treatments. He suggests parents adopt a case manager approach that will appeal to many parents.

The Misunderstood Child: Understanding and Coping with Your Child's Learning Disabilities (4th ed.) by Larry B. Silver (Three Rivers Press, 2006). This book, which is appropriate for parents and teachers, covers ADHD as well as LD. Its focus is to help parents become "informed consumers and assertive advocates." The book covers normal development, the effects of learning disabilities, current techniques for diagnosing learning disabilities, and current treatment approaches. It also covers federal law pertaining to education.

The Explosive Child: A New Approach for Understanding and Parenting Easily Frustrated, Chronically Inflexible Children by Ross W. Greene (Harper, 2010). This book addresses the explosive child—those with frequent, severe fits of temper, who have very low tolerance for frustration, change, and delay of gratification and who frequently have explosive verbal and/or physical outbursts. The author provides a conceptual framework for understanding the behavior and provides information on the neuroscience behind explosive behavior. It also provides tips on how to recognize when an explosion is impending, reduce tension, and lower frustration levels for the family.

New Skills for Frazzled Parents: The Instruction Manual That Should Have Come with Your Child by Daniel G. Amen. (MindWorks Press, 2000). This book covers parenting tips and explains how to use effective parenting techniques such as goal setting, establishing rules, and the need for consistency. It also provides a basic overview of ADHD.

The New Putting on the Brakes: Understanding and Taking Control of Your ADD or ADHD (2nd ed.) by Patricia O. Quinn and Judith M. Stern. (Magination Press, 2008). Parents often struggle to explain ADHD to their child. This book helps parents explain ADHD in simple language. It explains not only the nature of ADHD, but also how children and their parents can learn to manage it. It's intended for children in upper elementary through high school.

Distant Drums, Different Drummers: A Guide for Young People with ADHD by Barbara D. Ingersoll. (Cape Publications, 1995). This book presents a positive perspective on ADHD. It stresses the value of individual differences. The child with ADHD is portrayed as an adventurer and risk taker. This perspective helps children and adolescents struggling with ADHD to see themselves in a positive light (e.g., not hyperactivity but boundless energy).

FIGURE 6.1. Books for parents of children with ADHD.

www.nimh.nih.gov/health/topics/attention-deficit-hyperactivity-disorder-adhd/index.shtml

The National Institute of Mental Health is the government's lead agency for the treatment of mental illness. The ADHD section of its website has summaries of the disorder's core symptoms, a description of the ADHD diagnostic process, and links to research involving treatment of ADHD. The site also has a downloadable 28-page booklet on ADHD.

www.chadd.org

Children and Adults with Attention Deficit/Hyperactivity Disorder (CHADD) is a respected parent support group focused on helping children and adults with ADHD. The site offers information on parenting a child with ADHD, educational issues related to ADHD, and a professional directory search for medical and counseling professionals with backgrounds in treating ADHD. The site also hosts the National Resource Center on ADHD, which provides information on ADHD research.

www.ldonline.org/adhdbasics

LD Online is a website focusing on learning disabilities and ADHD. Its section on ADHD, titled ADHD Basics, has several pages that summarize many key aspects of the disorder. These pages include information on disorders commonly associated with ADHD, how families can effectively cope with the disorder, and advice for getting students with ADHD the educational assistance they require.

www.additudemag.com

This is the site of ADDitude, a quarterly publication dedicated to helping individuals and families cope with ADHD and learning disabilities. The site includes a section on parenting ADHD children, with subsections focusing on such issues as behavior and discipline, scheduling and organizing, and sports and hobbies. There are also sections on ADHD treatment and dealing with ADHD and learning disabilities in school.

school.familyeducation.com/learning-disabilities/add-and-adhd/34474.html

Part of the Family Education site focuses on ADHD. There are subsections dealing with understanding and diagnosing ADHD, ADHD treatment, ADHD in school, and ADHD outside of school. The section on ADHD in school has information on school issues, interventions, and ADHD and special education.

www.guilfordjournals.com/loi/adhd

Written by Russell A. Barkley and other leading experts, *The ADHD Report* examines the nature, diagnosis, and outcomes associated with the disorder, and provides a single reliable guide to the latest developments in the fields of clinical management and education. It includes research findings, as well as ongoing coverage of ADHD in the news.

FIGURE 6.2. Web-based resources.

Component	Description
Overview of ADHD	History of ADHD, medications, comorbidity, symptoms, how ADHD is diagnosed
Communication skills	Avoiding negative communication, focus on positive communication, giving effective directions
Behavior management	Principles of behavior management, understanding behaviors, reinforcement (e.g., praise, token economy), punishment (e.g., time-out, response cost)
Attending skills	Attending to positive behaviors, ignoring inappropriate behaviors
Problem-solving skills	Defining problem behaviors, brainstorming solutions, negotiating and deciding acceptable solutions, implementing solutions
Child-centered skills	Teaching the child a specific skill set (e.g., social skills, problem-solving skills)
Generalizing strategies	Modifying strategies for settings other than home
Planning responses for future use	Brainstorming ideas on how to handle future problems that may arise
School consultation and communication	How to talk to school personnel, working cooperatively with school personnel
Cognitive restructuring	Identifying and restructuring maladaptive thoughts or beliefs about parenting practices

FIGURE 6.3. Common components of parent education programs.

Parent Support Groups

As we noted earlier, parents of children with ADHD may experience high levels of stress and are at risk for depression or other mood disorders. They may question their parenting skills, and feel that their child's problems are insurmountable. For these reasons it is important for parents of children with ADHD to have an active support network. However, research has shown that many parents of children with ADHD tend to rely on small support networks, consisting mostly of kin, for concerns about their child's behavioral or emotional problems (Bussing et al., 2003). These support networks may not be able to supply parents with needed emotional supports or help with sound parenting advice because they lack knowledge of effective methods for dealing with problem behavior, and have not experienced the demands of a child with ADHD. Thus parents may feel the need for additional support. Parent support groups can help fill this need.

Parent support groups consist of parents with children with ADHD who meet on a regular basis to share their experiences dealing with ADHD. Parents can share their feelings, problems, or successes meeting the demands of a child with ADHD with others who can fully appreciate the experience. Support groups can also provide information and tips on dealing with common problems. Participation in a parent support group can lower stress levels, increase parents' sense of competence in their ability to work effectively with their child, improve their knowledge of ADHD, and result in a more proactive approach to parenting (Singh et al., 1997). Note also that there is evidence that support groups for children with ADHD can also be effective in increasing children's feelings of acceptance and self-worth (Frame, Kelly, & Bayley, 2003).

The largest and most well-established parent support group is Children and Adults with Attention Deficit/Hyperactivity Disorder (CHADD; *www.chadd.org*). CHADD is a national, nonprofit organization with chapters in most states. Unlike some other support groups, CHADD does not endorse specific medications, commercial treatment programs, or products on the website. The CHADD website is an excellent resource that provides up-to-date information on ADHD, recent research, recommended treatments (e.g., behavioral interventions, medication), legal rights, and working with schools. There is a locator service to help find local chapters; additionally CHADD provides information to help members locate health professionals in their area who work with children or adults with ADHD. CHADD also provide online forums for parents to discuss their experiences or problems. This can be valuable for parents who may not have ready access to a local support group (e.g., parents in rural areas). CHADD also offers "parent-to-parent" education programs in which specially trained parents teach classes on how to effectively manage ADHD. Parent-to-parent classes are also available online.

ENCOURAGING PARENTAL INVOLVEMENT

Teachers should strive to actively involve parents in their child's treatment. When parents are actively involved in their children with ADHD's treatment, the children benefit (Power & Mautone, 2008). There are three main types of parental involvement (Fantuzzo, McWayne, Perry, & Childs, 2004): school-based, which consist of activities parents engage in at school or in cooperation with the school (e.g., classroom volunteer, joining parent–teacher organizations, helping plan events); home–school communication, which consists of communications between school personnel and parents regarding the child's educational experience and progress (e.g., talking with parents about academic progress and difficulties); and home-based, which consists of actions parents undertake at home to improve behavior and promote a positive learning environment at home (e.g. providing learning opportunities at home, stressing the value of education). The time and effort teachers put into getting parents involved can pay big dividends down the road in terms of students' outcomes.

School-Based Involvement

School-based involvement is probably what first comes to mind when we think about parent involvement. Many schools have developed strategies to engage parents in school activities (e.g., signs stating that "This Is Our School," parent–teacher organizations, volunteer programs). One of the most effective means of increasing school-based parent involvement is to simply invite them by sending home announcements of opportunities to participate (Hoover-Dempsey et al., 2005). School-based involvement by parents is desirable because it is associated with improvements in attention and a reduced level of conduct problems (Fantuzzo et al., 2004). Why school-based involvement is effective is not yet understood. It's possible that the visible presence of the parents in the school may create a concrete connection for students between the school and home (Fantuzzo, Tighe, & Childs, 1999). Unfortunately, no research has addressed whether any specific activities (e.g., volunteer class aide, helping on field trips) are more effective than others, or the extent to which parents would need to be involved.

Home–School Communication

Parent–teacher interactions are a critical part of engaging parents. Parents are more likely to get involved in home-based and/or school-based activities if they are comfortable talking with the teacher, believe that the teacher cares about their child, and think that the teacher is interested in their ideas about how to work with the child (Hoover-Dempsey et al., 2005). Thus, effective home–school communications are critical for parent involvement. Unfortunately, lack of communication is a common complaint of parents of children with ADHD. They feel as if they are in the dark about how their child is doing, are unaware as to what interventions are being used in the classroom, and don't know whether the teacher is encountering any problems (Reid et al., 1996).

Teachers need to develop a home–school communication system and use the system consistently throughout the year (Bos, Nahmias, & Urban, 1999). The first step is to determine how best to communicate with parents (Knopf & Swick, 2008). For example, the teacher might send a note to the parents asking them how they would prefer to communicate (e.g., telephone, e-mail, home–school notes, parent–teacher conferences) and how frequently they would like to schedule communications (e.g., weekly, biweekly). Note that there is no "best" means of communication. How parents prefer to communicate depends on many factors. Some parents may see phone calls as intrusive while others may like to talk personally; some parents might relish the convenience of e-mail while others may not have access to e-mail. Home–school notes are an efficient means of communication, but for some students getting home–school notes to and from school consistently might be unrealistic. Some parents might prefer face-to-face meetings; others might not have time for regular conferences.

Next the teacher should establish a schedule for communication. After the schedule is established it is *critical* that the teacher maintain it. If a teacher fails to maintain the regular schedule it will likely undermine the teacher's credibility. Parents may perceive the communication as merely pro forma rather than as a real attempt to exchange information between the home and school that can help the child. For example, one parent expressed her frustration, "The teacher kept talking about sending notes home, and keeping in touch and he had a notebook that he was going to write in and we haven't brought it home once this year" (Reid et al., 1996, p. 79). Timely communication is also important. This can avoid letting small problems grow into big ones. One parent expressed her frustration about lack of timely communication, "Why didn't they come to us weeks ago when things were starting to deteriorate rather than wait until he was about ready to lose his field trip?" (Reid et al., 1996, p. 81).

Teachers also need to carefully consider the content and tone of communications. What teachers report to parents and how they report it is critical to effective communication. For example, sometimes all communication from the teacher pertains to problems. Thus, "all news is bad news." Some parents literally come to dread a call or note from the teacher. One parent whom we worked with described how she would get a knot in her stomach when the phone rang in the evening. Unfortunately, the "all news is bad news" trap is one that busy teachers can inadvertently fall into. Teachers don't intend to focus on the negatives, they simply forget that there are often positives. A related problem is that sometimes when teachers do communicate, they may inadvertently convey the impression that it is the parent's responsibility to deal with classroom behavior problems (e.g., "Karen won't stay at her desk. What can you do about it?'). Parents do not react well when they perceive that they are being blamed for a child's problems in school.

Tingley (2009) provides practical tips for teachers to communicate effectively with parents.

• *Be positive.* Teachers need to report problems. However, if communication is limited to a steady drumbeat of problems and inappropriate behavior, parents may simply tune it out. *Every child has strengths and positive traits.* It's important to convey this information to parents. Make sure to send home good news when it happens. For example, telling parents, "Karen got all her seatwork done Wednesday without any prompting!" is a victory. Both the parents and the child need victories. They are behaviors that parents can praise their child for. Parents of children with ADHD need opportunities for positive interactions with their child. Good news might be as simple as "Leslie is an excellent class helper" or "Steve has boundless energy." Remember that for children with ADHD an "uneventful" day or week could actually be very positive news. Note that remembering to include positive news gives the teacher credibility when he or she reports problems. Parents can see that the teacher is not solely focused on the problem behaviors.

• *Be specific.* Give parents the details of both positive and negative behaviors. For example, rather than saying "Roger acted out again," say "Roger did not comply with directions when told to stay in line." This gives parents more useful information. Similarly, rather than saying "Karin is doing better at her spelling," tell the parents "Karin got eight out of 10 on her weekly spelling test. She really studied hard!"

• *Be timely.* Let parents know immediately if a behavior begins to be a problem. Informing the parents immediately may allow the parents to intervene. Parents may also be able to provide insights into why a problem behavior is occurring (e.g., Roger has problems staying in line because a classmate teases him). If a small problem does develop into a large one, at least parents will be aware of what is occurring. This avoids parents being blindsided by a problem that from their perspective seemingly came from out of the blue.

• *Be judicious.* Teachers don't need to report everything, and it's not a good idea to report behaviors that are merely irritating to the teacher. For example, many children with ADHD fidget with objects (e.g., tapping their pencil) or squirm in their seat. The guiding principle should be whether a behavior would affect the academic, behavioral, or social functioning of the child.

• *Be proactive.* Teachers should anticipate possible problems and work with parents to deal with them. For example, if an upcoming field trip requires a permission slip that is signed by the parents, the teacher can inform the parents of this in advance and notify them again when the child will be bringing home the slip. Parents can then be sure to retrieve the permission slip and make sure it is signed and returned.

Home-Based Involvement

Establishing effective communication with parents is important; however, teachers should strive to enlist parents in home-based activities. When parents are involved in the home, they become active collaborators in treatment. Teachers should make the effort to engage parents in home-based activities because research suggests that family involvement in home treatment is *extremely effective* at reducing ADHD-related behavior problems at school (Fantuzzo et al., 2004), especially when combined with *school-based and home–school communication.* Ideally, teachers and parents can establish shared goals for the child, coordinate treatments across home and school, and monitor progress toward those goals across both school and home (Bos et al., 1999).

To engage parents as collaborators, teachers need to create a climate of collaboration and establish effective working relationships. Put simply, teachers need to communicate that parent involvement is both desired and valued (Knopf & Swick, 2008). There are two factors that affect the likelihood of parent–teacher collaboration: (1) parents' sense of shared responsibility for the child (i.e., both the teacher and the parents are necessary), and (2) parents' belief that their actions can help the child (Hoover-Dempsey et al., 2005). For this reason, teachers should stress a "we're in this together" team-based approach where parents are treated as equal partners in the process, and should project a "together we can do it" attitude (Cox, 2005). The most likely time to enlist parents as collaborators is during parent–teacher meetings (e.g., IEP meetings, parent–teacher conferences). Teachers should be aware of this and conduct meetings with an eye toward this goal. Note that in the case of students with ADHD it might be advisable to schedule a meeting very early in the school year. It may also be useful to schedule more frequent meetings. Figure 6.4 shows tips for how to hold effective meetings that can help engage parents as collaborators and establish effective working relationships.

Meeting time
Allow for flexible scheduling. Many parents have limited times when they are available. Allot sufficient time especially if it is the first meeting. Allow for a late start.

Meeting place
Whenever possible have the meeting in the classroom. Avoid impersonal conference rooms. Do not seat parents across the desk; this creates a psychological barrier between the teacher and parent. Instead, sit beside them at a table. Make sure there are adult-size chairs for everyone. Don't seat parents on child-size chairs!

Preparation
Have all relevant information (e.g., test scores, work samples, observation records) organized and at hand. Check with past teachers on what accommodation and interventions have been used and how effective they were. Check the parents' names. Joe Jones's mother may be Jessica Polipnik rather than Jessica Jones.

Setting the tone
Tell the parents that *you want to hear their thoughts, concerns, or ideas*. Ask if you can take notes (some parents don't like teachers to take notes). Demonstrate interest: face parents directly, make eye contact, ask questions, reflect on parents' comments (e.g., "So, social skills is an area of concern?").

Have clear goals
All meetings should have clear goals. Have an agenda that states the purpose of the meeting and goals for the meeting. The goal should be established prior to the meeting and communicated to all parties. Goals should be specific and relate to a defined problem. For example, a specific goal might be: "Increase the amount of seatwork Linda completes."

Stay objective
Focus on problems and solutions. Define problems in terms of specific behaviors (e.g., "Steve fails to return half his homework assignments."). Identify possible plans of action (e.g., homework chart, stickers for completed homework). Decide which plan(s) should be adopted, and who will implement the plan and how the effects will be monitored.

Be concrete
Have specific options ready (e.g., "Here are three possible ways we could address the problem."). Solicit parents' opinions on treatment options along with any ideas or modifications they might want.

Establish closure
At the end of the meeting *write out* what was decided. Make sure everyone agrees. If specific actions or activities were decided on, specify in writing who is responsible and establish time lines. If follow-up activities are indicated (e.g., monitoring homework completion), establish how this will be done and how information will be communicated.

FIGURE 6.4. Tips for meeting with parents. Based on Seplocha (2004), Bos et al. (1999), and Kroth and Edge (2007).

Teachers may also wish to ask parents questions that could clarify the parents' perceptions of the child's problems or needs, and provide information useful to treatment such as:

- "What are your child's areas of strength?"
- "In what areas would you like to see improvement?"
- "What concerns you most about school?"
- "What activities or hobbies interest your child?"
- "Is there any information that you feel I need to know about your child?"
- "Are you interested in sources of information about ADHD?"
- "Are you interested in learning more about how to work with your child?"
- "Would you be interested in meeting with other parents of children with ADHD?"

Teachers should be aware that there are considerable differences across parents in terms of their knowledge of ADHD and expertise in dealing with the problems posed by ADHD. Working with parents who have extensive background knowledge of ADHD and who have developed strategies for dealing with problem behaviors is much different than working with parents who are just beginning to realize that their child has ADHD, who may not understand the nature of the problems posed by ADHD, and who have not yet developed strategies for managing problem behaviors. Parents with extensive background knowledge of ADHD may be able to supply teachers with information on effective accommodations and interventions for the student. Even the parents with little knowledge may be able to supply useful information. Teachers should be sensitive to this—they should actively solicit parent input.

Teachers should also remember that parents of children with ADHD, like any other group of parents, differ in the degree to which they are willing and able to be involved. Some parents will actively seek out opportunities to collaborate; others may be reticent. Also remember that the degree to which parents are involved can change over time (e.g., parent involvement tends to decrease during adolescence) (Hoover-Dempsey et al., 2005). Teachers should also be aware of potential problems. Psychological distress and other stressors can affect parent–teacher interactions. For example, parents with ADHD can have problems with organization. They may show up late for meetings or miss meetings entirely. They may forget to bring forms or other important information. They may have problems with follow-through if they are involved in treatment (e.g., forgetting to give a child a reward when appropriate). During a meeting their attention may wander, or they may abruptly shift topics or interject off-topic comments (Weiss et al., 2000). Parents with depression could appear resistant to involvement because they may feel powerless. Feelings of helplessness or despair are symptomatic of depression. High levels of anxiety and stress can increase treatment seeking (Bussing et al., 2003). If a parent makes unrealistic requests for services or continually seeks new services, this attitude could be related to anxiety or high stress levels. Note that this should *not* be confused with the services and accommodations students are entitled to under law. Finally, teachers should be sensitive to factors such as single parenting or economic distress (e.g., working two jobs). These can make attending a meeting difficult.

HOME–SCHOOL ACTIVITIES

There are many ways for parents and teachers to collaborate in treatment. Some activities are home-based. Others involve both home and school and require collaboration between parents and teachers. In this section we discuss general home-based activities, one specific home-based activity—helping with homework, and one effective home–school intervention—the daily report card.

Home-Based Activities

A number of simple home-based activities can promote learning and improve school behavior. For example, Power and Mautone (2008) reported that parents could:

- *Communicate the importance of education*. Stress the need to succeed in school and the value of an education. Parents should demonstrate to the child that school is important.
- *Schedule family reading time to stress the value of independent reading*. Demonstrate that reading is important by modeling the behavior for the child. For younger children, parents might read to or with the child.
- *Be available to assist if a child experiences problems with schoolwork*. Assist when needed (but only when needed). Children with ADHD have problems persisting with difficult tasks; appropriate assistance can improve homework completion.
- *Communicate reasonable expectations for academic success*. Set goals for academic progress and discuss them with the child. Make sure the goals are realistic and meaningful.
- *Monitor academic and behavioral progress*. Communicate knowledge of school successes (and failures). This demonstrates parents' interest in school activities and the importance of school activities.
- *Limit television, video games, and recreational computer activities*. There is evidence that limiting these activities can improve behavioral and academic functioning. Use these activities as rewards for appropriate behavior or academic accomplishments.

Homework

Students with ADHD commonly have problems with homework completion (DuPaul & Stoner, 2003). They often fail to write down assignments, rush through schoolwork, experience high levels of stress and frustration, and make careless mistakes. They also have problems beginning tasks in a timely manner, staying on-task, remembering assignments, organizing materials, and managing their time. Homework problems increase as the child progresses through grades because in middle and high school students are expected to become more independent learners (Meyer & Kelley, 2007). This can result in family conflict as parents fight the nightly "homework battle." Addressing homework problems effectively requires both home-based activities and school-based activities.

Home-Based Activities to Improve Homework Completion

To help parents deal with homework problems, teachers should first be sure that parents are aware of the school's homework procedures (Margolis & McCabe, 1997). For example, some schools require parents to sign a form indicating that the student has shown them a list of assigned homework. Some schools require students to use homework organizers or logs. Teachers need to communicate any special procedures to the parents. Teachers should also indicate roughly how much time students should spend on homework. Parents can also help to create an environment that is conducive to homework completion. There are a number of recommended actions that parents can take to improve homework completion. These include:

- *Establish a homework location.* Make sure your child has a quiet, well-lit place to do homework. Do not allow the child to do homework with the television on or in places with other distractions, such as people coming and going. Note that for some students, background noise (e.g., music or white noise) can be helpful (Zentall, 2006).
- *Make sure the materials your child needs, such as paper, pencils, or a dictionary, are available.* Ask your child if special materials will be needed for some projects and get them in advance.
- *Establish a homework routine.* Establish a set time each day for doing homework and *stick to it*. Don't let the child put off homework until just before bedtime. Think about using a weekend morning or afternoon for working on big projects, especially if the project involves getting together with classmates. Praise compliance with homework routine.
- *Help with time management.* Monitor progress with homework assignments. Set times for completion (e.g., 10 minutes for spelling practice). Use a timer to help the student's awareness of time spent on activities.
- *Help the child figure out what is hard homework and what is easy homework.* Have the child do the hard work first. This will mean the child will be fresh and alert for the most difficult work.
- *When the child asks for help, give only as much as needed.* Parents should not do homework for the child. Giving answers means the child will not learn the material. Too much help might teach the child that when the going gets rough, someone will do the work for him or her.

- *Watch for signs of failure and frustration.* If the child begins to get frustrated or has a problem focusing on the task, allow a short break. It may be useful to schedule short breaks at regular intervals (e.g., every 30 minutes there's a 5-minute break).
- *Reward progress in homework.* Praise the child for successful homework completion. Parents should stress that they appreciate that the child has worked hard. After consistent successful completion or finishing long or difficult assignments, celebrate success with a special event (e.g., pizza, a walk, a trip to the park) to reinforce effort (U.S. Department of Education, 2003).

School-Based Activities to Improve Homework Completion

Teachers' practices can directly affect the likelihood of homework completion. Teachers should address three main areas: organization, appropriate assignments, and feedback and reinforcement. Well-organized homework procedures are extremely important. Teachers should develop and follow regular rules and procedures for assigning, collecting, correcting, evaluating, grading, and returning homework assignments (Epstein, Polloway, Foley, & Patton, 1993). The rules and procedures for homework should be taught to the students and periodically reviewed if necessary (e.g., the student fails to follow procedures). Teachers should also provide students with organizational supports such as an assignment notebook in which they can record homework assignments (Zentall, 2006). Note that simply providing a notebook isn't sufficient. Teachers need to instruct the students in how to use the notebook to keep track of assignments, cue them to use their notebook (e.g., by directly asking the student if he or she wrote down the assignment), and provide practice sessions in how to use the notebook (Margolis & McCabe, 1997). Teachers should also brainstorm with students on how they can ensure that homework will be returned and handed in (e.g., "As soon as each piece of homework is done, put it in your backpack. When you get to school, immediately put the homework in the homework box"). Finally, teachers should also monitor student's use of the notebook (e.g., Is the student using it consistently? Does the student write down assignments correctly?).

One documented problem with homework completion is that homework may simply be too difficult for the student (Salend & Schliff, 1989). Students with ADHD are unlikely to complete homework that is at their frustration level. Teachers should take care to match the difficulty level of the homework to the student's level of competence. For example, readings should be at or near the student's independent reading level (i.e., the student should be able to read almost all words with no difficulty). Initially assign homework that should be very easy to complete, then gradually increase difficulty. Begin assignments in class, if students experience difficulty, then modify the assignments. Discuss any aspects of an assignment that might be confusing and make sure the student understands expectations (Margolis & McCabe, 1997).

Teachers should also be sensitive to the amount of homework assigned. Even in the best of circumstances, students with ADHD have problems maintaining effort for long periods of time. If students perceive the amount of homework as overwhelming, they may not even attempt to complete it. Reducing the amount of homework assigned is often a good idea for students with ADHD; "less is more," especially if the student has a comorbid learning disability (Zentall, 2006). Students should not spend hours doing homework that other students do in a fraction of the time (Margolis & McCabe, 1997). Remember that school can often be stressful for students with ADHD. They need down time at home to "unwind." A good guideline for the amount of homework that is appropriate for typically achieving students is the "10-minute rule" (Cooper, 2007). That is, for a first grader no more the 10 minutes of homework per night, for a second grader no more that 20 minutes, and so on up to a maximum of 2 hours in high school. These amounts would likely be high for students with ADHD. To help determine how much homework to assign students with ADHD, teachers can ask parents to estimate how much time the student can spend on homework before it becomes unproductive. Teachers can also help by varying homework assignments. Introducing novelty can improve the performance of students with ADHD. For example, teachers might give students a choice between two or three different assignments, or allow students to practice a different way (e.g., use a computer game to practice math facts) (Zentall, 2006).

Providing students with ADHD ongoing feedback on their efforts is extremely important. Students with ADHD can be extremely insensitive to their performance levels (Barkley, 2006). This is also true of their academic performance. Teachers should provide students with written feedback on homework that notes what the student did well and what specific actions students could take to improve their performance (e.g., "Good job remembering your math facts! Be careful to keep the numbers lined up correctly in the problems or you'll make a mistake."). Teachers can also use charts or graphs to provide feedback to students on their performance over time. For example, a teacher might graph the percent of homework a student completed each day, or the percent correct on math homework. Feedback of this sort gives students valuable, ongoing feedback on their performance, and also can be extremely motivational.

In summary, teachers should be sensitive to potential problems with homework. Dealing successfully with homework requires both home- and school-based activities. Parents need to establish a suitable environment for homework completion and a homework routine. Teachers need to ensure that assignments are at the appropriate level of difficulty and length. There are other techniques teachers can use to help with homework completion (e.g., homework completion strategies, self-monitoring) that are discussed in subsequent chapters.

Daily Report Card

The daily report card (DRC) is an effective, widely used, home–school intervention that can enhance teacher–parent communication and improve problem behavior

(Cox, 2005; Pelham, Wheeler, & Chronis, 1998). DRCs have been used widely in the schools, are simple to use, and require minimal time investment on the teacher's part after initial planning (Murray, Rabiner, Schulte, & Newitt, 2008). To use DRCs, the teacher creates a "report card" that includes daily performance objectives (see Figures 6.5 and 6.6 for examples). Note that initially the teacher should focus on one or two objectives that are most important in terms of the student's classroom functioning. The teacher grades the student on his or her performance daily, and sends the DRC home to the parents. Parents then discuss the DRC results with the student and provide specific rewards based on the student's performance level. Procedures for implementing DRCs are well established and detailed descriptions of DRCs along with extensive support materials are available online (Pelham, 2002). Steps for implementing a DRC (Pelham, 2002) are as follows:

1. *Select areas for improvement.* Parents and teachers collaboratively establish areas for improvement. Teachers and parents determine the areas in which the child is most impaired and decide on specific areas that need improvement. Areas such as improved peer relations, improved academic work, and increased rule following/ compliance are areas commonly targeted.

2. *Define target behaviors.* Identify specific target behaviors that can be changed. Target behaviors should be (a) *meaningful*—behaviors should be ones that will significantly impact the child's functioning in the classroom, (b) *well specified*—behaviors should be objectively defined (e.g., completes all assigned seatwork or stays in seat for the whole period), (c) *observable*—behaviors should be ones that the teacher can directly observe to see whether or not the target behavior occurred, and (4) *easy to assess*—behaviors should be easy to measure or count.

3. *Select behaviors and set criteria for target behaviors.* Decide which target behaviors will be included on the DRC. It's a good idea to start with at least a few behaviors the teacher and parents judge to be amenable to change. This way the child is likely to experience immediate success and receive rewards; this will increase the likelihood of other behaviors improving. After the target behaviors are selected, the teacher needs to determine the criterion level (i.e., how well the child must perform the behavior to receive a reward). For example, staying in seat for 10 minutes, copying spelling words three times, or completing all math problems would be examples of criteria for behaviors. To establish the criterion level for behavior, first establish current levels of the behavior by observing, estimating, or checking records. Then set a criterion level for the behavior (e.g., How long does Steve stay in his seat? How much seatwork does Karin complete?). Criterion levels need to be set carefully. The criterion level should be set at a level that the child can reasonably attain. Initially, it's probably better to err on the side of setting the criterion too low than too high. If the level is too high the child won't receive a reward, and thus there is unlikely to be a behavior change. Additionally, when starting a DRC, criteria should be set for several parts of the day (e.g., one period or a portion of one period) rather that the whole day. This allows a student to earn rewards based on a portion of the day.

Name: _____

Date: _____

	Specials	Language Arts	Math	Reading	Science
Raises hand and waits to be called on.	Y N	Y N	Y N	Y N	Y N
Finishes assignments within the designated time.	Y N	Y N	Y N	Y N	Y N
Hands in all assignments.	Y N	Y N	Y N	Y N	Y N
Follows instruction the first time without arguing (two or fewer instances of noncompliance).	Y N	Y N	Y N	Y N	Y N
Keeps hands and feet to self.	Y N	Y N	Y N	Y N	Y N

Total number of yeses _____

Total number of nos _____

Percentage _____

      90–100% = 3 STARS

      80–89% = 2 STARS

      70–79% = 1 STAR

Teacher's initials: _____

Comments: _____

_____

_____

_____

_____

_____

_____

_____

_____

_____

_____

_____

FIGURE 6.5. Daily report card (1).

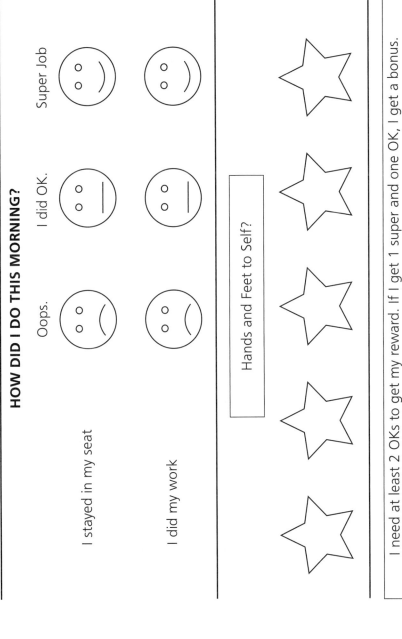

HOW DID I DO THIS MORNING?

	Oops.	I did OK.	Super Job
I stayed in my seat	☹	😐	☺
I did my work	☹	😐	☺

Hands and Feet to Self?

★ ★ ★ ★ ★

I need at least 2 OKs to get my reward. If I get 1 super and one OK, I get a bonus. I get 3 minutes of computer time for each star I have left.

FIGURE 6.6. Daily report card (2).

Meeting goals for an entire day would likely be too difficult for many students, at least initially.

4. *Explain the DRC to the child*. Meet with the child and explain the DRC. Show the DRC to the child. Explain to the child that he or she will be able to earn rewards based on behavior. Make sure the child understands the target behaviors that will be used and the criterion levels. Explain that the teacher will mark the DRC each period. The DRC form provides performance feedback. This is valuable because many children with ADHD are unaware of how well or how poorly they are performing. Note that for young children more graphic forms may be appropriate. Explain to the child that she or he will take the DRC home each day and that there will be rewards based on how well he or she performs the target behaviors.

5. *Establish home-based rewards*. Create a "rewards menu" in consultation with the parents. The rewards menu should consist of activities or tangible items that the parents and teacher believe would be desirable to the child (e.g., extra story time, a special dessert, playing a computer game). Parents may wish to allow the child to create his or her own rewards. For example, one child created the "drive about" game where the child was allowed to direct her mom where to drive the car for a set period of time. Allow the child to select rewards from a rewards menu. Note that it's important for the child to select the reward; *the value of the rewards is in the eye of the child*. Otherwise the rewards might not reinforce the child for reaching criterion levels. See Figure 6.7 for example rewards. Rewards should be arranged by level—more desired rewards could be earned with higher levels of performance. Label the reward levels (e.g., one-star rewards, two-star rewards). See Pelham (2002) for an extensive list of possible rewards.

6. *Monitor performance and modify if needed*. Record the child's daily performance (e.g., how many yes's received). If the child begins to meet a criterion level regularly, raise the criterion; conversely, if the child regularly fails to meet a criterion, it should be lowered. When a child regularly meets the criterion level for a behavior, and the criterion is at an acceptable level for the classroom, drop the behavior from the DRC and replace it with another if necessary. Be sure to tell the child why the behavior is being dropped and stress that it is because of improvement. If the child's daily performance is consistently at criterion for all target behaviors, move to a weekly report system. Again inform the child why and stress that this is a positive change. If the child begins to consistently function appropriately for the classroom for a period of time, the DRC may be discontinued. The DRC can be reinstated if problems reoccur.

7. *Troubleshooting*. If the DRC does not affect the child's behavior, try to determine whether there is a problem. Figure 6.8 shows common problems that can occur. One serious problem is if parents forget to follow through with home-based rewards. If this occurs teachers should switch to school-based rewards. The child can continue to use the DRC, as it would still serve to help inform the parents on the student's school behavior.

Three-star rewards
- Going to the video arcade at the mall
- Going fishing
- Going shopping/going to the mall
- Going to the movies
- Bowling, miniature golf
- Having friend over to spend night
- Going to friend's house to spend night
- Choosing family movie

Two-star rewards
- Having a friend come over to play
- Allowance bonus
- Special activity with mom or dad
- Earn day off from chores
- Game of choice with parent/family
- Making popcorn
- Going to the park
- Getting ice cream

One-star rewards
- Staying up *X* minutes beyond bedtime
- Educational games on computer for *X* minutes
- Choosing family TV show
- Talking on phone to friend (local call)
- Video game time for *X* minutes
- Playing outside for *X* minutes
- Listening to radio/stereo for *X* minutes

FIGURE 6.7. Examples of home rewards. From Pelham (2002). Reprinted with permission from William E. Pelham, Jr.

SUMMING UP

In this chapter we outlined techniques that teachers can use to involve parents in their child's education and ADHD treatment. Parental involvement is highly desirable. When parents and teachers communicate effectively and work together toward shared goals, student's outcomes are likely to improve. Here are some major points to remember:

✓ Parents of children with ADHD may be under a lot of stress. Parents themselves may have ADHD. Maybe parents are experiencing psychological distress. Be sensitive to these possibilities.

✓ Be aware of resources for parents should they indicate a need. Develop a list of informational resources, and seek out information on local parent education programs and parent support groups.

Problem	Solution
• Is the child taking the report card home?	• Ensure that the child has a backpack or special folder in which to carry DRC. • Have the teacher for last class of the day prompt the child to take DRC home. • Parents should assume the child received a negative report if he or she does not have DRC. • Parents should implement positive consequences for bringing home DRC.

• Are the target behaviors appropriate?
  ○ Are the target behaviors clearly defined for the child?
  ○ Are the target behaviors meaningful/socially valid?
  ○ Can the target behaviors be reasonably attained in the classroom context?
	• Redefine the target behaviors for the child.
	• Change the target behaviors.
	• Modify the target behaviors or class context (i.e., "gets along with peers" should not be a target if the class structure does not provide the opportunity for peer interactions).

• Does the child remember the target behaviors throughout the day?	• Implement a system of visual prompts (e.g., put task sheet on desk).
• Are the criteria for success realistic (i.e., not too high or too low relative to baseline)?	• Make the criteria easier or harder for the child as necessary based on performance.
• Is something interfering with the child reaching the criteria (e.g., child does not complete assignments due to messy, disorganized desk)?	• Work on removing the impediment (e.g., work on improving organizational skills, modify class schedule or structure).

• Does the child understand the system?
  ○ Can the child accurately describe the target behaviors and criteria for positive evaluations?
  ○ Can the child accurately describe the relationship between the criteria and the rewards?
	• Implement a system of visual prompts, if necessary.
	• Review system with child until child can accurately describe system. Increase frequency of reviewing if child continues to have difficulty.
	• Explain the DRC system to the child again. Simplify the DRC system if necessary.

• Is the monitoring system working properly?
  ○ Have the target behaviors been sufficiently clearly defined that the teacher can monitor and evaluate them?
  ○ Is the monitoring and recording process sufficiently efficient that the teacher is doing it accurately and consistently?
	• Clarify the definitions of the target behaviors.
	• Provide visual or auditory prompts for recording. Simplify the monitoring and recording process.

• Can the child accurately monitor his or her progress throughout the day?	• Design and implement a monitoring system that includes a recording form for the child (may include visual or auditory prompts).

(cont.)

FIGURE 6.8. Troubleshooting a daily report card. From Pelham (2002). Reprinted with permission from William E. Pelham, Jr.

Problem	Solution
• Is the child receiving sufficient feedback so that he or she knows where he or she stands regarding the criteria?	• Modify teacher's procedures for providing feedback to the child (e.g., provide visual prompts, increase immediacy, frequency, or contingent nature of feedback).
• Is the home-based reward system working properly? o Are the home-based rewards motivating for the child? o Do parents deliver rewards when the child did not earn them? o Are the parents delivering the rewards reliably? o Can the child delay gratification long enough for home-based rewards to be effective?	• Change the home-based rewards (e.g., increase the number of choices on menu, change the hierarchy of rewards). • Review reward procedures with parents again and ensure that reward is provided only when child has earned it. • Modify the procedures for delivering the home-based rewards (e.g., visual prompts) or the nature of the home-based rewards. • Design and implement procedures for providing school-based rewards.

FIGURE 6.8. *(cont.)*

✓ Successful communication is critical to parent involvement. Teachers should set up a communication system and maintain a regular schedule.

✓ When communicating with parents avoid the "all news is bad news" trap.

✓ Effective meetings are needed to engage parents in home-based and home–school involvement.

✓ Remember that parents differ in the degree to which they can be involved. Remember too that involvement levels may change over time

✓ Give parents tips for helping their child complete homework.

✓ Be sure to give an appropriate amount of homework at the appropriate difficulty level.

✓ Use effective home–school interventions such as the DRC when feasible.

CHAPTER 7

Medication

It is easy to get a thousand prescriptions
but hard to get one single remedy.
—CHINESE PROVERB

Medication is one of the more controversial, highly charged aspects of ADHD. The controversy surrounding medication use may be due in part to the attention given to medication treatment in the popular press (Jackson & Peters, 2008). For example, medication is a regular cover story in national news magazines and has received prominent coverage by network and public television. Medication has been termed "education's fix-it drug" by social critics (Divoky, 1989) and has been attacked by religious groups as being tantamount to mind control (Barkley, 2006). Some have suggested that we are "medicating for social disadvantage" (Isaacs, 2006); others suggest the medication is a middle-class phenomenon (Diller, 1996). There are also widespread claims of overprescription of medication for ADHD (Safer & Malever, 2000).

Moreover, there is an informal but very active "grapevine" that serves to perpetuate information, misinformation, and perhaps "disinformation" about the use of medication treatments with children with ADHD. Claims of miraculous changes in behavior, academic achievement, and social functioning abound, alongside stories of children in a zombie-like haze and parents (or schools) who push medication to avoid dealing with problem behavior. There are also growing concerns about medication misuse and abuse (students selling medication or using it to "get high"). Sorting through these conflicting claims is difficult for parents and educators.

Medication has been, and continues to be, the most widespread treatment for ADHD; it is now considered by some to be the first-line treatment for ADHD (e.g., Pelham, 1993; Spencer, Biederman, Wilens, & Faraone, 2002; Waschbusch, Pelham, Waxmonsky, & Johnson, 2009). Medication use for children with ADHD has increased dramatically in the past three decades. In the 1980s, fewer schoolchildren received medication for ADHD (Mayes, Bagwell, & Erkulwater, 2008). For example, in 1987 an estimated 750,000 school-age children received medication for ADHD (Safer & Krager, 1988). During the 1990s medication use expanded greatly to an estimated 1.8 million (Diller, 1996; Olfson, Marcus, Weissman, & Jensen, 2002). By 2003, an estimated 2.5 million children received medication for ADHD (Centers for Disease Control and Prevention, 2005). This translates to 4.5% of school-age youth. In practical terms, this means that most classrooms will have at least one child who is receiving medication for ADHD (Mayes et al., 2008). Because medication is now widely accepted and used by health professionals to treat ADHD, and because new medications for use with children with ADHD continue to appear, it's unlikely that there will be any marked declines in its use.

Although educators obviously will not prescribe medication, there are medication-related issues that affect them. Because educators will regularly work with children who receive powerful prescription medications, they should be involved in monitoring the effects of medication (Barkley, 2006; Forness, Kavale, & Davanzo, 2002). They will be in the best position to accurately assess the effectiveness of medication during the school day. Further, there is an ethical and professional responsibility that school personnel who work with students who receive medication be aware of potential side effects of medication (Council for Exceptional Children [CEC], 2009). Educators may also be called on to dispense medication during school hours. Thus, policies and procedures for storing and administering medication in the schools are necessary. Because the medications used for ADHD are often controlled substances, educators must have a mechanism to ensure communication between all involved parties, such as fellow educators, parents, and health professionals, in order to assure all medication is properly accounted for (CEC, 2009). Since parents often have questions or concerns about medication, educators also should be able to serve as a source of accurate information for parents.

While it is important for educators to have a sound working knowledge of medications used to treat ADHD, many educators receive little if any professional development in the area of medication either in teacher preparation programs or as in-service staff development. This is a long-standing problem. For example, in 1992 one study found that 96% of teachers reported they had received little or no training on medication, and 50% of teachers did not know that side effects could occur as a result of medication (Kasten, Coury, & Heron, 1992). Recent studies investigating teacher's knowledge of medication found that both general education teachers (Snider, Busch, & Arrowood, 2003) and special educators (Ryan, Reid, & Ellis, 2008) rated their knowledge level as low, and were surprisingly uninformed about even the most commonly prescribed ADHD medications. Educators themselves were aware of this knowledge gap. Nearly all of the special educators who were surveyed (92.8%) expressed a desire to increase their knowledge of medication therapy (Ryan, Reid, & Ellis, 2008).

In this chapter we discuss educators' roles and responsibilities in working with children receiving medication. First, we address what can and cannot be expected from medication and common concerns about using medication. Second, we provide an overview of medications used with students with ADHD. Third, we outline educators' role in the medication process, when students are initially prescribed medication and afterward. Finally, we discuss issues related to parents.

WHAT CAN EDUCATORS EXPECT FROM MEDICATION?

The effects of medication are one of the most thoroughly researched aspects of ADHD. There have been well over 200 randomized clinical trials that assessed the effects of medication and even more small-scale studies. In fact, there are literally too many studies for all of them to be considered separately (Swanson et al., 1993). As a result, the effects of medication are well established. Medication is effective for most students: around 80% of students respond positively. For these students, medication can have a pronounced, positive effect on their ability to function effectively in the school environment. If a student responds positively, educators can expect to see (Barkley, 2006; DuPaul & Stoner, 2003):

• *Significant reductions in ADHD symptoms.* Students should show increased attention, and they should be able to better maintain effort and focus on school-related tasks, especially those that are difficult or tedious. Impulsive behaviors (e.g., calling out) and disruptive physical behaviors associated with hyperactivity (e.g., fidgeting with objects) should also be greatly reduced. Often students demonstrate increased compliance with requests and decreases in aggressive behaviors.

• *Improved academic functioning.* Students often show improved cognitive functioning (e.g., better short-term recall, improved retrieval of verbal information). Academic work (e.g., seatwork) often improves in terms of the amount completed and overall accuracy. However, *there is no evidence of long-term improvement* in learning as measured by standardized tests.

• *Improved social functioning.* Reductions in negative social interactions between the student and teacher are common. This is likely due to increases in compliance (e.g., prompt and positive response to requests). Peer relations may also improve due to reductions in impulsive behaviors, and students may be more accepted by their peers.

The benefits of medication for many students are indisputable; however, educators must understand some important facts about medication. First, medication is not a cure. Medication does not suddenly eliminate all of a student's problems. Students will still have problems with ADHD-related behaviors. Only the degree or frequency of problems will be reduced. *Students will still need accommodations, behavior management, and other interventions.* Educators must avoid the perception that medication alone is sufficient. That is seldom, if ever, the case. Moreover, some research suggests that the effects of medication are enhanced when it is combined with other interventions such as behavior management or self-regulation strategies (DuPaul & Stoner, 2003). Second, educators must understand that the effects of medication *are temporary.* When the effects of medication wear off, the ADHD-related problems will return. Finally, it is critical for educators to understand that medication is not a long-term solution for many students. Research shows that around 50% of students will discontinue medication after 1–2 years (Bussing et al., 2005; Reid, Hakendorf, & Prosser, 2002). Moreover, there is evidence that the effectiveness of medication may decrease markedly after 2–3 years for some students (Gilchrist & Arnold, 2005). In summary, educators need to understand that medication is not a panacea. Medication is an effective, beneficial treatment. For some students medication can literally be the factor that allows them to function in the school environment. However, medication is not the proverbial "magic bullet" that will eliminate all the problems associated with ADHD.

MEDICATIONS USED WITH ADHD

There are literally too many medications used for ADHD to discuss each in any detail. Instead we discuss the major types of medication. Readers who wish a more comprehensive discussion should consult a more comprehensive source such as Dulcan's guide (2007). There are two types of medications most commonly used with children with ADHD: stimulants and antidepressants. A third type, antihypertensives, are less commonly prescribed, but are used frequently enough to warrant discussion. In this section we discuss each in turn. For more detailed information on specific medications, see the U.S. Food and Drug Administration (FDA) website which contains detailed information on medication including manufacturers' guidelines for medication use (*www.fda.gov/Drugs/DrugSafety/ucm085729. htm*).

Stimulants

Figure 7.1 lists some of the stimulants commonly prescribed for ADHD and their potential side effects. Both the trade name (the name used by the manufacturer to market the drug), and the generic name (the name that describes the chemical composition) are included, as both are commonly used by health professionals. Note that the stimulants used for ADHD are a controlled substance. Possession without a valid prescription is a crime. Stimulants are the most commonly prescribed

Trade name/(*generic name*)	Some common side effects	Some less common but more serious side effects

Adderall/Adderall XR *(amphetamines)*
Daytrana *(methylphenidate)*
Desoxyn *(methamphetamine)*
Dexedrine *(dextroamphetamine)*
Dextrostat *(dextroamphetamine)*
Focalin/Focalin XR
  (dexmethylphenidate)
Metadate ER/Metadate CD
  (methylphenidate)
Ritalin/Ritalin SR/Ritalin LA
  (methylphenidate)
Vyvanse *(lisdexamfetamine
  dimesylate)*
	• Stomachache
	• Headache
	• Nausea
	• Decreased appetite
	• Trouble sleeping
	• Nervousness
	• Dizziness
	• Heart palpitations
		• Heart-related problems such as chest pain, shortness of breath, or fainting
		• Acting subdued or withdrawn
		• Feeling helpless, hopeless, or worthless
		• New or worsening depression
		• Thinking or talking about hurting self
		• Extreme worry, agitation, panic attacks
		• Irritability
		• Aggressive or violent behavior
		• Extreme increase in activity or talking
		• Frenzied, abnormal excitement

FIGURE 7.1. Some stimulant medications used with ADHD. This is not a complete list of side effects. Data from *www.fda.gov/downloads/Drugs/DrugSafety/ucm085910.pdf.*

medication for ADHD: around 80% of students who receive medication for ADHD receive stimulants. The use of stimulants with children with ADHD-like symptoms is not new. Stimulants have a long history of use with children with ADHD. The first study using stimulants for children with ADHD occurred in the 1930s (Bradley, 1937), and methylphenidate was approved for use for hyperactivity-related problems by the U.S. Food and Drug Administration in 1961 (Mayes et al., 2008). Stimulants are also the most well researched of medications used for ADHD. They have been studied for over half a century, and there have been hundreds of studies investigating the effectiveness of stimulant medications with children with ADHD. The research clearly shows that stimulants are effective in ameliorating the core symptoms of ADHD. Stimulants can improve attention span and increase persistence on tasks; they also decrease distractibility and impulsivity.

Teachers should be aware of two practical issues related to stimulant use. First, the effects of stimulant medication are not immediate—it typically takes around 30 minutes for meaningful effects to be noticeable, and around 60 minutes for the maximum effects to be apparent. Second, the duration of effects varies greatly across different stimulants. The effects of some stimulants such as Ritalin SR or Adderall last only around 4–5 hours. With these stimulants multiple doses (i.e., a morning and an afternoon dose) may be needed. Other stimulants are time-release formulations and can last 8 hours or longer, which would effectively cover the entire school day. Examples of time-release stimulants are Metadate ER, Focalin XR, Ritalin LA, and Concerta. The time needed for medication effects to occur and the duration of effects have practical ramifications. For example, if students take medication when they arrive at school, the maximum effects likely would not be realized until their second class period. Hopefully students can receive core academics during the time period when their medication is at maximum effectiveness. Teachers should also be aware of "rebound" effects experienced by some students. Rebound occurs when the effects of stimulant medication are wearing off (Barkley, 2006). When rebound occurs, problem behaviors may actual return with increased intensity. Educators should be aware of the duration of medication effects so as to accommodate potential problems with rebound. The last 30–60 minutes when medication is wearing off is a good time for undemanding, nonstressful activities (e.g., story time, word finders, fun reading) if possible.

Antidepressants

Figure 7.2 lists some antidepressants commonly prescribed for ADHD and their potential side effects. Although the effectiveness of antidepressants in reducing ADHD symptoms is well documented (e.g., Spencer et al., 2002), antidepressants generally are not the first choice of medication for ADHD. This is because potential side effects of antidepressants can also be more serious than those for stimulants. They are typically used with individuals who do not respond to stimulants or who cannot tolerate stimulants.

Trade name/(*generic name*)	Some common side effects	Some less common but more serious side effects
Atypical antidepressants Effexor *(venlafaxine)* Serzone *(nefazodone)* Wellbutrin *(bupropion)* **Tricyclic antidepressants** Anafranil *(clomipramine)* Pamelor or Aventyl *(nortriptyline)* Tofranil *(imipramine)* **SNRIs** Strattera *(atomoxetine)* Edronax *(reboxetine)* **SSRIs** Celexa *(citalopram)* Luvox *(fluvoxamine)* Prozac *(fluoxetine)* Zoloft *(sertraline)*	• Dry mouth • Constipation • Blurred vision • Drowsiness • Headaches • Nausea • Sleeplessness or drowsiness • Agitation (feeling jittery) • Sweating • Diarrhea • Tremors • Anxiety • Agitation • Apathy/loss of affect	• Suicidal thoughts • Confusion • Hallucinations • Increased activity (e.g., rapid speech) • Irritability • Motor tics • Seizures • Severe change in behavior • Difficulty urinating • Irregular heartbeat • Severe dizziness/nausea • Abnormal bleeding • Severe allergic reactions

FIGURE 7.2. Some antidepressants used with ADHD. This is not a complete list of side effects. Data from *www.fda.gov/downloads/Drugs/DrugSafety/ucm085910.pdf.*

There are four different types of antidepressants used with ADHD: tricyclic antidepressants (TCAs), atypical antidepressants, selective norepinephrine reuptake inhibitors (SNRIs), and selective serotonin reuptake inhibitors (SSRIs). The TCAs, atypicals, and SNRIs are useful in reducing symptoms of ADHD. The use of tricyclics has decreased in recent years because of the possibility of cardiac side effects. Atypical antidepressants are often used when students have comorbid disorders (e.g., depression); however, they may not be as effective as stimulants at reducing ADHD symptoms (Spencer et al., 2002). SNRIs are newer and are seen as promising in reducing ADHD symptoms (Spencer et al., 2002). Strattera (atomoxetine), an SNRI, is now a commonly prescribed ADHD medication. SSRIs have little effect on ADHD symptoms; they are typically used to treat comorbid depression (Spencer et al., 2002). SSRIs are often prescribed in combination with stimulants. Teachers should be aware that there is a major difference between stimulants and antidepressants in terms of the time required for therapeutic effects to appear. Unlike stimulants in which effects are seen quickly (i.e., within hours), the effects of most antidepressants on ADHD symptoms are not immediate. It typically takes several weeks for the effects of antidepressants to become apparent. SNRIs are the exception. Their effect may be apparent in as little as 1 day.

Antihypertensives

Antihypertensives are not a first-line medication for ADHD, but they are prescribed frequently enough that educators are likely to encounter students who are prescribed antihypertensives. Clonidine (Catapres) and guanfacine (Tenex) are two antihypertensives used commonly with ADHD. Both clonidine and gaunfacine are effective at reducing ADHD symptoms (Spencer et al., 2002). They may be prescribed for students who have motor tics or who have problems with anger or oppositional behavior. They may also help with insomnia. Clonidine may be administered via tablets or a skin patch. Guanfacine is available only in tablet form. These medications *should not be discontinued abruptly* because serious rebound problems may occur. Some common side effects include fatigue, sleepiness, dry mouth, dizziness, and constipation. Some less common but more serious side effects include irregular heartbeat, severe dizziness or fainting, difficulty breathing, and severe allergic reactions (e.g., rash, itching, or swelling of the face, tongue, or throat). If dosage is too high students may have difficulty staying awake or appear to be dazed.

EDUCATORS' ROLE IN MEDICATION TREATMENT

Most school district and states have established policies for administering medication (Center for Health Care in Schools, 2007). Educators should be familiar with their state and district policies. They should also ensure that the policies meet best practice standards. There are several tasks that educators or other school personnel will be required to attend to when a student begins a course of medication for

ADHD. These include properly dispensing medication, establishing channels of communication, helping to evaluate a student's response to medication, and monitoring for side effects.

Dispensing Medication

The number of students who need to receive medication for ADHD during school hours appears to be declining (DuPont, Bucher, Wilford, & Coleman, 2007; Ryan, Reid, Gallagher, & Ellis, 2008). This may be due to the increasing popularity of time-release stimulant medications that can be administered by parents at home. However, there are still a significant number of students who receive medication at school. Dispensing medication during school hours is a legal requirement. Both IDEA and Section 504 require schools to accommodate students by administering medication needed to manage their conditions (e.g., ADHD). This includes determining students' need for administration of medication, administering medication at school if indicated, supervising administration of medication, training personnel to administer medication, and communicating with the health professional who prescribed the medication (Copeland, 1995). Note also that under IDEA students have the right *not* to receive medication. Students cannot be required to obtain a prescription as a condition for attending school, receiving an evaluation, or receiving any type of special education or related services (Ryan & Katsiyannis, 2009). Before medication is dispensed at school, educators should ensure that all staff members involved with dispensing medication are properly trained, all necessary information is on hand, and appropriate procedures for dispensing and accounting for medication are in place.

Staff Training

The American Academy of Pediatrics (AAP; 2009) policy statement on administration of medication in schools recommends that only trained staff members administer medication. Ideally this should be a school nurse. Realistically, this is not possible given that many school nurses now are assigned to two or more schools. As an alternative, unlicensed assistive personnel (UAP) who have been trained in medication procedures may administer medication under the supervision of a licensed registered nurse. The UAP should be a staff member (e.g., a health assistant/aide) who is knowledgeable about district health procedures and who is trained in basic first aid. Training should be regularly updated. Untrained staff (e.g., a school secretary) should never administer medication to students (AAP, 2009). This creates risks for students and also exposes the school to possible medical liability.

Obtaining Information

Before dispensing medication, the following information should be on hand (AAP, 2009; CEC, 2009):

- A written authorization form signed by the health care provider and parents giving permission for administering medication.
- Written authorization to communicate with the health care provider who prescribed the medication.
- The name and contact information of the prescribing health care provider.
- The prescribed dose and administration time(s).
- Which behaviors or symptoms should be affected.
- A list of any potential side effects (this can be obtained from the medication guidelines that come with the medication).
- Information on how to properly store and (if necessary) dispose of medication.

Establishing Channels of Communication

It is critically important for educators to be able to communicate with parents and health care providers. Before administering medication, educators should obtain written permission from the parents to communicate with the health care provider. This can be obtained along with the authorization to administer medication. Procedures for communicating information should also be in place. Educators should be able to easily share information on the effectiveness of medication and on side effects should they occur (evaluating effects of medication and monitoring for side effects are discussed in the following section). If an educator has reason to suspect a medication-related problem, she or he should know exactly who to contact and how to contact them. Research shows that if a breakdown in communication occurs, it is likely to be due to the lack of an established procedure for information exchange (Sprague & Ullman, 1981).

Educators must also be sensitive to students' privacy rights. Educators should be mindful that the fact that a student is receiving medication is confidential. An educator should never publically call attention to the fact that a student is receiving medication (e.g., by asking a student if he or she has taken his or her pill in front of the class). Under the Family Education and Privacy Rights Act (FERPA) of 1974 students' educational records are considered confidential. Similarly under the Health and Insurance Portability and Accountability Act (HIPAA) of 1996 students' medical information is considered privileged; parental permission is required for health professionals to communicate information with schools (Ryan & Katsiyannis, 2009).

Administering Medication

The school is required to have a procedure to ensure that students receive their medication as prescribed (Reid & Katsiyannis, 1995). It's not enough simply to say "Remember to take your pill." Procedures should ensure that medication is safely maintained, that the medication regimen is adhered to, and that all medication can be accounted for. Recommended practice for dispensing medication (AAP, 2009; CEC, 2009) include the following:

- Medication must be provided to the school in its original container. Parents should deliver the medication. This eliminates any possibility of diversion (discussed below). The insert (which contains medication guidelines) should be included.
- Medication should be stored in a locked cabinet. Remember that many of the medications used for ADHD are controlled substances!
- Medication should only be administered by qualified personnel.
- There should be a procedure to ensure that the student receives medication as prescribed (e.g., one dose each morning). This information should be communicated to the classroom teacher. Failure to adhere to the medication regimen can have negative consequences in the classroom (e.g., attention problems, noncompliance).
- Personnel administering the medication should make sure that the student actually swallows it. Some students are reluctant to take medication and may only pretend to actually ingest it.
- There should be procedures in place to deal with errors such as an accidental overdose, a case where a child misses a dose, or a case where a child is given the wrong medication.
- To avoid students receiving incorrect medication, tape a photograph of the student to the container.
- The personnel responsible for administering medication should maintain a log of the time and date of all medication dispensed. This allows for all medication to be accounted for. There should also be procedures to notify parents when it is time to renew supplies of medication.
- A school nurse or school physician should review all medication orders to ensure that the medication is appropriate for the student and dosages are within recommended ranges. This is to ensure that a student does not receive inappropriate medication or excessive dosage due to an error (e.g., an incorrectly filled prescription). The nurse should document the concern and contact the provider to resolve the problem.

In the case of some medications (e.g., asthma inhalers) it is considered appropriate for responsible students to carry and self-administer their medication. In our opinion, a student with ADHD should never be allowed to carry or self-administer medication for ADHD in the school or to and from school. Stimulant medications, used with the great majority of students, are controlled substances. A minor should never have unsupervised possession of or access to a controlled substance. Moreover, students with ADHD are frequently the target of classmates who wish to obtain medication for recreational purposes (Wilens et al., 2008). Diversion of medication for misuse (e.g., getting high) is a serious concern; educators should not exacerbate the problem with policies that make diversion easier.

GETTING STARTED ON MEDICATION

Twenty-five years ago it was not unusual for the first indication that a student was starting medication was when he or she showed up at the school with a bottle of pills. Luckily this phenomenon is now rare as guidelines for medication have been developed by professional organizations such as the American Academy of Child and Adolescent Psychiatry (AACAP; 2007, 2009) and health professionals are much more sensitive to the need for input from educators when medication is being considered. Currently it is considered best practice for the health professionals to contact the school prior to the start of any medication. As we noted earlier, children may take medication at home and/or at school. Regardless of where the child receives the medication, educators have a responsibility to monitor the effectiveness of medication and monitor for possible side effects.

Evaluating Response to Medication

For most of us, our experience with taking medication runs something like this: (1) a doctor gives us a prescription, (2) we take the medicine, and (3) we get better. If only it were so simple for ADHD! There are so many variables such as metabolism and possible comorbid conditions that a health professional can't just write a prescription and solve the problem. What's right for one student might not even affect another. To further complicate the issue, too high a dose of medication can actually have a detrimental affect on cognitive performance (e.g., overfocusing) and too low a dose may have little or no effect on any behavior. In addition, the effects of medication may differ across behaviors. For example, the dosage that results in optimal performance in academics may be different from the dosage that results in the maximum time on-task (e.g., Rapport, Denney, DuPaul, & Gardner, 1994). Most importantly, the health professional isn't able to directly assess the effects of medication.

How educators go about evaluating a student's response to medication depends to some extent on the practices of the health care provider who prescribes the medication. Interestingly, health care providers tend to weight evidence from teachers highly when evaluating the need for medication and a child's response to medication (AACAP, 2007). Health care providers' practices vary widely from almost no communication or follow-up to a high degree of involvement. Best practice requires the health care provider to collect (1) baseline information on students' behavior when they are not medicated, (2) information on behavior changes after medication begins, and (3) periodic assessment of maintenance (AACAP, 2007, 2009). However, educators should collect this information *regardless* of whether the health professional requests it. Remember that the child is under the care of educators, and as such the educators are responsible for the student's well-being and safety. The fact that some providers do not follow best practice does not mean that the school should follow suit.

Step 1

The first step in the process is to collect baseline data (i.e., measures of the student's behavior when he or she is not receiving medication). This is crucial. Baseline data provides a point of comparison to determine whether or not and to what degree medication affects problem behavior. Without this data it would be impossible to objectively determine whether problem behavior improved. Health care providers often ask educators and parents to fill out ADHD behavior rating scales (described in Chapter 3). These scales are commonly used to evaluate the effects of medication and are sensitive to the effects of medication (i.e., changes in behavior will be reflected by changes in ratings). Educators may have already collected some of this information during the ADHD assessment process. In addition, we would recommend that educators collect information on the student's academic performance. This is critical information that is not addressed by the behavior rating scales used to assess ADHD.

Educators should collect work samples, noting how much seatwork (e.g., arithmetic problems on a worksheet) a student completes, and monitor homework completion. This type of data has the advantage of high validity and is easy to collect. There are instruments specifically designed to assess the academic performance of students with ADHD such as the Academic Performance Rating Scale (APRS; DuPaul, Rapport, & Perriello, 1991; see Figure 7.3). These instruments can help educators identify problem areas. Behavioral observations can be extremely useful and we urge educators to do them (see Maag, 2004, for a guide to behavioral observations). They provide the most detailed information on the child's most important behavior problems because the behaviors observed are the specific ones that school personnel have selected as problematic. They are also the most ecologically valid indicators you can collect. It may be difficult to gauge the practical significance of a change on a behavior rating scale, and in truth it may have little noticeable effect; however, a 60% reduction in "being out of seat" is an obvious and quite meaningful improvement.

Step 2

The second step begins when the health professional starts the student on medication. When medication is started, recommended practice is for the health professional to start the student on a low dosage of medication. After the student has been on the initial low dose for a period of time (at least 1 week) educators (and the parents) should again collect information on the student's behavior by readministering the behavior rating scales. To determine whether medication is improving a student's behavior, the student must be observed over a period of time—usually at least a week—in both the home and the school environments (AACAP, 2007).

The health professional and educators can then compare results from baseline and the initial medication level to determine what effects medication had on the

For each of the below items, please estimate the student's performance over the past week. For each item, please circle *one* choice only.

	0–49%	50–69%	70–79%	80–89%	90–100%
1. Estimate the percentage of written math work *completed* (regardless of accuracy) relative to classmates.	1	2	3	4	5

	0–49%	50–69%	70–79%	80–89%	90–100%
2. Estimate the percentage of written language arts work *completed* (regardless of accuracy) relative to classmates.	1	2	3	4	5

	0–49%	50–69%	70–79%	80–89%	90–100%
3. Estimate the *accuracy* of completed written math work (i.e., percent correct of work done).	1	2	3	4	5

	0–49%	50–69%	70–79%	80–89%	90–100%
4. Estimate the *accuracy* of completed written language arts work (i.e., percent of correct work done).	1	2	3	4	5

	Consistently poor	More poor than successful	Variable	More successful than poor	Consistently successful
5. How consistent has the quality of this child's academic work been over the past week?	1	2	3	4	5

	Never	Rarely	Sometimes	Often	Very often
6. How frequently does the student accurately follow teacher instructions and/or class discussion during *large-group* (e.g., whole-class) instruction?	1	2	3	4	5

	Never	Rarely	Sometimes	Often	Very often
7. How frequently does the student accurately follow teacher instructions and/or class discussion during *small-group* (e.g., reading group) instruction?	1	2	3	4	5

	Very slow	Slow	Average	Quickly	Very quickly
8. How quickly does this child learn new material (i.e., pick up novel concepts)?	1	2	3	4	5

	Poor	Fair	Average	Above average	Excellent
9. What is the quality or neatness of this child's handwriting?	1	2	3	4	5

(cont.)

FIGURE 7.3. Academic Performance Rating Scale. From DuPaul, Rapport, and Perriello (1991). Copyright 1991 by the National Association of School Psychologists, Bethesda, MD. Reprinted with permission of the publisher *www.nasponline.org*.

	Poor	Fair	Average	Above average	Excellent
10. What is the quality of this child's reading skills?	1	2	3	4	5

	Poor	Fair	Average	Above average	Excellent
11. What is the quality of this child's speaking skills?	1	2	3	4	5

	Never	Rarely	Sometimes	Often	Very often
12. How often does the child complete written work in a careless, hasty fashion?	1	2	3	4	5

	Never	Rarely	Sometimes	Often	Very often
13. How frequently does the child take more time to complete work than his/her classmates?	1	2	3	4	5

	Never	Rarely	Sometimes	Often	Very often
14. How often is the child able to pay attention without you prompting him/her?	1	2	3	4	5

	Never	Rarely	Sometimes	Often	Very often
15. How frequently does this child require your assistance to accurately complete his/her academic work?	1	2	3	4	5

	Never	Rarely	Sometimes	Often	Very often
16. How often does the child begin written work prior to understanding the directions?	1	2	3	4	5

	Never	Rarely	Sometimes	Often	Very often
17. How frequently does this child have difficulty recalling material from a previous day's lesson?	1	2	3	4	5

	Never	Rarely	Sometimes	Often	Very often
18. How often does the child appear to be staring excessively or "spaced out"?	1	2	3	4	5

	Never	Rarely	Sometimes	Often	Very often
19. How often does the child appear withdrawn or tend to lack an emotional response in a social situation?	1	2	3	4	5

FIGURE 7.3. (*cont.*)

student's behavior. Because students are typically started on a low dosage, initial responses may be minimal. Usually the health professional will then gradually increase the dosage (AACAP, 2009). After each dosage increase, data are collected and evaluated. The dosage is increased until clear effects on behavior are noted (i.e., ADHD-related problems decrease) and further increases in dosage do not result in improvements, or it is clear that the student either is not responding or cannot tolerate the medication (e.g., high levels of side effects occur and do not subside). This is a simple, straightforward, and effective procedure. It is, however, critical for educators to monitor medication effects. Around 25% of children will not respond to medication (Barkley, 2006) and others may respond only minimally. Therefore it's important to document whether and how much medication affects a child. Otherwise students may receive medication when they shouldn't or they may not receive full benefits of medication.

Step 3

The final step is ongoing monitoring. Monitoring involves periodic collection of information on the student's behavior using the same procedures used to assess medication effects. This information should be collected monthly (AACAP, 2007). Ongoing monitoring is necessary because the effects of medication may change over time due to changes in the student (e.g., changes in metabolism) or environment (e.g., a more stressful environment). It is also possible that a student might develop new symptoms (e.g., aggression, depression). This in turn might require dosage adjustments, adding another medication, or a change to a different medication.

Side Effects

In addition to monitoring the effectiveness of medication, educators also should monitor for the appearance of side effects. All educators who work with students who receive medication should be informed that the student is receiving medication and be provided information on possible side effects. This includes both the common and relatively minor side effects and the uncommon but much more serious side effects. Figures 7.1 and 7.2 show some of the possible side effects for some stimulants and antidepressants commonly used with students with ADHD.

Educators should know that some side effects are potentially life-threatening. The FDA has issued a black-box warning for both stimulant and antidepressant medications used with students with ADHD. A black-box warning is a statement that must be included with the medication guidelines that accompany the medication. It is the strongest action that the FDA takes short of disapproving the use of a medication. In the case of stimulants, heart-related problems have been reported. The FDA warning states that the health professional should be called if "signs of heart problems such as chest pain, shortness of breath, or fainting" occur while taking stimulant medication. In addition, psychiatric side effects have been reported. The FDA warning notes that "new psychotic symptoms (such as hearing voices, believing things that are not true, are suspicious) or new manic symptoms" may occur. In the case of antidepressants, the FDA warns that "antidepressant medicines may increase suicidal thoughts or actions in some children, teenagers, and young adults within the first few months of treatment." The most dangerous times are when medication is begun or when the dosage is changed. Students who have (or have a family history of) bipolar disorder or suicidal thoughts or actions are at increased risk. If a student is receiving medication, *educators should be sensitive to any unusual changes in behavior*, especially any sudden changes, in mood, behaviors, thoughts, or feelings. If these occur educators should notify parents and appropriate health professionals immediately.

Reading the list of side effects in Figures 7.1 and 7.2 along with the black-box warnings might make educators nervous about working with students who receive medication or wonder if the student is in danger of serious harm. Let's try and put the danger of side effects in perspective. Here is a list of side effects for another medication. Does it sound alarming?

- Severe allergic reactions (rash; hives; itching; difficulty breathing; tightness in the chest; swelling of the mouth, face, lips, or tongue)
- Black or bloody stools
- Confusion
- Diarrhea
- Dizziness
- Drowsiness
- Hearing loss
- Ringing in the ears
- Severe or persistent stomach pain
- Unusual bruising
- Vomiting

Most readers have probably taken this medication many times without any problem and without worrying about serious side effects—it's aspirin. Note that we *are not* equating aspirin to medications used with ADHD. The point of this example is that it's important for educators to maintain an appropriate perspective on side effects. There are side effects, some potentially life-threatening, for the vast majority of medications, even over-the-counter medications such as aspirin. It would make little sense to deny oneself the benefits of a medication because of the unlikely event of side effects. A much more sensible approach is to weigh the risks versus the benefits of medication. We make risk-versus-benefits decisions every day. For example, most of us drive to work every day despite the risk associated with driving a car (e.g., over 30,000 highway deaths each year). It's true that risks associated with medication include potentially serious side effects; however, these are extremely uncommon. In contrast, the benefits are significant improvements in students' ability to function in the school environment. Medication is used safely every day with literally millions of students with ADHD. The key is for educators to be aware of possible side effects and to know what to do if side effects occur.

PARENTS AND MEDICATION

Most parents agonize over the decision to medicate their child. Parents report conflicting emotions over whether to medicate, fears about the effect of medication, pressure from family and friends to refrain, guilt that medication means they are bad parents, and, unfortunately, pressure from educators to start (or to avoid) medication (Bussing & Gary, 2001; Jackson & Peters, 2008; Singh, 2004). In our opinion, educators *should never suggest medication* or pressure parents to medicate (or not medicate) their child. Few if any educators are qualified to make that determination, and the ultimate decision is one that should only be made by the parent in conjunction with a health professional.

Parents commonly report seeking advice and information on medication from educators (Bussing & Gary, 2001; Jackson & Peters, 2008). We believe that when a parent broaches the subject of medication, educators should refrain from advocating for or against medication. Instead they should *ask the parents about their concerns* and thoughts about medication, provide accurate information about their concerns, and perhaps reassure parents that their concerns are normal and shared by many parents. There are some concerns that occur commonly.

- *"Medication changes children's personality."* Parents sometimes fear that medication will drastically alter their child's personality. Some parents have expressed the fear that a child will become "crazy," "walk around like a zombie," or become a "criminal" or a "lunatic, killing people 10 years from now" (Bussing & Gary, 2001). It is true that children with ADHD and comorbid conduct disorders are at risk for later delinquency, but this is largely due to the comorbid conduct disorders (Bernfort, Norfeldt, & Persson, 2008). We are not aware of any evidence that links medication with delinquency or criminal behavior. In contrast, there is substantial evidence demonstrating that medication actually reduces antisocial behaviors (e.g., aggression, swearing) associated with delinquency (e.g., Connor, Glatt, Lopez, Jackson, & Melloni, 2002; Klein et al., 1997). It is possible for a child whose dosage is much too high to exhibit extremely overfocused ("zombie") behavior. This problem should be quickly detected and can be easily corrected by adjusting dosage or switching to a different medication. The bottom line is that medication should have little if any discernable effect on a child's personality.

- *"ADHD medication is a 'gateway' drug."* Concerns have been raised regarding the relationship between medication for ADHD and later substance use disorders

(Wilson, 2007). In fact, there is good evidence that suggests receiving medication for childhood ADHD actually lowers the likelihood of later substance use (Lynskey & Hall, 2001). The fear is, however, that the experience with medication will lead to later substance use (e.g., alcohol, tobacco, marijuana). It is true that ADHD is a risk factor for later substance use disorders; for example, individuals with ADHD have higher rates of smoking and cocaine use than individuals without ADHD (Wilson, 2007). Once again the presence of comorbid conduct disorders is a critical factor in later substance use. These children are at greatest risk. However, the idea that medication leads to later substance use disorders is incorrect.

- *"Giving my child medication makes me a bad parent."* When parents first consider medication as a treatment, they often report feelings of guilt (Jackson & Peters, 2008; Singh, 2007). They feel that medicating their child means that they are ineffective or incompetent parents who cannot manage their child's behavior. Parents also report that friends or family members often characterize the decision to medicate their child as selfish. The implication is that parents who medicate their children are only thinking of their own needs; medication is seen as an easy way out or a quick fix made by parents in a casual fashion solely to make their own lives easier (Jackson & Peters, 2008; Singh, 2007; Taylor, O'Donoghue, & Houghton, 2006). This common misperception that medication in some way equates to selfish or lazy parents is fueled by media mischaracterization of ADHD medication and the overall lack of knowledge of ADHD on the part of the public (Kennedy, 2008; McLeod, Fettes, Jensen, Pescosolido, & Martin, 2007). In fact, the decision to medicate is not made quickly or casually; most parents commonly report considerable soul searching (Jackson & Peters, 2008). It is true that medication can make parents' life easier, but medication can also dramatically improve the quality of life for a child. This is the reason most parents decide to try medication. Trying to improve the quality of life for one's child hardly makes one a "bad parent." Moreover, medication is seldom sufficient in isolation—many challenges remain.

- *"My child will get 'hooked' on ADHD medication."* Some parents are concerned that their child will develop a dependence on medication used for ADHD (Leslie, Plemmons, Monn, & Palinkas, 2007). It is true that stimulant medications are chemically similar to amphetamines that do have potential for dependency and abuse. Luckily the problems with dependency and abuse do not appear to be present in children who receive stimulants for ADHD. Research has shown that children and teenagers with ADHD who take stimulants do not report getting high, feelings of euphoria, or other subjective feelings associated with substance abuse or dependency (Kollins, 2007, 2008). Note that dependency or abuse are not an issue for antidepressants and antihypertensives—only for stimulants.

- *"Medication will stunt my child's growth."* The effect of stimulant treatment on children's growth has long been a concern (AACAP, 2007). Initially, researchers believed that stimulants had no effects on children's growth; however, more recent research has shown that stimulants do have an effect on some children's growth (e.g., MTA Cooperative Group, 2004; Zachor, Roberts, Hodgens, Isaacs, & Merrick, 2006). In these studies children's height and weight gains were less than would have been projected. However, we would stress that *the effects on growth were not extreme.* For example, the children receiving medication grew around and inch and a half less than would be expected and gained about 5 pounds less than expected over a period of 3 years (AACAP, 2007). Additionally, children were *still in the average range* for height and weight (Zachor et al., 2006). The growth suppression appears to be most pronounced during the first year (AACAP, 2007). Many of the children studied were on high dosages of medication; it's possible that high dosages could have affected their growth rate. The AACAP now recommends that children's height and weight be monitored on an ongoing basis to assess whether medication is having an effect on growth.

CULTURAL FACTORS IN MEDICATION TREATMENT

Medication treatment is effective for all cultural groups; there is no evidence to suggest that any group does not respond or responds differently to medications commonly used for ADHD (Miller, Nigg, & Miller, 2009). However, educators should be aware that there are well-documented differences in the rate of medication use across different cultural groups (Rowland et al., 2002; Safer & Malever, 2000; Stevens, Harman, & Kelleher, 2005). Compared to Caucasian students, African American and Hispanic students are significantly less likely to receive medication for ADHD. There are several possible reasons why these students are less likely to receive medication. Parents may be reluctant to seek medication treatment (Leslie et al., 2007; Miller et al., 2009), and physicians may be less likely to make an ADHD diagnosis and prescribe medication (Stevens et al., 2005). There are also practical problems. Many parents may lack health insurance. In addition, they may not have a regular health care provider, or may lack transportation to travel to a health care provider (Leslie et al., 2007).

Although more research is needed, educators should be aware of the possibility that cultural factors may affect parents' decision to use medication. Some research suggests that Hispanic and African American parents may resist an ADHD diagnosis and medication treatment; additionally, African American parents in particular may tend to have a more negative perception of medication than Caucasian parents and worry more about side effects (dosReis et al., 2003; Leslie et al., 2007). Knowledge about ADHD may also play a role in lower rates of medication. African American and Hispanic parents are less aware of ADHD, have lower levels of knowledge about ADHD, and are more likely to believe that ADHD is not a "real" disorder (McLeod et al., 2007). They are more likely to view ADHD as a temporary problem or to see the behavior as normal, and are less likely to consider ADHD as a medical or biological problem. This could make them less likely to consider medication (Bussing, Gary, Mills, & Garvan, 2003; Bussing, Schoenberg, Rogers,

Zima, & Angus, 1998). African American and Hispanic parents also are less likely to receive information on ADHD from teachers (Bussing et al., 2007; McLeod et al., 2007). Thus parents may not have a source of accurate information that could provide an accurate perspective on ADHD and potentially change their views on medication.

If any child has an ADHD diagnosis or parents ask about ADHD, educators should be prepared to supply parents with information on ADHD or refer them to community resources. This may be even more important in the case of African American or Hispanic parents. Medication can be an important factor in ADHD treatment. The evidence suggests that many African American and Hispanic students who could benefit from medication are not receiving it, and that the decision to forgo medication may be based on misconceptions about ADHD. The decision whether or not to medicate should be the parents' and their decision should be respected, but educators should make every effort to ensure that parents make *an informed decision*. Otherwise students may not have access to treatment that could significantly improve the quality of their school experience.

SUMMING UP

In this chapter we presented information on medication treatment for students with ADHD. Educators will work with students who are receiving medication for ADHD on a regular basis so it's important to have a basic working knowledge of medications, their effects, and their side effects. Here are some major points to remember:

- ✓ Medication is a beneficial treatment for many students with ADHD, but it's not a "magic bullet."
- ✓ Medication should not be the only treatment. It should be used along with classroom accommodations, behavior management, and other supports (e.g., counseling) at school and at home.
- ✓ Medications differ in duration of effects. Educators should be aware of duration and try to schedule core academics during times of peak effectiveness.
- ✓ Some students will receive medication during school hours. Educators should establish policies and procedures for administering medication.
- ✓ Medication should only be administered by trained personnel.
- ✓ Educators should monitor the effectiveness of medication on an ongoing basis.
- ✓ Educators should be aware of common and less common side effects of medication prescribed for their students. They should monitor for side effects. There should be an established procedure for reporting any suspected side effects.

- ✓ Parents often agonize over whether or not to try medication with their child. Educators should refrain from encouraging or discouraging medication. Instead educators should provide accurate information on medication, and urge the parent to seek the advice of a qualified health professional.
- ✓ Educators should be aware of some of the myths about medication and be prepared to provide accurate information.
- ✓ Educators should be sensitive to cultural factors that might affect parents' decision to refrain from seeking medication.

CHAPTER 8

Functional Behavioral Assessment

Environment affects behavior.
—B .F. SKINNER

Over the last several decades our society has increasingly embraced a medical perspective on psychological disorders. This is understandable given the great strides made in medical science, which have led to increased understanding of the basic mechanisms underlying both physical and psychological disorders. From a medical perspective, disorders (either physical or psychological) are caused by an underlying biologically based factor. Thus a head cold is the result of a virus, and depression is the result of a neurotransmitter imbalance in the brain. ADHD is commonly viewed from a medical perspective. This is understandable.

There is now compelling evidence from numerous fields (e.g., biochemistry, genetics, neuropsychiatry) that ADHD is a disorder with a biological basis. That is, individuals with ADHD have a predisposition to exhibit behaviors that we would describe in terms such as inattentive, impulsive, or hyperactive, and the inattentive, impulsive, or hyperactive behaviors are the result of factors that lie within the individual. Unfortunately, viewing ADHD from a strictly medical perspective can have unintended consequences. For example, if we see Linda fidgeting with her pencil, Stevie jumping out of his seat, or Paul talking out in class, we may see the behavior as "ADHD coming out." While this may be literally true, it is a dead-end street for educators in terms of addressing problem behaviors because educators can literally do nothing to address the underlying biological bases of ADHD.

Seeing problem behavior as "ADHD coming out" also runs the risk of ignoring a very important and often overlooked factor in problem behavior: the environment. It is critically important to assess behavior in the context of the environment in which the behavior occurs. Even small changes in environment can sometimes have dramatic effects on behavior. For example, even small changes in the difficulty level of seatwork can dramatically affect the frequency of disruptive behaviors (DePaepe, Shores, Jack, & Denny, 1996). Note that "environment" refers to much more than just the physical layout of the classroom space. It also includes curriculum, instructional practices, and teacher—student interactions. Awareness of the effects of environment on behavior is crucial because educators *can change the environment.*

To work effectively with students with ADHD, educators should adopt a functional perspective on ADHD. That is, educators must be aware of the interaction between ADHD-related behavior and the environment, and realize that many classroom problems are the result of the classroom environment. Rather than seeing problem behavior as "ADHD coming out," educators should examine the environment for factors that can serve to trigger or maintain problem behavior. To accomplish this, educators must be able to systematically examine problem behaviors in terms of the context in which they occur. One way to do this is through functional behavioral assessment (FBA). FBA is a structured assessment process designed to help educators determine why problem behaviors occur and to identify effective interventions that will prevent or reduce the occurrence of problem behaviors. Research has demonstrated that FBA can help educators deal effectively with the academic and behavioral problems associated with ADHD and even add to the effectiveness of medication. In this chapter first we provide an overview of FBA and discuss the legal requirements of FBA. Next we discuss the FBA process and what is entailed at each step in the process. Finally, we provide examples of how educators can adopt a functional perspective on problem behaviors that can help them proactively address these behaviors

OVERVIEW OF FBA

FBAs were mandated by the 1997 amendments to the Individuals with Disabilities Education Act (IDEA). The intent of the law was to help provide a balanced approach to students with behavior problems that both reflects the need for a safe and orderly school environment and protects the rights of students to receive a free and appropriate public education (Drasgow & Yell, 2001). The concern was that problem behaviors should be addressed in a preventive or proactive manner through the provision of behavior interventions and supports, rather than in a manner that relied primarily on punishment. FBAs are intended to help educators understand the causes and purposes of problem behaviors. An FBA should be conducted if a student exhibits disruptive behavior that negatively affects classroom instruction, noncompliance, verbal or physical abuse, property destruction, or aggression toward students or school staff (Drasgow, Yell, Bradley, & Shriner, 1999). An FBA must be conducted if a student has been suspended or placed in an alternative setting for 10 or more consecutive days, if a student has been placed in an interim alternative setting for 45 days due to misconduct involving weapons or drugs, or if it has been determined that the student is a danger to self or others.

There has been some confusion over exactly what an FBA entails. In part this is due to the fact that exactly what constitutes FBA is not explicitly stated in IDEA. Drasgow and Yell (2001, p. 242) suggested that the following five components of an FBA are required to meet the intent of the law:

1. A clear description of the problem behavior.
2. Identification of the events, times, and situations that predict when the behavior will and will not occur.
3. Identification of the consequences that maintain the problem behavior.
4. Development of one or more summary statements or hypotheses that describe the behavior and its function.
5. Collection of direct observation data.

Another cause of confusion is that FBA has been described in different terms in the literature, including functional analysis, experimental analysis, functional assessment, descriptive analysis, and structural analysis (Lewis & Sugai, 1996). However, despite the different nomenclature, the underlying assumptions and procedures are consistent. For simplicity, we use the term FBA throughout.

THE FBA PROCESS

FBA is based on three assumptions (Dunlap, Kern-Dunlap, Clarke, & Robbins, 1991). First, behavior is not random. Rather behavior is purposeful and serves a function for the student. The student receives some benefit or reinforcement from performing a behavior (e.g., a child may perform a behavior to escape from an unpleasant situation, to gain attention, or to reduce anxiety). Second, behavior is caused by the interactions of environmental factors (i.e., setting events, antecedents, and consequents) that occur in the classroom or other school environments and factors inherent to the student (e.g., academic skill level). Third, the identification of these factors can help educators develop effective interventions to alleviate behavior problems. The goal of FBA is to identify a functional relation between problem behaviors and environmental events or consequents. In short, FBA attempts to find what environmental factors serve to trigger or maintain problem behaviors.

In essence, the FBA process consists of a series of hypothesis-development and hypothesis-testing sequences (Elliott, Gresham, & Heffer, 1987). Hypotheses are created based on available information, and assessments are conducted specifically to determine possible relations between a child's behavior and environmental factors.

For example, a teacher may observe that a student frequently interrupts peers' conversations or activities (one of the diagnostic criteria for ADHD). The teacher could simply conclude that the inappropriate behavior was the result of ADHD and that nothing could be done. In contrast, from a FBA perspective the teacher might hypothesize that a student interrupts others because it results in attention from peers. This reinforcement serves to maintain the behavior. From this general information, more specific hypothesis can be generated and tested. For example, the teacher might manipulate the composition of the peer group to determine if the interruptions occur with some peers but not others. Alternatively the teacher might reinforce peers for ignoring the student's inappropriate behavior and provide positive reinforcement when the student engaged in appropriate behavior. If the manipulations reduce or eliminate the inappropriate behavior, then the teacher can conclude that there is a functional relation between interrupting others and peer attention.

Another example might be a case in which a student becomes disruptive and noncompliant during writing instruction. The teacher might hypothesize that the problem behavior was due to difficulty with the writing process. For example, the student might not know how to write a story, or might have problems with handwriting such that producing text resulted in frustration. In this case the teacher might check the student's writing to see if there were problems with the work (e.g., missing important elements, very short text, or laborious handwriting). The teacher can then develop and implement effective interventions based on this knowledge. The teacher might then teach the student a story-writing strategy and work to make handwriting easier. If the students' behavior improved, then there was a functional relation between the problem behavior and the difficulties with the writing process. We would stress that for students with ADHD *academic difficulties frequently serve to trigger behavior problems* and teachers should be sensitive to this fact. A task that is too difficult or demanding can result in problem behaviors that serve to allow a student to escape the task. In cases such as this, teachers must provide instructional accommodations (e.g., shorter assignments, simpler assignments, extra instruction on how to accomplish the task, teaching a strategy to accomplish the task). Note that these examples were very straightforward; it's possible for more than one function to support behavior. For example, if the student in the previous example received attention from classmates when he was disruptive this might also have served to maintain the behavior.

The classroom teacher should be an integral part of the FBA process; however, few teachers have the training or expertise to independently conduct a FBA. In most cases teachers will work with a behavior specialist or school psychologist. In the next section, we describe the FBA process. There are several different approaches to conducting FBA. We describe a framework for FBA developed by Dunlap and Kern (1993) that has been successfully used in the classroom in numerous studies. Their FBA process consists of three stages: (1) hypothesis development, (2) hypothesis testing, and (3) intervention development.

Hypothesis Development

To begin the process of developing hypotheses about the function of a behavior, it is necessary to (1) precisely define the behavior of concern, (2) collect information on the conditions under which the behavior occurs, and (3) analyze the information for patterns that might be indicative of a functional relation.

Defining a Behavior

Precisely defining the behavior of concern (i.e., developing an operational definition) is a critical step in the FBA process. There are three reasons why a behavior must be precisely defined (Alberto & Troutman, 2006).

1. It allows all parties involved to share the same definition and accurately collect data on the same behavior. If definitions differ, then there cannot be an accurate and consistent description of the occurrence or nonoccurrence of the behavior.
2. It allows for confirmation by a third party. That is, a person who is not acquainted with the student should be able to determine whether or not the behavior is occurring. This allows independent confirmation of changes in behavior.
3. It allows for continuity across time and settings. The student will likely need interventions to continue across school years and possibly across different settings where the behavior occurs.

To precisely define a behavior, the operational definition should focus on the observable and measurable aspects of the behavior and eliminate as much ambiguity as possible. For example, "on-task" is a behavior that concerns every educator. However, if this was the extent of the definition it is likely that there would be considerable variability across observers because being "on-task" is ambiguous and difficult to accurately measure. A better definition might be: "On-task behavior occurs when the student is at his or her desk, oriented toward the teacher or task, working on the assigned activity, using appropriate materials, or asking for assistance by raising a hand." The elements of this definition are all observable and measureable.

Educators should also carefully consider the type of behavior that would be the focus of FBA. Educators sometimes become fixated on a behavior that bothers them, but has no adverse effect on students' learning or functioning in the classroom. The "So What" test (Kaplan, 1995) helps to avoid focusing on these types of behaviors. The "So What" test suggests that educators ask themselves, "So what if the behavior continues?" If a behavior will not negatively impact a students' academic, social, or behavioral functioning, then it's not one that should be considered for an intervention or a FBA. For example, so what if a student fidgets with objects if the student manages to complete assigned work and classmates are not distracted by this behavior. This behavior would not be worth the time and effort needed for an FBA. On the other hand, if the fidgeting prevented the student from completing work and disrupted peers, then it would be a candidate for an FBA. Remember that students with ADHD may have many behaviors that could be a potential target for intervention, but educators have limited time and resources. Only the behaviors that most meaningfully affect functioning in school should be targeted for FBA.

Information Collection

The goal of FBA is to understand the conditions under which a student's behavior occurs. There are a variety of environmental conditions that interact with a child's behavior: teacher tolerance levels, classroom arrangement, curriculum and instructional variables, peers' reactions to a child, and task difficulty, to name but a few. Given this list of factors, collecting information can appear to be a daunting task. However, there are a number of techniques for collecting information on behavior: interviews, direct observation, rating scales, and archival records (Dunlap et al., 1991; Dunlap & Kern, 1993). Of these techniques, interview and direct observation are probably the most reliable sources of information and should be included in any FBA. However, before implementing these approaches, it may advantageous to examine archival records and complete behavior rating scales. Archival records such as psychological reports, standardized testing, office referrals, student assistance team reports, and IEPs may provide useful background information on the history of a problem and on interventions that have been used in the past. Rating scales are less useful because they provide only general information on broad problem areas.

The next step is to conduct interviews. Dunlap and Kern (1993) recommended that at least two school personnel involved with the student be interviewed. The purpose of interviewing multiple people is to determine if certain behaviors occur in some, but not other, contexts and conditions. They recommended that an interview should focus on two core questions: (1) Under what conditions or circumstances is the behavior most likely to occur? and (2) Under what conditions or circumstances does the behavior rarely or never occur? Figures 8.1 and 8.2 provide sample interview forms for teachers and students. The information garnered through interviewing is relatively global and often appears in nonbehavioral terms. For example, one teacher may say a child is off-task during most of the independent seatwork activity while another teacher may say that the child is inattentive during lectures. "Off-task" and "inattentive" are not specific behaviors. Nevertheless, this information can help to formulate hypotheses.

Next, direct observations would be conducted. Direct observation allows for a fine-grained assessment of environmental factors that may be acting to either maintain inappropriate behavior or prevent the performance of appropriate behavior. The process of defining target behaviors, observing and recording their occurrence or nonoccurrence in the natural environment, and analyzing the data is the most

How long have you known/taught _____?

1. What do you see as the major problems? Prioritize problems from most to least severe.

2. In what situations do these behaviors occur?

3. In what situations is behavior most appropriate?

4. What are the student's greatest strengths?

5. What are the student's greatest weaknesses?

6. Why do you think the students acts in the way he/she does?

7. What do you think needs to be done to help the student? How?

8. What does the student like the most?

9. What does the student like the least?

10. What events or actions seem to trigger inappropriate behavior during:

teaching   lunch

recess   unstructured time

11. What can be done to increase the likelihood of appropriate behavior during:

teaching   lunch

recess   unstructured time

FIGURE 8.1. FBA interview form. From Reid and Maag (1998). Copyright 1998 by Taylor & Francis. Reprinted by permission. *www.informaworld.com.*

Student: _____ Interviewer: _____ Date: _____

Section 1

1. In general, is your work too hard for you?	Always	Sometimes	Never
2. In general, is your work too easy for you?	Always	Sometimes	Never
3. When you ask for help appropriately, do you get it?	Always	Sometimes	Never
4. Do you think work periods for each subject are too long?	Always	Sometimes	Never
5. Do you think work periods for each subject are too short?	Always	Sometimes	Never
6. When you do seatwork, do you do better when someone works with you?	Always	Sometimes	Never
7. Do you think people notice when you do a good job?	Always	Sometimes	Never
8. Do you think you get the points or rewards you deserve when you do good work?	Always	Sometimes	Never
9. Do you think you would do better in school if you received more rewards?	Always	Sometimes	Never
10. In general, do you find your work interesting?	Always	Sometimes	Never
11. Are there things in the classroom that distract you?	Always	Sometimes	Never
12. Is your work challenging enough for you?	Always	Sometimes	Never

Section 2

1. When do you think you have the fewest problems with [target behavior] in school? Why do you not have problems during this/these time(s)?

2. When do you think you have the most problems with [target behavior] in school? Why do you not have problems during this/these time(s)?

3. What changes could be made so you would have fewer problems with [target behavior]?

4. What kind of rewards would you like to earn for good behavior or good schoolwork?

5. What are your favorite activities at school?

6. What are your hobbies or interests?

7. If you had the chance, what activities would you like to do that you don't have the opportunity to do now?

(cont.)

FIGURE 8.2. Student-assisted functional assessment interview. From Kern, Dunlap, Clarke, and Childs (1994). Copyright 1994 by the Hammill Institute on Disabilities. Reprinted with permission from Sage Publications, Inc.

Section 3

Rate how much you like all the following subjects:

	Not at all	Fair	Very much
Reading			
Math			
Spelling			
Handwriting			
Science			
Social Studies			
English			
Music			
P.E.			
Computers			
Art			

Section 4

What do you like about reading?   What don't you like about reading?

What do you like about math?   What don't you like about math?

What do you like about spelling?   What don't you like about spelling?

What do you like about handwriting?   What don't you like about handwriting?

What do you like about science?   What don't you like about science?

What do you like about social studies?   What don't you like about social studies?

What do you like about English?   What don't you like about English?

What do you like about music?   What don't you like about music?

What do you like about P.E.?   What don't you like about P.E.?

What do you like about computers?   What don't you like about computers?

What do you like about art?   What don't you like about art?

FIGURE 8.2. *(cont.)*

direct and ecologically valid FBA technique (Elliott et al., 1987; Feindler & Ecton, 1986). Collecting direct observations of students' behavior serves two purposes (Dunlap & Kern, 1993). First, direct observation serves to objectively confirm (or deny) a relation between behavior and environmental events. Second, it provides quantifiable baseline (pretreatment) information that can be used to gauge the magnitude of the problem behavior and the effects of accommodations or interventions. FBA often uses antecedent–behavior–consequence (A-B-C) analysis (Alberto & Troutman, 2006). Antecedents are events that precede a behavior and may serve as a prompt, or cue, for behavior to occur. Consequences occur after a behavior and serve to maintain, increase, or decrease the future probability of the behavior occurring. There are three types of A-B-C analyses.

First, an anecdotal record can be kept such as the one appearing in Figure 8.3. An anecdotal record is compiled by turning a piece of paper horizontally and making three columns labeled with the words *antecedents, behavior,* and *consequences.* Observations are then numbered and recorded according to their occurrence under the three columns. Note that the consequence of a given behavior can become the antecedent for a succeeding behavior. Second, antecedents, behavior, and consequences can be compiled using structured observation forms such as the one appearing in Figure 8.4. In this particular observation form, various tasks and activities are listed along the vertical axis. Certain types of appropriate and inappropriate behaviors appear along the horizontal axis. By marking an "X" in the box that intersects a certain task/activity and behavior, a general pattern emerges of the antecedent conditions that prompted certain behaviors to occur.

Third, the scatterplot method, illustrated in Figure 8.5, can be used to collect direct observations of behavior (Touchette, MacDonald, & Langer, 1985). In this

Antecedent	Behavior	Consequence
1. Teacher: "Time for spelling practice." Teacher begins handing out sheets.	2. Steve gets up to sharpen his pencil.	3. Karen laughs when Steve bumps her desk.
4. Teacher asks Steve what he is doing.	5. Steve makes a face. Linda giggles.	6. Steve sits down and begins tapping his pencil.
7. Teacher: "Please stop that, Steve."	8. Steve turns around to talk to Linda.	9. Teacher tells Steve to turn around.
10. Steve begins tapping his pencil again.	11. Teacher: "Steve, how many times do I have to remind you not to do that!"	12. Karen giggles.
13. Teacher: "Have you started your spelling yet, Steve?"	14. Steve: "I don't want to. It's boring."	15. Teacher: "You have to or else you'll be in from recess."

FIGURE 8.3. Example A-B-C analysis.

Student: _____   Date: _____

Observer: _____

Material/task	Appropriate student behaviors						Inappropriate student behaviors				
	Answer question	Ask question	On-task	Work finished	Ask for help		Aggression	Off-task	Out of seat	Defiant	Talk-out
Paper and pencil											
Listen											
Class discussion											
Workbook											
Individual											
Group											
Transition											

FIGURE 8.4. Observation form. From Reid and Maag (1998). Copyright 1998 by Taylor & Francis. Reprinted by permission. *www.informaworld.com.*

Student: Leslie Dates: 11/1 to 11/15

Behavior: Talking without permission; noncompliance

Observer: Mrs. Smith

X = 3 or more   O = 1 or 2   blank = behavior absent

Activity	Time	M	T	W	TH	F	M	T	W	TH	F
									Days		
Warm Up	8:30–9:00	O		O			X	O			
Reading Groups	9:00–9:30	O					X				
Spelling	9:30–10:00	X					O				
Recess/Story	10:00–10:30										
Math	10:30–11:00	X	O		X	X	X		O		O
Lunch	11:00–11:30										
Free Read	11:30–12:00	X					O				
Social Studies	12:00–12:30						X				
Art/Music/Health	12:30–1:00									O	
Phys. Ed.	1:00–1:30		O								
Science	1:30–2:00				O						
Catch Up	2:00–2:30	X					O				
Prepare for Home	2:30–3:00										

FIGURE 8.5. Example of a completed scatterplot. From Reid and Maag (1998). Copyright 1998 by Taylor & Francis. Reprinted by permission. *www.informaworld.com.*

approach, the school day is divided into units (e.g., class periods) that are listed on the vertical axis. The days of the week are listed on the horizontal axis. This process results in a grid in which instances (or noninstances) of a behavior can be charted over a period of weeks, thereby making it possible to identify certain patterns. For example, an examination of the scatterplot in Figure 8.5 suggests that math period seems to be a particularly important antecedent for problem behavior occurring, so time of day or problems with math may be important. This information suggests that it would be a good idea to do an anecdotal A-B-C analysis during math time to determine specific antecedents or consequences related to the inappropriate behavior. It also appears that more inappropriate behavior occurs on Mondays than any other day of the week. There may be some event(s) that occur on Monday that is related to the problem behavior. The teacher might want to check with the parents to see if there is something different in the student's routine on Monday. It's also possible that the student may not receive medication on Monday for some reason.

Hypothesis Generation

Once information is obtained about the environmental factors that may be related to a student's inappropriate behavior, the focus shifts to hypothesis generation. Information from multiple sources is synthesized to try to determine the functional relation between the behavior the student exhibits and the outcome that the behavior achieves (Neel & Cessna, 1993). Remember that from the FBA perspective, when a student exhibits a behavior, it serves a function, that is, it is exhibited to achieve a result. All behaviors, even those considered inappropriate, are purposeful and achieve an outcome for students. It's not just "ADHD coming out." Figure 8.6 shows common behavioral functions. These functions describe the "payoff" that a student's behavior achieves. For example, consider a student who often acts out during math class and is sent to the office. The student may have acted out to avoid

Outcome	Description
Escape/avoidance	When a child's outcome is to avoid a task, activity; escape a consequence; terminate or leave a situation.
Attention	When a behavior results in the student becoming the focus of a situation; draws attention to self; puts the student in the foreground of a situation.
Stimulation	When a behavior allows the student to access sensory stimulation.
Tangible	When a behavior results in access to an object, activity, or event.

FIGURE 8.6. Common functions.

the math class. Thus the behavior served to allow the student to escape from an unpleasant situation.

Dunlap and Kern have developed guidelines for developing hypotheses (Dunlap & Kern, 1993; Kern, Childs, Dunlap, Clarke, & Falk, 1994). They suggest that:

- Hypotheses should be based on at least two sources and be based on observed data.
- Hypotheses must be stated in terms of observable classroom variables (i.e., antecedents/consequents).
- Hypotheses must be directly testable.
- Both teacher and the FBA team must agree that hypotheses are reasonable (note that the teacher may make hypotheses independently).
- Hypotheses must lead directly to an intervention that can be implemented without excessive effort or disruption to instructional routine.

Some examples of acceptable hypotheses would include:

- Michael's on-task behavior will increase if task length is shortened and he is given opportunities to choose assignments.
- Paul's outbursts will decrease when he is provided with specific praise and staff ignore undesirable behavior.
- Heidi's oppositional behavior will decrease when she is given specific examples in long division prior to seatwork.
- Jessica's rate of assignment completion will increase when she is not in close proximity to Katy, when she is given regular attention, and when she self-monitors assignment completion.
- Fred's talk-outs will decrease when he is allowed to respond frequently and use a word processor for writing tasks.

Hypothesis Testing

The next step, after forming functional hypotheses, is to test them. Testing consists of establishing conditions where the antecedents and/or consequents thought to be related to the behavior can be controlled and manipulated directly (Karsh, Repp, Dahlquist, & Munk, 1995). The student is observed performing the target behavior in the natural environment where the target behavior occurs, while the educator systematically controls or manipulates environmental factors thought to be related to the target behavior. For example, assessment could be used to test the hypothesis that a behavior served to gain a student teacher attention. The teacher would systematically attend to the student when the target behavior occurred or attend to the student when the target behavior did not occur. The practitioner would note changes in the target behavior depending on whether attention was provided contingent on the target behavior. These observations could be recorded on a chart similar to the one appearing in Figure 8.5. If the frequency of the target behavior increased when attention was provided, then there is a functional relation between attention and the target behavior. Note that several observations would be required in order to determine the validity of the hypothesized functional relation. Hypothesis testing can be time-consuming and educators may be tempted to omit this step. However, the time involved in testing hypotheses may pale in comparison to the time, effort, and expense of implementing ineffective accommodations or interventions. Dunlap and Kern (1993) provided three reasons why hypothesis testing is desirable. First, it is possible to determine which environmental variables have the greatest impact upon a child's behavior. Accommodations and interventions can then be developed around those variables. Second, manipulating variables helps narrow the selection of potentially effective accommodations and interventions and provides information on how best to implement them. Third, testing allows a teacher to evaluate the effects of interventions relative to the amount of effort required for implementation. Note also that hypothesis testing is in effect a mini-intervention. The same (or very similar) manipulation used in hypothesis testing will be used in interventions.

Implementing Accommodations or Interventions

During the third stage, information derived from testing hypotheses is translated into accommodations and/or interventions (Dunlap & Kern, 1993). The antecedents and/or consequents identified from testing hypotheses are used to develop specific accommodations and interventions. Umbreit's (1995) study of an 8-year-old boy with ADHD who displayed disruptive behavior provides an excellent example of how hypotheses can be translated into interventions approach. Data from A-B-C analyses indicated that the disruptive behavior was maintained by the student's desire to escape from an activity and to receive peer attention. Umbreit generated two hypotheses from this information: (1) Corey's behavior during independent work would improve if he was seated away from others and (2) Corey's behavior in group work would improve if his group did not contain friends. These hypotheses were confirmed during testing. The following four interventions were then implemented: (1) Corey was assigned a special work area away from peers; (2) Corey worked in groups that did not contain his friends; (3) Corey was taught to request a break when needed; and (4) instructional staff ignored his disruptive behaviors. The results of the intervention were striking: disruptive behavior was reduced to zero.

Similarly, Stahr, Cushing, Lane, and Fox (2006) worked with a fourth-grade student with ADHD who exhibited high rates of off-task behavior that in turn created a disruption in the classroom. They hypothesized that the student's off-task behavior served a dual function: it was maintained by reinforcement in the form of teacher attention and by escape from independent tasks. Three interventions were implemented to address the problem. First, the teacher instigated a card system so that the student could signal when he needed help with his work. A green card indicated he was able to work independently and did not need assistance with the task. During these times the teacher praised his on-task behavior. A yellow card indicated that he was trying to do the work, but would need assistance soon. The teacher or paraeducator would respond to this card within 5 minutes. A red card indicated that the student was feeling either anxious or angry and needed immediate assistance. The teacher or paraeducator would respond to a red card within 1 minute. The student was reinforced for each appropriate use of the cards.

Second, self-monitoring was used to help the student monitor his own on-task behavior. The self-monitoring checklist included six items that the student should monitor: (1) "I am listening," (2) "My hands and my feet are still," (3) "I am seated in my seat," (4) "I understand the directions," (5) "I am using my cards correctly," and (6) "I am doing what I am supposed to be doing." The checklist contained two columns, one for the student to indicate whether he thought he was on-task and a second column for the teacher to confirm the accuracy of the student's responses. Third, the student received attention from the teacher or paraeducator only when he used the card system and/or made appropriate verbal requests. Otherwise the adults ignored any attempts to obtain attention. After implementing these interventions, the student's on-task behavior increased dramatically. The results of these study illustrate the potential of FBA to help students with ADHD function better in the classroom. As yet, there are no validated rubrics for matching interventions to functions. DuPaul (personnel communication) has developed some guidelines based on his previous research (DuPaul & Ervin, 1996). For example, if the function of a behavior is escape, teachers can:

- Reduce task demands (e.g., make the task simpler or shorter)
- Make the task more stimulating (e.g., each math problem completed provides a clue to the location of a treasure chest).
- Allow a choice of tasks (e.g., students can choose seatwork from a "menu").
- Provide breaks at set intervals contingent on remaining on task (e.g., after every 10 spelling practices the student gets a 2-minute break).

If the function of the behavior was attention, the teacher can:

- Ignore off-task behavior.
- Attend to on-task behavior.
- Reinforce peers for ignoring off-task behavior.
- Use peer tutoring.

Although FBA is not a trivial undertaking, it can be well worth the effort. The key point is to view the assessment and intervention components as reciprocal. Educators often view assessment as a process distinctly separate from, and occurring prior to, an intervention. In a traditional sense (e.g., achievement testing), this may be true. However, from a FBA, generating hypotheses and testing them are not separate from, but rather are an integral part, of the intervention process since the antecedents and consequents that serve to maintain a behavior will be used in the actual intervention(s) developed.

THINKING PRACTICALLY ABOUT FBA

FBA is an effective method for addressing classroom behavior problems, and research suggests classroom teachers view FBA procedures as acceptable (Packenham, Shute, & Reid, 2004). However, there are serious concerns regarding the practical reality of implementing FBA in the classroom (Reid & Nelson, 2002). First, many educators are not trained in FBA procedures. Second, the time required for a full FBA, which could require several weeks to complete, could be a problem for a classroom teacher. Third, many problems that students with ADHD exhibit may not be serious enough to warrant a full FBA. Luckily, it may be possible for educators to use the principles of FBA in a more timely and less labor-intensive manner. In this section we discuss how educators could use a more efficient approach to analyzing problem behaviors in the classroom.

Streamlining the FBA Process

One promising approach to FBA is to greatly streamline the process by truncating the hypothesis development stage. Recall that one labor-intensive step in the hypothesis development process is to observe the problem behavior to determine when, where, and under what circumstances it occurred most frequently. In practice, it may be possible to shorten this process by taking advantage of the fact that the classroom teacher has already had a great deal of prior experience with the student and has observed the problem extensively. Thus, it's possible that a classroom teacher may already be well aware of the topography of the problem behavior. What is necessary is to provide the teacher with a framework to organize the knowledge so that hypotheses can be generated. Packenham et al. (2004) demonstrated how a truncated FBA could be accomplished in practice with two students, Michelle and Jack, who exhibited disruptive classroom behavior.

In the first step, the teacher was interviewed using an instrument devised by Larson and Maag (1998) to determine the circumstances under which the behavior was most likely and least likely to occur. After the interview the teacher and the researcher noted information that could be functionally related to the behavior. Next the teacher compared each student's behavior to descriptions of behaviors indicative of attention-related functions and escape-related functions (see Figure 8.7) and decided which behavior pattern most resembled the behaviors of each student. Based on the descriptions the teachers decided that one student's behavior was attention-related and the other student's behavior was escape-related. Next the teacher generated hypothesis statements for each student using guidelines developed by O'Neill et al. (1997). The statements were:

Escape/avoidance

This pattern of behavior results in the student escaping the performance demands established by the teacher by engaging in behaviors to get him/her to remove or lower the requirements of the demand. In essence the student is saying " I won't do this" or "Back off." Examples include:

- Behavior occurs following a request to perform a difficult task.
- Behavior is designed to push you away when you are trying to get him/her to do what you ask.
- Behavior decreases when you aren't making demands of him/her.
- Behavior occurs when any request is made of him/her.

Attention-seeking behavior

An attention-seeking behavior pattern is one in which the student engages in behaviors that cause the teacher to interact with him/her. In essence the student is saying "Get over here now." Examples include:

- Behavior causes you to spend some time with the student.
- Behavior is designed to pull you to the student when you are not paying attention to him/her.
- Behavior occurs when you are not attending to him/her.
- Behavior occurs in response to your talking to other students.

FIGURE 8.7. Guidelines for identifying the function of a behavior. From Packenham, Shute, and Reid (2004). Copyright 2004 by West Virginia University Press. Reprinted by permission.

> During silent reading time, Michelle will engage in inappropriate behaviors in order to gain teacher attention.
>
> When given a written task, Jack will engage in off-task behaviors in order to avoid the task.

Next, the teacher selected appropriate interventions using the guidelines developed by DuPaul and Ervin (1996). Because Michelle's behavior appeared to be attention-related, the teacher focused on making attention contingent on appropriate behavior. Michelle was provided with a card that she could place on her desk if she wanted to speak with the teacher during silent reading. The card could be used only once during the silent reading period. The teacher told Michelle that she could come to his desk provided that she read silently until she was called. In Jack's case the teacher made three simple accommodations (i.e., modifications to antecedents). First, he met briefly with Jack before a writing task to clarify instructions and expectations. Second, Jack was given shorter writing assignments. Third, Jack was shown exactly how much writing was needed to accomplish the assignment (e.g., write at least three sentences) and his work was checked at 5–10 minute intervals. Additionally, Jack was provided with reinforcers for completing work satisfactorily.

The results of the interventions were quite positive. Disruptions decreased to near zero and Jack's work completion improved significantly. The hypothesis generation and intervention selection processes were accomplished in under 2 hours. The classroom teacher did not perceive the process as overly time-consuming or intrusive, and he was pleased with the results of the interventions. The classroom teacher had no difficulty in identifying the time and the context in which problem behaviors were most likely to occur and then matching the behavior to a function (i.e., attention or escape). In fact, he indicated that he had already noted this information. What he lacked was a framework that allowed him to respond to the function and match it with an appropriate intervention. All told, the results of the study suggests that with only minor support a classroom teacher can identify the function of a problem behavior and develop effective interventions or accommodations.

Setting a Focus

Classroom teachers have many demands placed on them. Thus they need to be sure to focus their efforts in the most efficient and effective manner. With regard to FBA, researchers have suggested that teachers should focus on antecedents because often simple changes in the classroom can prove extremely effective in reducing inappropriate behaviors and increasing desired behaviors (Dunlap & Kern, 1993). As we noted earlier, many FBA studies show that there were functional relations between factors related to instruction and problem behavior. This often took the form of escape-related behavior when academic tasks were too difficult or demanding. There is good reason to believe that task difficulty can be directly related to disruptive behaviors. For example, DePaepe and colleagues found that task difficulty (i.e., high-difficulty and low-difficulty tasks) was directly related to disruptive behavior (DePaepe et al., 1996). Even a small increase in task difficulty could cause an increase in disruptive behaviors. Moreover, simple curricular modifications can result in dramatic behavior changes. For example, with some students the opportunity to choose their assignments can positively affect behavior (e.g., Powell & Nelson, 1997). This suggests that academic performance problems merit particular attention. Figure 8.8 shows examples of instructional factors that research has shown can be functionally related to problem behaviors.

SUMMING UP

The most critical aspect of a functional approach to problem behaviors is to adopt a functional perspective. Behavior problems should not be seen as the result of a disorder that is inherent to the student. Instead, behavior problems should be viewed as the result of environmental factors that serve to cue or maintain the behavior. This change in perspective is critical. We can do nothing about problems inherent to a student; however, we can alter the environment. Note that this change in perspective serves to empower educators. Rather than taking a reactive stance where the focus is on dealing with problem behaviors after they occur, the focus shifts to preventing the occurrence of problem behaviors. And, as the old saying goes, "An

Type	Examples from research
Physical environment	
Location in room	Dunlap et al. (1993); Kern, Childs, et al. (1994); Umbreit (1995)
Group/individual); peers	Dunlap et al. (1993); McAfee (1987); Umbreit (1995)
Temporal (time of day or week)	Umbreit (1995)
Task/materials	
Feedback (high/low/none)	Barkley (1990)
High or low stimulation	Kern, Childs, et al. (1994)
Response mode (e.g., written, oral, typed, active, passive)	Karsh et al. (1995); Kern, Childs, et al. (1994)
Structure (high–low)	Barkley (1990)
Interest level/preference	Cooper et al. (1992); Dunlap et al. (1991, 1993); Foster-Johnson, Ferro, & Dunlap (1994); Kern-Dunlap, Clarke, & Dunlap (1990)
Instructional	
Lesson length, lesson format, lesson difficulty	Dunlap et al. (1991, 1993); Kern, Childs, et al. (1994); Carr & Durand (1985); Cooper et al. (1992); DePaepe et al. (1996); Durand & Carr (1991)
Transitions	Lalli, Browder, Mace, & Brown (1993); Singer, Singer, & Horner (1987)
Opportunity to respond	Barkley (1990); Cooper et al. (1992); Dyer, Dunlap, & Winterling (1990); Dunlap et al. (1991, 1993, 1994)
Choice of activity	

FIGURE 8.8. Instructional factors functionally related to problem behaviors.

ounce of prevention is worth a pound of cure." Educators should think of FBA as an investment. A little time put into FBA has the potential to save much more time in the future. Here are some points to remember:

✓ Behavior is not random. Even problem behaviors can serve a function. Finding the function a problem behavior serves is the first step in interventions that can prevent or greatly reduce future occurrences.

✓ FBAs should be conducted for students who display chronic behavior problems that disrupt the classroom environment in a manner that affects their learning or that of their classmates.

✓ FBA must be conducted for students who have been suspended for more than 10 days or exhibited misconduct involving weapons or drugs.

✓ Environmental factors can serve to trigger or maintain problem behavior.

✓ Behaviors should be well defined and pass the "So What" test.

✓ Hypotheses should be based on observational data and lead to an intervention.

✓ Interventions selected should be acceptable to the classroom teacher.

✓ Teachers can use functional approaches without conducting a full FBA. Teachers may often be aware of the function of a behavior.

✓ Altering antecedents can often be the most efficient and effective way to deal with problem behavior.

✓ Proactive teacher actions (e.g., providing a strategy, giving extra instructions, providing supports such as a worked example of a long division problem) are critically important.

CHAPTER 9

Behavior Management

One size does not fit all.
—GEORGE DUPAUL

Let's suppose that a new student moved into your school district. Katy is a third grader who has cerebral palsy. Her motor movements are so uncoordinated that for the most part she is confined to a wheelchair. Her speech is intelligible, but it is very slow and laborious. She can write, but because her coordination is so poor making the letters takes a great deal of time. Additionally her handwriting is very large. It's literally impossible for her letters to fit on standard lined paper. Her cognitive abilities, however, are not affected; in fact she is quite talented and excels at math. Katy is also fiercely independent—she likes to do things on her own whenever possible. She will be in a third-grade general education classroom, but obviously she will have tremendous difficulty functioning in a typical classroom environment. How could we ensure that Katy has the same chance at an education as the other students? The answer is straightforward: we would need to change the classroom environment.

The first thing we might do is to ensure that the student had physical access to the school. Actually this probably has already been attended to, because under the Americans with Disabilities Act most schools now have ramps to ensure that they are wheelchair-accessible. Of course we would also need to examine the classroom setup. The aisles would need to be wide enough for the wheelchair to pass through. Frequently used materials should be on shelves that Katy could reach. We would need to provide a table for her to work at because she can't use a standard desk. A lapboard could be useful also. We might also want to give Katy a buddy who could help out with tasks she couldn't manage (e.g., sharpening a pencil). We would also need to attend to the instructional environment. For example, during class discussions we would need to give Katy plenty of time to respond orally. Because Katy can't raise her hand we might need to establish some way for her to signal a need for attention. If an activity required writing, we might need to make it easier for Katy by taping paper to her table (or lapboard), blowing up worksheets to accommodate her larger printing, and minimizing the amount of text she needs to produce. We might even allow Katy to dictate answers to a paraeducator or study buddy. All of the accommodations are commonsense, simple, and practical. They can all easily be implemented in the classroom. And, most importantly, they systematically alter the classroom environment to help the student function better.

The same principle applies to students with ADHD. Teachers can systematically alter the physical and instructional environment in their classrooms to adapt to the needs of students with ADHD. Barkley (1997a) terms this process the creation of "prosthetic environments." Just as a wheelchair ramp would allow Katy access to the school and the benefits of education, so simple, straightforward changes in the classroom environment combined with well-established behavior management techniques would allow students with ADHD the opportunity to better function in the classroom and profit from an education. Unfortunately, many educators do not have the same reaction to alterations for students with behavioral problems—such as ADHD—as they would for students such as Katy. In fact, suggesting changes to accommodate students with ADHD could even evoke a negative reaction. As we discussed in Chapter 1, there is the notion that all students are simply supposed to "behave themselves," follow rules, and comply with teachers' requests as a matter of course. If students fail to behave appropriately the typical reaction is punitive— punish the student (Maag, 2001). Making alterations can be perceived as "special treatment" or construed as "rewarding misbehavior." Alternatively there may be fears that alterations will stigmatize students with ADHD or even encourage misbehavior on the part of other students (Pfiffner et al., 2006).

The difference in the reaction to alterations is striking. Consider this: If there was no ramp for Katy, would we punish her for excessive absenteeism? Would we give her detention for not sitting at a desk? Would we lower her class participation grade because she couldn't speak as much? Would we fail her on an assignment because she was unable to produce text that fit on standard lined paper? Would we have concerns that if we provided Katy a paraeducator that every student would want one? Would we be worried that giving Katy a table to work at would somehow stigmatize her? We seriously doubt that any educator would agree with any of these hypothetical reactions. In fact, we believe that most educators would be horrified and would consider the reactions either nonsensical or terribly unfair. After all, who would knowingly penalize or punish a student for something beyond her control?

The same argument applies to students with ADHD: punishing students for a problem that they have little control over is equally unfair. The only difference is that Katy has a disability that affects her physical activities, but students with ADHD have a disability that affects their behavior. Moreover, punishment is unlikely to be successful. For example, giving Katy a failing grade on written assignments because her letters don't fit between the lines won't help her handwriting. The same is true for students with ADHD. Keeping them in from recess because they didn't finish an assignment won't help them complete the next assignment. In fact it could even make it less likely!

The evidence is clear that using accommodations and behavior management techniques can significantly reduce problem behaviors (e.g., disruptions, noncompliance) and increase appropriate behaviors (e.g., time on-task, assignment completion; Pelham & Fabiano, 2008). They should be a part of any treatment program for students with ADHD. Behavior management techniques can also enhance the effectiveness of medication and enable students to receive lower dosages of medication (Fabiano et al., 2007). In this chapter, we describe how educators can create a classroom environment that can help children with ADHD function better. First, we provide an overview of principles of behavior management and discuss specific considerations for students with ADHD. Second, we discuss how to structure the classroom and classroom management procedures useful with students with ADHD. Finally, we present an overview of three effective interventions and provide step-by-step instructions on how to implement them in the classroom. Note that instructional practices are also a critical aspect of the classroom environment. They are discussed in Chapter 10.

BEHAVIOR MANAGEMENT

Teachers of students with ADHD often grow frustrated because students with ADHD don't "play by the rules." Techniques that work with other students may not work with students with ADHD. In this section, we discuss how teachers can effectively use behavior management with students with ADHD. We begin with an overview of terminology. Next we discuss specific considerations for students with ADHD that can affect behavior management in the classroom. Space prohibits an extensive discussion of this topic; for an approachable but comprehensive treatment, see John Maag's (2004) book on behavior management.

Terminology

From a strictly behavioral perspective, all behavior occurs because of reinforcement. By definition, reinforcement is something that changes the likelihood of the occurrence (or frequency or duration) of a behavior. Reinforcement is used when it is necessary or desirable to increase a behavior. The term "reward" is often used synonymously with reinforcement. This is not technically correct. For example, if we gave Heidi $50.00 for each time she raised her hand and waited to be called on, she would definitely be rewarded for the behavior. However, unless the frequency of the behavior changed (i.e., Heidi increased the number of times she raised her hand and waited to be called on) the $50.00 would not have served as a reinforcer. Put more simply, a student must see the reinforcer positively for it to change behavior. There are many forms of reinforcement including social (e.g., a smile or a compliment), tangible (e.g., a sticker or a toy), and activity (e.g., the opportunity to play a game or read a book). All of these types are useful for students with ADHD.

There are two types of reinforcement: positive and negative (Maag, 2004).

1. *Positive reinforcement* occurs when a behavior is followed by a consequence that in turn results in an increase in the rate at which the behavior occurs. For example, a teacher who smiles at Heidi for raising her hand is using positive reinforcement (as long as Heidi likes having the teacher smile at her). Positive reinforcement is awarded after a behavior occurs. The teacher must have control of the reinforcer. Students should receive the reinforcer only when they perform the behavior that the teacher wished to increase.

2. *Negative reinforcement* occurs when a behavior is followed by the removal or prevention of an unpleasant event or condition. For example, if John started his homework to stop his mom's constant annoying reminders, this would be negative reinforcement. After he starts his homework his mom's reminders cease. In negative reinforcement when the behavior occurs the undesirable stimulus goes away.

Sometimes it is necessary or desirable to reduce the frequency of a behavior. This is termed punishment. Punishment occurs when a behavior is followed by consequence that results in a decrease in the rate of the behavior. Punishment is intended to eliminate or greatly reduce the occurrence of a behavior. There are two types of punishment (Maag, 2004).

1. *Type I punishment* (application of contingent stimulation) occurs when a stimulus is applied after the behavior. The stimulus is aversive or unpleasant to the student. For example, Max talked back to the teacher and was told to "Stop that immediately!" If this caused Max to stop or lower the rate of backtalk, then the verbal reprimand served as a punisher.

2. *Type II punishment* (contingent withdrawal of a stimulus) occurs when a reinforcer is removed following the occurrence of a behavior. For example, Skip did not do his seatwork so his teacher required him to complete his work during the daily free time. Removal of free time as result of an inappropriate behavior constituted the punishment. Note that this type of punishment is only effective if what is withdrawn is a reinforcer. If free time is not a reinforcer for Skip, then withdrawing it would not be effective. It's important to distinguish between negative reinforcement and punishment. Going back to the example of John, if he started his homework and finished on time, it would be negative reinforcement at work. If he did not and as a result lost his TV viewing privileges, it would be Type II punishment.

As a general rule teachers should *always* try positive reinforcement before considering negative reinforcement or punishment. Teachers should focus on teaching and reinforcing appropriate classroom behaviors that allow a student to function effectively in the classroom. In general, punishment should be used sparingly and reserved for serious behaviors. Note also that punishment *does not create new and appropriate behaviors*; it only reduces or eliminates undesirable behaviors. Additionally, if punishment is applied too frequently to reduce one behavior, other undesirable behaviors are likely to appear (DuPaul & Stoner, 2003). Note that if punishment is effective after an initial period, *it will seldom need to be used* because the frequency of the problem behavior should diminish dramatically.

Behavior Management with Students with ADHD

Behavioral management can be effective for students with ADHD; however, students with ADHD may not respond in quite the same manner as other students. Teachers may need to alter their existing behavior management schemes and style of student–teacher interaction to deal with students with ADHD. There are well-established guidelines for using behavioral interventions with students with ADHD (DuPaul & Stoner, 2003; Pfiffner et al., 2006).

Powerful Reinforcement

Students with ADHD *are less sensitive* to reinforcement than their peers. Reinforcers that are commonly used in the classroom (e.g., being the line leader, teacher praise) and that are effective in maintaining appropriate behaviors for many children may not be sufficient in isolation for students with ADHD. These students often will require additional and more powerful reinforcement over and above what is provided through normal classroom management to provide sufficient reinforcement to alter behavior.

Frequency

Students with ADHD will typically require *more frequent* reinforcement than their peers. Teachers need to attend very carefully to a student's behavior and be sure to provide reinforcement for every instance of the behavior. If reinforcement is provided sporadically or inconsistently it is unlikely to be effective.

Timing

Reinforcement should be provided *as soon as possible* after the behavior has occurred. This is especially important in the case of younger students. It's critical for students to associate the behavior with the reinforcer. This is important for any student, but is critical for students with ADHD. For these students, delays in reinforcement are likely to render interventions ineffective. Telling Rhonda that she will receive her reinforcer "later" may decrease or eliminate any change in behavior. Note that the same principle also applies to punishment.

Satiation

Satiation refers to a situation in which a reinforcer loses its effectiveness and thus awarding the reinforcer no longer results in a change in behavior. This is a common occurrence for students with ADHD who tend to reach satiation more quickly than their peers. This means that teachers will need to change reinforcers more frequently for students with ADHD. One way to deal with the problem of satiation is to create "reward menus" (discussed shortly) that provide a number of possible rewards from which students can select. To determine what is reinforcing for students, teachers can ask students directly and/or observe students' preferences when they have free access to potential reinforcers. For example, if Dexter chooses to read a graphic novel during free time, this could be a potential reinforcer for him.

Negative Reinforcement/Punishment

Teachers often use negative reinforcement or Type I punishment with students with ADHD (Pfiffner et al., 2006). This often takes the form of commands for performance, reprimands, or admonishments (e.g., giving a student a lecture about inappropriate behavior). Teachers need to be careful in how they use negative reinforcement and punishment for two reasons. First, many students with ADHD have few positive interactions with teachers. If the only attention they receive is likely to be negative reinforcement or punishment, they may see the teacher or school environment negatively. This is not a desirable situation. Second, as we noted in the previous chapter, teacher attention can actually serve to maintain inappropriate behaviors.

STRUCTURING THE CLASSROOM

To help children with ADHD cope with the demands of the school environment teachers must be aware of how the physical setup of the classroom can affect behavior (Reid, 1999). Changes in physical setup can have dramatic effects on behavior. Note that there is also a potential for synergy. For example, changing the physical setup may make classroom management easier or more effective.

Physical Setup

Physical setup refers to the actual classroom layout, and the students' locations within the classroom. Children with ADHD can be easily distracted by extraneous stimuli. The physical layout of the classroom is an important factor in reducing or eliminating potential distractions. Physically enclosed classrooms (i.e., classrooms with four walls) are more appropriate for students with ADHD than open classrooms because open classrooms provide many more opportunities for distraction (e.g., the child may be distracted by another class's activities or by children coming and going) and may be noisier (Pfiffner et al., 2006). For children with ADHD, these types of distractions can result in decreases in time on-task and an increase in other problem behaviors (Whalen, Henker, Collins, Finck, & Dotemoto, 1979). Note, however, that it is *not* necessary (or desirable) to create a minimally stimulating environment (Abramowitz & O'Leary, 1991). The idea is to minimize outside distractions. Class size is also important. An overcrowded classroom will result in more distractions for the student and less individual time with the teacher.

Physical changes can also help children who need physical activity. Reid (1999) suggested that for these students, teachers should consider providing two desks in the front of the room (one on each side). Whenever the student needs physical activity, he or she simply moves to the other desk. The student is also taught the appropriate manner of moving from one desk to another (e.g., take all work/materials necessary, move directly to the new desk, don't speak to other students while making the move). Another simple accommodation for children who need more physical activity is a stand-up desk. A stand-up desk is a desk that has been raised to approximately chest height, allowing the child to stand and work. This can be done quite simply by extending desk legs to the maximum or by placing the desk on blocks. Stand-up desks allow for more physical movement during independent work. It may also be desirable to combine various types of seating arrangements for a student. For example, a child might have one normal desk and one stand-up desk.

The student's physical location in the classroom is also important. The student's desk should be away from high-traffic areas and potential distractions such as the doorway, window, or pencil sharpener (Bender & Mathes, 1995). It's best to seat a student with ADHD near the teacher. The teacher's physical proximity can have a positive effect on students' behavior. It also allows for easier and more frequent monitoring and feedback. Students with ADHD should be monitored often to ensure that they are engaging in appropriate behaviors and to prevent minor misbehavior from escalating. Research is clear that students with ADHD perform best when they are regularly monitored and given frequent feedback on their performance (DuPaul & Stoner, 2003).

Unfortunately, busy teachers may forget to monitor. There are several effective means for teachers to cue themselves to monitor a student and provide feedback (Pfiffner et al., 2006). One simple method involves the teacher placing a number of coins in one pocket and transferring a coin to another pocket each time he or she monitors the student and provides feedback. Another method involves the use of a timer or taped tones that occur at random intervals every few minutes. When the timer goes off the teacher is reminded to monitor behavior and provide feedback. This method can also serve as a precursor to self-regulation interventions (discussed in Chapter 11).

Seating arrangements and instructional grouping can also affect students with ADHD because of proximity to other students who may serve as potential distractions or may unwittingly reinforce inappropriate behavior. Ideally, students with ADHD should have individual desks (Pfiffner et al., 2006). Arranging desks in rows (as opposed to clusters of desks) *during independent or large-group work*, and surrounding the child with students who maintain effort and who ignore inappropriate behaviors can help decrease potential distractions and help the student with ADHD maintain focus (Bender & Mathes, 1995; Pfiffner et al., 2006). It's appropriate to group desks in a cluster during small-group activities when the activity demands student-to-student interaction. Small-group activities may also present problems for children with ADHD. These children may perceive small-group activities as an opportunity for social interaction or attention. The composition of groups can sometimes cause this problem. Peer attention can serve to trigger or maintain inappropriate behavior of children with ADHD (Lewis & Sugai, 1996; Northrup et al., 1995; Umbreit, 1995). One straightforward solution is to place the child with ADHD in a group that does not include his or her friends (Umbreit, 1995).

CLASSROOM MANAGEMENT

Classroom management is often construed as dealing effectively with misbehavior. This is an important aspect of classroom management, but it is only half of the story. The most important aspect of effective classroom management is actually to manage the classroom in such a way as to systematically instill appropriate behaviors and increase their frequency. The logic is simple: when appropriate behavior increases inappropriate behavior decreases. Good class management is critical if teachers are to successfully work with children with ADHD in any instructional environment (i.e., either special education or general education). The ability to behave appropriately within the constraints of the classroom is a necessary prerequisite for academic success for any child. For children with ADHD this may be an impossible task if the classroom is noisy, disorderly, or lacking clear consistent routines and expectations. For children with ADHD to succeed, teachers need to (1) create and maintain stable, predictable classroom routines, (2) create effective rules, and (3) interact effectively.

Creating Routines

A stable, predictable classroom routine is important because it helps children know what they should be doing now, and what they will be doing next. The rationale for classroom routines is simple. When children do not know what they should be doing there is little chance that they will do it. When children do not know what they will be doing next, they may be unprepared or have difficulty shifting to a new task. Creating a stable, predictable classroom routine is simple and straightforward. It involves making a written schedule of daily activities in which the school day is divided into blocks of time; posting it prominently (typically on a designated spot on the blackboard); and maintaining this daily routine (Bender & Mathes, 1995; DuPaul & Stoner, 2003). Within each block of time, the daily schedule should clearly state what activities will occur and what tasks students will need to perform. The schedule starts from the time students first enter the classroom and ends when the students leave at the end of the day.

For students with ADHD, simply posting the schedule may not be enough. The teachers should literally teach the schedule so that the students understand that the schedule tells them what they should be doing. Teachers should also provide reminders and cues about what is needed to start/complete activities (e.g., "You need to have your math worksheet and a pencil.") before starting the activities. It's also important to have well-specified procedures for activities that commonly occur as a part of classroom activities, such as getting a drink, using the bathroom, distributing materials, going to the cafeteria, or sharpening a pencil (Paine, Radicchi, Rosellini, Deutchman, & Darch, 1983). Teachers shouldn't assume that a student with ADHD simply knows how to perform these tasks appropriately or "will pick up" the knowledge by being in the classroom. Teachers should teach these tasks in the same manner as they would teach reading or math because in a very real way appropriate classroom behavior is a part of the curriculum in schools. For example, here is how a teacher might teach a procedure for sharpening a pencil.

- Tell the students that you are going to show them what to do when they need to sharpen their pencil.
- Tell them why it's important that they do it correctly (e.g., they don't waste time, they don't bother others).
- Ask when it's appropriate to sharpen pencils (e.g., during seatwork or small groups) and when it's not appropriate (e.g., when the teacher is talking to the whole class).
- Model how to move from their desks to the pencil sharpener and back (e.g., go straight to the pencil sharpener, be quiet while moving and don't interrupt or talk with other students, sharpen the pencil quickly, and then go directly back to their desks).
- Ask a student to model the appropriate procedure and describe what he or she is doing aloud to the class. Then ask another student to model inappropriate behaviors (e.g., wandering around the room) and discuss why it is not desirable.

After teaching procedures, remember to reinforce students for using the procedures correctly (e.g., "Luke, I like the way that you went straight to the pencil sharpener and then right back to your seat."). One concern that often arises about spending time teaching procedures to students is that it is taking away time that could be used in teaching content. This is actually a false economy. It's better to think of teaching procedures as an investment that prevents disruptions and that actually saves more time in the future. Note that this will likely be beneficial to many students, not just students with ADHD.

The time when various instructional activities occur is an important factor. Teachers should schedule core academics and/or content that might be most cognitively challenging during the morning hours, and "hands-on" or less demanding activities in the afternoon because research indicates that the behavior of children with ADHD often deteriorates over the course of the day (Pfiffner et al., 2006). For this reason, it is best to fit the instructional schedule to the periods when the student is able to perform at his or her peak whenever possible. A final consideration in scheduling pertains to preferred versus nonpreferred activities. It's best to schedule nonpreferred activities *before* preferred activities, and to make preferred activities contingent upon successful completion of nonpreferred activities. For example, math seatwork would be scheduled (and should be completed) before the student could participate in a 15-minute free-reading period.

Notice that many of the situations above involve *transitions*. A transition is the interval between two activities. Transitions are important because if they are not done properly they result in lost instructional time, and that means less learning. Transitions can be very difficult for students with ADHD and behavior problems are more likely when students with ADHD are preparing for a transition (Whalen et al., 2006). If a student with ADHD is required to wait for a prolonged period of time, he or she is likely to grow frustrated and exhibit problems. Note that "prolonged" is relative. Some transitions may also be inherently more difficult for students with ADHD. For example, for elementary school students with ADHD, transitioning from the unstructured environment of the playground, where activity is relatively uninhibited, to the highly structured and regulated classroom can be difficult (Pfiffner et al., 2006). Before beginning instruction, teachers may want to schedule a brief low-stress activity (e.g., reading a short story to the class) to allow the student to settle into the classroom environment. Here are some guidelines for smooth, efficient transitions (McIntosh, Herman, Sanford, McGraw, & Florence, 2004; Paine et al., 1983; Walker, Shea, & Bauer, 2004):

- *Teach transitions.* Establish procedures and communicate exactly what students are to do in transitions and then teach students what to do. To teach transitions, teachers should tell students why the skill is important, model the skill, teach students what is appropriate and inappropriate during the transition, and practice the transition.

- *Signaling transitions.* Cue students before a transition is going to occur so they can be ready for it. For example, a few minutes before the time allotted for math practice is up tell the students that they need to finish up in 2 minutes. Signaling transitions establishes readiness.

- *Gain attention before starting.* Before the transition actually begins, make sure that you have the students' attention. For students with ADHD it may be useful to use proximity to ensure that you have gained attention.

- *Reminders.* At least initially, it's useful to remind students about what is expected of them during transitions (e.g., "Remember to go straight to your learning station."). This should only encompass brief remarks or, if possible, noting good student models.

- *Traffic rules.* Establish procedure for movement or give *explicit* directions at the time the transition occurs. For example, "All the people wearing blue jeans line up at the door." You need to tell *who* is to move and *where* they are to go.

- *Reinforce good transitions.* Appropriate behavior should be reinforced. Communicate this to the class. For example, if the class saves time by making good transitions, then the extra time is their time and can be used for fun activities. This gives students an incentive to make efficient, appropriate transitions.

Rules

Good rules are crucial for a smoothly running classroom. Rules help to set expectation and should communicate to students the behaviors that they *should be* performing. Figure 9.1 shows guidelines for creating effective class rules (Paine et al., 1983). Note that students with ADHD may need additional prompts or cues to remind them of rules. Teachers can help make rules more salient by taping a prompt card listing important behaviors to the student's desk (e.g., "Am I doing my work? Am I listening to the teacher?"). These prompts can serve to remind students what they should be doing and may help students to redirect their behavior. Regular reviews of the rules can also be beneficial (Pfiffner et al., 2006). It's also important to systematically reinforce students for following the rules. One effective means of reinforcing compliance is teacher praise. Teacher praise can be an effective means of increasing appropriate behaviors and decreasing inappropriate behaviors. It is especially important that students with ADHD be systematically praised for complying with rules and for other appropriate behavior (e.g., maintaining effort, starting a task immediately with a reminder). Unfortunately, teacher praise is often underused and applied ineffectively (Brophy, 1981). To use praise effectively teacher should (Brophy, 1981):

- Praise students only after they have performed an appropriate behavior (e.g., when a student with ADHD performs an appropriate transition). Random praise is not only ineffective, it could also be counterproductive as it may serve to reinforce inappropriate behaviors.

- Specify exactly what was praiseworthy. For example, "Luke, I like how you went straight to your desk and got to work." would be effective whereas "Great job Luke!" would not be because the teacher did not specify the behavior for which the student was being praised.

- Link praise to performance criteria and to effort. For example, "Steve, you practiced all your spelling words in 10 minutes just like we talked about. You really stayed at it. Great work." Note that this can also be appropriate for effort. For example, "Steve, I really like how you worked on your spelling words for the whole 10

Establish a few good rules.
In most classrooms three to five rules that cover a broad range of behaviors is best. If students cannot remember the rules, they are unlikely to follow them.

Keep rules short and simple.
Keep rules brief and state them simply. If students cannot understand rules they cannot follow them. It also makes it easier for the teacher to praise students for following the rule or to correct violations.

Keep rules positive.
Rules should stress what the children should do as opposed to what they should not do (e.g., "Keep hands and feet to myself" instead of "No hitting").

Post rules prominently.
Rules should be displayed. Post rules where children are likely to see them (and thus be reminded). Refer to the posted rules when pointing out infractions.

Teach the rules.
Treat class behavior as another important aspect of curriculum. Teach the rules. Discuss the meaning of rules and why they are necessary. Ask students to point out and model behavior that exemplifies following (and not following) rules.

Establish consequences.
There must be consequences (mild punishment) for rule violations. Consequences should be enforced for all violations.

Reinforce compliance.
Teachers should systematically monitor compliance and reinforce students for following the rules. Rule violations should result in consequences (e.g., mild punishment or reprimands).

FIGURE 9.1. Guidelines for effective class rules. Based on Paine, Radicchi, Rosellini, Deutchman, and Darch (1983).

minutes, and you got eight of 10 practiced. If you keep at it like that I bet you will get all 10 next time."

• Praise should be sincere and for meaningful accomplishment. Praise must be credible to be effective. The student must believe that the teacher's praise statement reflects the teacher's honest appraisal. Praise also should be reserved for accomplishments that demonstrate progress or real achievement. Note that "commonplace" activities can often be real achievements for students with ADHD. For example, "Doug, you raised your hand and waited to be called on. That's great!" would be meaningful if the student had not done this previously. On the other hand, "Lynn, it was so great how you picked up that pencil." would be meaningless empty praise.

We would caution teachers that some students *do not like* to be publicly praised. They may feel singled out or feel anxiety when praised publicly. If this is the case, develop a system to praise the student privately (e.g., a signal such as a pat on the shoulder, eye contact).

Consequences for rule violations are a critical component of good rules, especially for students with ADHD. Consequences should be clearly spelled out and communicated to students. There are three keys to effective use of consequences (Pfiffner et al., 2006). First, consequences should be clearly posted and communicated to students. This is especially true for students with ADHD. Second, it is important for teachers to administer consequences consistently and quickly. Consistent enforcement of rules is critical. Students must know that if they violate a rule, consequences will inevitably follow. Teachers should closely monitor rule adherence. For students with ADHD, letting rule violations "slide" sends mixed messages and is likely to result in more violations. It is also important for consequences to be administered as quickly as possible following the violation. If consequences are delayed, the student may not associate the consequence with the rule violation or effects may be weakened. This is especially important in the case of younger students. Finally, consequences should be reasonable—the punishment should fit the crime. Unreasonable severe consequences are unlikely to actually be administered (e.g., keeping a student after school for a month for disobedience) and extremely mild consequences are unlikely to be effective. Note that effective class rules alone are not sufficient. For students with ADHD effective rules should be combined with teacher praise/positive reinforcement for compliance with rules, and mild reprimands (or punishers) for rule violations (Acker & O'Leary, 1987; Pfiffner & O'Leary, 1987; Pfiffner, Rosen, & O'Leary, 1985). Effective reprimands are discussed below.

Effective Interactions

Teachers should be sensitive to the nature of their interactions with students with ADHD. When teachers interact with students with behavior problems, such as some students with ADHD, interactions often are either neutral or negative. Additionally, these students typically receive more teacher attention following inappropriate behavior than following appropriate behavior (Moore Partin, Robertson, Maggin, Oliver, & Wehby, 2010). This can have the effect of actually increasing inappropriate behavior. There are two types of commonly occurring interactions that can be a problem for teachers of students with ADHD (Reid, 1999): giving effective directions and giving effective reprimands.

For students to understand what they are expected to do and successfully accomplish it, teachers must be able to convey directions clearly and effectively. When giving directions to students with ADHD, teachers should be sensitive to potential problems with working memory and attention. Working memory (discussed in more detail in Chapter 10) refers to the ability to hold information in memory and manipulate it in order to perform tasks (Baddeley, 2000). Many students with ADHD experience difficulty with working memory (Martinussen & Tannock, 2006).

In practice, this means that students with ADHD may have difficulty keeping the steps of instructions in their memory, especially if the directions are complex or involve multiple steps. Attention may be a problem because students may not focus on the teacher or may become distracted when instructions are given. Note also that there is evidence that suggests that when students' working memory is challenged (e.g., when directions are complex or there are a number of steps to remember) inattentive behavior increases (Kofler, Rapport, Bolden, Sarver, & Raiker, 2009). Some tips for giving effective directions include (Reid, 1999):

• *Get attention before giving directions.* Don't assume that students are attending even if they are making eye contact. Use physical proximity, touch, and eye contact to ensure attention.

• *Keep directions short and to the point.* Long, involved directions are difficult to remember and will cause children with ADHD to lose focus. Avoid giving multistep directions all at once. Instead break up directions into shorter chunks (e.g., "Get out your math book and turn to page 45."), wait for compliance (and reinforce it) and then continue with the next step.

• *Keep directions explicit.* Use simple appropriate language, provide examples, or model the task when possible. Refer to the specific behavior the student must perform (e.g., "Put your books in your desk and your workbook in your cubby." rather than "Clean up your desks.").

• *Give directions multiple times.* For example, first, give directions, second, paraphrase the directions, third, provide an additional cue/reminder by writing the directions on the blackboard or overhead. The written reminder eases the burden on working memory because students don't need to maintain directions in memory.

• *Check for understanding.* Ask the student to repeat the directions or to perform a part of the task (e.g., the student shows that she has the correct page open, and works one problem).

Many students with ADHD will exhibit some degree of problem behavior even under the best of circumstances. When this occurs teachers need to be able to administer effective reprimands (e.g., admonishments) and redirect students' behavior. Effective reprimands and redirection (Abramowitz & O'Leary, 1991):

• Should be delivered in a calm, unemotional manner (preferably privately, not publicly).
• Should be firmly stated (e.g., "Start your work now.").
• Should be brief and to the point, otherwise the attention may actually serve to reinforce the inappropriate behavior or draw attention from other students.
• Should be given as closely as possible after occurrence of the inappropriate behavior.
• Should avoid mixed messages (i.e., some praise and some reprimand) as this may actually reinforce the inappropriate behavior.

Note that the effectiveness of reprimands may be increased by use of close proximity, eye contact, and physical contact (e.g., a hand on the shoulder).

Sometimes even appropriate reprimands or redirections do not result in compliance. When a student does not respond quickly, exhibits resistance, or ignores the reprimand or redirection, teachers often make the mistake of repeating it, often multiple times (Barkley, 1997b). As the process repeats itself, teachers often grow frustrated and angry. Teachers then attempt to apply pressure by threatening negative consequences. Threatened consequences may be exaggerated because of anger, and students rarely comply. Teachers may also raise their voice or yell. Yelling is equally ineffective and actually tends to reduce the chances of compliance (Kapalka, 2005). Barkley (1997b) recommends that if a student is initially noncompliant, teachers should (1) repeat the reprimand or redirection one time, (2) warn the student of the consequences of noncompliance one time only, and (3) administer consequences if the student has not complied. Adopting this procedure helps teachers to remain calmer, and prevents a minor incident from escalating. Teachers are also more likely to select a plausible consequence that could actually be administered. Ideally, the consequences for noncompliance would be established beforehand (e.g., failing to comply would result in loss of computer free time). Research suggests that this procedure can significantly reduce noncompliant behaviors in the classroom (Kapalka, 2005).

INTERVENTIONS

Most students have little difficulty behaving appropriately in the classroom. For these students, the naturally occurring reinforcements in the classroom (e.g., teacher praise, a "gold star" on a paper) are sufficient to support and maintain appropriate behavior. This is not the case for students with ADHD. These students often will need additional behavioral interventions. Unfortunately many teachers have only limited training in the use of behavioral interventions and as a result the effects of their interventions may be limited (Fabiano & Pelham, 2003; Pfiffner et al., 2006). For these teachers who work with students with ADHD, additional training can increase confidence in their ability to successfully implement behavioral interventions (Arcia et al., 2000; Fabiano & Pelham, 2003). Note that under IDEA teachers have the right to receive training to develop the skills to work effectively with students with disabilities such as ADHD. In this section we present three interventions that can be effective with students with ADHD: token economy, response cost, and time-out.

Token Economy

A token economy (also referred to as "token reinforcement") is a positive reinforcement system that has demonstrated effectiveness for students with ADHD in the classroom (DuPaul & Weyandt, 2006). In a token economy, a child is given a token such as a poker chip or a tally mark when a desired behavior(s) occurs. Tokens can be exchanged later for a variety of tangible, social, or activity backup reinforcers. Note that, *in theory*, there is nothing inherently reinforcing about receiving a token. Tokens are analogous to money. Money has no intrinsic value itself; however, money can be exchanged at a later time for desired objects and activities. In practice, however, some students appear to find the actual tokens reinforcing and don't want to spend them. Token economies are practical for classroom use and can be maintained for long periods of time (Pfiffner et al., 2006). They are particularly well suited for students with ADHD because they allow teachers to provide reinforcers as soon as a behavior occurs. This eliminates any lag time between a student performing a behavior and him or her receiving reinforcement. We describe procedures for establishing a token economy based on those developed by Cooper, Heron, and Heward (2007).

Select Tokens

Frequently used tokens include washers, marbles, coupons, poker chips, tally marks, teacher initials, or punch cards. There are several criteria for selecting tokens. First, the token should be safe—it should not be harmful to the student. Avoid objects that a young child could swallow. Second, the teacher should control the tokens—students should not be able to bootleg tokens. Third, tokens should be durable because they may have to be used for an extended period of time, and they should be easy to handle. Fourth, tokens should be readily accessible to the teacher so that they can be dispensed immediately after the behavior occurs. A prospective token should be easy for the teacher to carry and handle.

Select Target Behaviors

There are several considerations for selecting target behaviors. First, behaviors should be well described using specific language so that they can be easily observed and counted. Second, the criterion for acceptable performance (task standard) should be stated so as to avoid any confusion or arguments between teacher and student as to whether the behavior was performed. Third, begin with a small number of behaviors. One or two is fine, and certainly no more than three to five. Targeting more behaviors may be confusing for a student and difficult for a teacher to manage. Be sure to include at least one or two behaviors that are easy for students to perform. It's critical for students to receive reinforcers frequently early on. This also lays the groundwork for including more difficult behaviors later. Fourth, ensure students have the prerequisite skills for performing the targeted behaviors or that the behaviors are already being performed at least to some extent. Remember that a token economy does not create new behaviors; it only changes the frequency of existing behaviors.

Make Rules and Post Rules

For a token economy to be effective, students must know the rules. There are several rules that should be stated in a token economy. First, procedures for dispensing tokens should be specified. For example, teachers may state that they circulate around the room and dispense tokens (or points) or may award them at specified times (e.g., at the end of each period). Second, teachers should describe how tokens are to be exchanged for backup reinforcers. For elementary students, this may entail having a "store" with backup reinforcers displayed at the end of every hour (this might be needed initially for young students), 15 minutes before lunch, 15 minutes at the end of the day, or 15 minutes at the end of the day on Friday. Note that reinforcers do not have to be tangible. Activity reinforcers (e.g., free reading, extra computer time) are also appropriate. For secondary students, a menu can be developed similar to ones used at restaurants. Third, consequences for students "bootlegging" tokens should be described. The most common way to deal with this problem is to confiscate a certain number of tokens. Fourth, in the case of younger students, inform students that they can play with the tokens for a specified amount of time, for example, the first 5 minutes of the day. This establishes the tokens as reinforcers. Later, a storage system can be used. Fifth, inform students of the policy for purchasing backup reinforcers. Sometimes students won't purchase backup reinforcers for a variety of reasons. Assuming that the backup items are reinforcing, a student may not purchase items because they don't have enough tokens. In this situation, state that items can be purchased on "layaway." Establish a "bank" where students may save their tokens until they are able to purchase the backup reinforcer. Conversely, for some students receiving tokens appears to be reinforcing in and of itself. These students enjoy "hoarding" tokens more than spending them. If receiving tokens maintains appropriate behavior, we do not see this as a problem. Hoarding could be a problem if a student earned enough tokens early in the day to purchase a backup reinforcer. The student could misbehave for the rest of the day yet still purchase a reinforcer. This problem can be dealt with by specifying that after the store is closed, everyone begins with zero tokens.

Establish Backup Reinforcers

Most token economies can use naturally occurring activities and events as backup reinforcers. For example, tokens can be used to buy time with a popular game, listening to music, having lunch with a favorite teacher or peer, or writing and delivering a note to a friend. A way to establish backup reinforcers is to use a reward menu. Two of the easiest and most effective ways to develop a menu of backup reinforcers is to ask students what they would like and to identify what students do when they have free access to do whatever they want. Students should be permitted to suggest items for a reward menu. Students should not be permitted to debate the cost (number of tokens) of the various rewards after prices have been established. Enlist students' participation in revising the reward menu frequently. Students can become bored with the same reinforcers day after day. Figure 9.2 shows an example of a reward menu.

Establish "Prices"

Initially the price of backup items should be low to provide immediate reinforcement for students. This is especially important for students with ADHD. Later on, the price of reinforcers can be raised. There are several considerations when setting the prices for reinforcers. First, make sure that the prices are low enough that students can buy at least some of the reinforcers. Second, some students may earn enough tokens to purchase backup items and still have tokens left over. Teachers may establish a "bank" where students can "deposit" leftover tokens. Students can be allowed (or encouraged) to save up for special "big ticket" items. Note that this can be an excellent learning activity. As the number of tokens students earn increases, the number of "big ticket" backup activities should also increase. Note that teacher should never loan students tokens! This is giving students a reward before they perform the desired behavior.

Field Test the System

Before actually implementing a token economy system, teachers should field test it. Over a period of 2 or 3 days teachers can tally the tokens they would award if the system was implemented. This will help teachers decide how many tokens to award for a behavior and to establish prices at an appropriate level.

Reinforcer	Time	Cost
Extra free time	10 minutes	20 tokens
Listening to music	10 minutes	20 tokens
Cutting and pasting	5 minutes	10 tokens
Art project	12 minutes	25 tokens
Borrowing a CD	48 hours	35 tokens
Watching a video	15 minutes	30 tokens
Playing a computer game	10 minutes	15 tokens
Line leader	—	10 tokens
Lunch with the teacher	10 minutes	25 tokens
Extra free-reading time	20 minutes	30 tokens
Putting on a puppet show	10 minutes	30 tokens
Choosing a game for the class	—	10 tokens

FIGURE 9.2. Sample reinforcer menu.

Implement the Token Economy

It's best to start with a few behaviors (even one behavior) and a simple system of awarding and redeeming tokens. Teachers can then build on firm understanding. Explain the system to students, be patient, and answer all students' questions. It is better to delay implementation than create confusion and frustration. Teachers should evaluate the effectiveness of the token economy. If there is no change in behavior, teachers should reconsider the target behaviors and/or the available reinforcers.

Response Cost

Response cost is an intervention that has been used successfully in the classroom with students with ADHD and is effective in reducing or eliminating inappropriate behaviors (Pelham & Fabiano, 2008; Pfiffner et al., 2006). It can be used alone or in combination with positive reinforcement-based interventions such as token economies. In response cost students lose a specific amount of a reinforcer as a consequence of performing an inappropriate behavior. Response cost is analogous to a traffic ticket (Maag, 2004). If you exceed the speed limit (the inappropriate behavior), you lose a specific amount of money (the reinforcer). A variation of response cost that is also useful is bonus response cost. In bonus response cost the student is given extra reinforcement (e.g., an extra 10 minutes of computer time at the end of the day). Every instance of the problem behavior results in the loss of a specified amount of the extra reinforcement (e.g., each time Fowler refused to comply with a request he loses 2 minutes of the extra computer time). Procedures for implementing response cost systems are straightforward. The steps are as follows (Cooper et al., 2007):

• *Conference with the student.* Tell the student that there is a problem with his or her behavior. Establish the specific behavior that is causing the problem. Remember that the student has to know the exact behavior that will result in a fine.

• *Establish the amount of the fine.* Tell the student how much the fine for each instance of the behavior will be. For example, each time Elwood fails to comply with an instruction he will lose 2 minutes of computer time or three tokens.

• *Establish means to communicate the fine.* The student must know when he or she has been fined. There are many ways to do this. For example, put 10 stars on the blackboard. Each time the student is fined, erase one star. Another means is to take a piece of paper and cut strips on one end. Each time a fine occurs you simply tear off one strip. Fines should be administered immediately following the inappropriate behavior. When a fine is administered it should be done in matter-of-fact, unemotional manner; this avoids inadvertently reinforcing the student by providing attention (Pfiffner et al., 2006).

- *Ensure reinforcement reserve.* Remember that student should not lose all reinforcement. It's desirable (but not always possible) for students to receive more reinforcers than they lose. If students' lose all reinforcement they have no reason to behave appropriately. However, students should not go below zero.

- *Evaluate effectiveness.* Keep records of the amount of problem behavior exhibited each day and graph the results. The effects of response cost should be apparent quickly. If there is not a rapid change in behavior within a week, teachers should examine their procedures to determine if response cost has been implemented correctly and consistently. If so another technique should be adopted. Therefore it's important to keep records to evaluate effectiveness.

Teachers also need to be aware of possible problems with response cost (Cooper et al., 2007; Maag, 2004). Sometimes teachers who use response cost can become overly focused on fining students and ignore or fail to reinforce appropriate behaviors. Some students may overreact to the loss of reinforcement. Response cost may not be appropriate if there is a potential for aggressive outbursts. Teachers also need to be aware that students may seek to avoid the situation where they lose reinforcement. For example, Jackie may resist or avoid group work because she loses tokens for arguing with group members. In cases like this, teachers should make sure that Jackie receives positive reinforcement for appropriate behavior she exhibits during group time. Sometimes communicating the fine can actually focus attention on the student and thus serve to maintain or actually increase the behavior. For example, each time Jordan leaves his seat without permission the teacher removes one poker chip from Jordan. The other students see this and make remarks or giggle. This attention could actually serve to increase the behavior. In cases like this teachers need to examine procedures carefully to ensure that they don't inadvertently reinforce inappropriate behaviors. Alternatively, the teacher could reinforce the class for ignoring or not reacting when Jordan loses tokens.

Time-Out

Time-out is an intervention that is commonly included as a component of treatment programs for students with ADHD (Fabiano et al., 2004). Note that time-out is shorthand for time-out from reinforcement. In time-out, a student is denied access to the opportunity to receive reinforcement for a set period of time (e.g., teacher or peer attention, tokens, being in the classroom). There are a number of different types of time-out procedures that have been used with students with ADHD (Pfiffner et al., 2006). Figure 9.3 shows descriptions of time-out procedures For more detailed descriptions, see Cooper et al. (2007) or Maag (2004). Time-out is typically reserved for behaviors that are serious problems to the classroom environment such as aggression or disruptive behavior (Pelham & Fabiano, 2008; Pfiffner et al., 2006). To implement time-out, Cooper et al. (2007) recommend the following procedures:

Seclusion
The student is removed from the classroom and placed in a specially designed isolation room or cubicle for a short period of time.

Exclusion
The student is removed from the classroom and placed outside (e.g., in the hallway), in a corner of the classroom, or in a carrel for a set period of time.

Contingent observation
The student is removed from, or not allowed to participate in, a class activity for a fixed period of time. The student remains in a position to observe the class but may neither participate nor receive any form of reinforcement.

Good behavior clock
The student has the opportunity to earn reinforcers for his- or herself and the class while a special "good behavior clock" is running. The clock runs when the student is on-task and otherwise behaving appropriately. If the student exhibits inappropriate behavior, the clock is stopped and the student cannot earn reinforers for a set period of time.

Planned ignoring
The student receives no attention (i.e., any physical, verbal, or visual interaction) for a set period of time following an inappropriate behavior.

Do a task
The student must go to an isolated desk facing a wall and complete a set amount of academic work (e.g., copying a passage). The teacher sets the amount of work (e.g., "Give me three sheets.") After the student completes the work he or she places it on the teacher's desk and rejoins the class.

FIGURE 9.3. Time-out procedures.

• *Ensure that the classroom has reinforcement value.* For time-out to be effective it is critical that time-in be reinforcing. If the student receives little or no reinforcement for being in the classroom, then time-out will have no effect in reducing behavior because the student is not being removed from reinforcement. Before implementing time-out teachers need to ensure that the student is receiving regular reinforcement. One way to do this is to systematically reinforce an appropriate behavior that is incompatible with the problem behavior. For example, for each 10-minute interval that Joe keeps his hands and feet to himself and refrains from aggressive verbal challenges he receives five tokens (along with regular teacher praise).

• *Decide on the type of time-out.* Determine the appropriate type of time-out procedure. Note that the exclusion and seclusion levels should be reserved for very serious behaviors. These levels of time-out require additional safeguards and include addressing legal, administrative, and ethical practice concerns (see Cooper et al., 2007; Maag, 2004).

- *Communicate the problem behavior.* Meet with the student and explain the behavior that is a problem. It is important that the student understands exactly what behavior(s) will result in a time-out. Use specific examples and nonexamples. For example, yelling "Get out of my face!" would result in a time-out, but saying "Please stop." would be appropriate.

- *Establish time-out procedures and rules.* After the student understands the problem behavior the teacher explains time-out procedures and rules. The time-out procedures refer to how the time-out will be implemented. For example, the student will go to the time-out carrel in the back of the room. No materials (e.g., books, pencils, or potential playthings) are allowed. The student sits facing the back of the carrel. The student is not to turn around to face the class, call out, or talk. After the student is seated, the teacher starts a timer. When the timer goes off the student may rejoin the class. If the student violates procedures the timer is restarted and the time-out begins over.

- *Evaluate effectiveness.* Teachers should assess whether time-out is effective at reducing problem behavior. Teachers should keep records of the frequency of the problem behavior before and after time-out. If time-out is effective there should be a rapid decrease in the frequency of the problem behavior. The teacher should also keep a time-out log (Nelson & Rutherford, 1983) that includes (1) the student's name, (2) a description of the problem leading to time-out, (3) the time of day the student was placed in time-out, (4) the total duration of each time-out, (5) the type of time-out employed, and (6) a description of the student's behavior in time-out. It's very important that teachers monitor how frequently time-outs are administered. If time-out is effective, then the number of time-outs administered should *decrease*. If the time-out procedure is not reducing the problem behavior *it should be discontinued*.

There are potential problems that can occur when implementing time-outs. Students may resist complying (e.g., refuse to go to the time-out carrel) or not follow time-out procedures (e.g., talks with classmates). If this occurs teachers should consider (1) reducing the length of time-out for complying with procedures or providing a reinforcer for compliance; (2) adding additional time for additional infractions (e.g., calling out to classmates results in an additional 2 minutes); (3) adding response cost so that the student loses other reinforcers for noncompliance; or (4) the student serves the time-out after school (assuming school personnel are available to supervise and the student is timed-out of a desirable activity; Pfiffner et al., 2006). Time-out should be used consistently. When the problem behavior occurs, time-out should be administered. If time-out is used inconsistently students may be confused about whether the behavior is acceptable or not (Cooper et al., 2007). Time-out can be misused. Teachers may use time-out for minor behavior problems (e.g., talking out; Maag, 2004). Because this has the effect of removing the student from the classroom, time-out may actually serve as a reinforcer for the teacher.

Remember that time-out should only be used for serious behavior problems that can't be ignored or dealt with by other means. Finally, time-out may not be appropriate for cases in which the student refuses to perform academic tasks (Pfiffner et al., 2006). As we noted in the previous chapter, in these situations, time-out may result in students being able to avoid the task and thus actually serve to reinforce the behavior.

SUMMING UP

Educators often make a point of how unique all students are. Unfortunately, in practice all too frequently this does not extend to the classroom. Instead there is a "one size fits all" mentality that requires students who vary dramatically on numerous factors (e.g., academic skills, attention span, compliance, activity level, ability to focus) to function within a standardized setting despite the fact that this desire is unrealistic in many cases. There is clear evidence that students with ADHD can function effectively in the classroom when provided accommodation and effective interventions. Here are some points to remember.

- ✓ Behavior management techniques are effective with students with ADHD in reducing problem behaviors and increasing appropriate behaviors.
- ✓ Start with positive reinforcement first. Try to catch students being good and reinforce the behavior. Remember that the goal should be to teach students appropriate behaviors and increase their frequency.
- ✓ Negative reinforcement (e.g., reprimands, admonishment) is necessary, but should be used sparingly and effectively.
- ✓ Punishment is often needed, but should be used judiciously for serious problem behaviors. Remember that punishment doesn't create new appropriate behaviors.
- ✓ Students with ADHD need powerful reinforcers that are frequently delivered in close proximity to the behavior. To avoid satiation, teachers need to rotate reinforcers or provide a number of options (reinforcement menus).
- ✓ Make the physical environment more conducive by reducing potential distractions and enabling appropriate physical activity. Monitor students frequently and provide them with feedback on their behavior.
- ✓ Set up stable, predictable classroom routines and maintain them. Teach the routines and reinforce students for compliance. Establish procedures for everyday activities; teach the procedures and reinforce students for performing activities correctly.
- ✓ Use class rules to establish expectations. Make sure students know the rules and understand them. Reinforce students for following rules. Consequences for rule violations should be swift and sure.

✓ Effective reprimands and redirections are brief and to the point. Don't repeat reprimands, yell, or get angry and allow a minor problem to escalate. Warn students of consequences and administer consequences immediately if the student fails to comply.

✓ Don't assume students with ADHD heard or understood directions. Remember that problems following directions may be related to forgetting directions.

✓ Interventions such as token economy, response cost, and time-out are often necessary.

CHAPTER 10

Academics and ADHD

If you give me a lever and a place to stand
I can move the world.
                                    —ARCHIMEDES

Academic deficits are commonplace among students with ADHD. They are evident early and tend to persist throughout students' academic careers (Breslau et al., 2009; Galéra, Melchior, Chastang, Bouvard, & Fombonne, 2009). The deficits are often pronounced. On average, the academic progress of children with ADHD is about 25% lower than their peers in reading and math (Frazier et al., 2007). Many possible explanations for these deficits have been proposed. The association between LD and ADHD no doubt accounts for some of the deficits (Cantwell & Baker, 1991). The high incidence of language impairments, which affects students' ability to quickly and efficiently process verbal information, could also negatively affect academic outcomes (Schnoes et al., 2006).

It's also possible that ADHD itself does not interfere with the ability to learn, but instead affects the "availability for learning" (Silver, 1990, p. 396). That is, inattention and impulsivity interfere with students' ability to concentrate, maintain effort, and reflect before acting, and thus adversely affect learning (Breslau et al., 2009; Currie & Stabile, 2006). Associated emotional and behavioral problems may also interfere with learning. It's also possible that the relationship between ADHD and academic difficulties is due to the fact that school-related problems are required for a diagnosis of ADHD; thus students with serious academic difficulties are more likely to be referred and diagnosed as having ADHD (Loe & Feldman, 2007).

Academic underachievement has serious consequences. Students who fail to master basic skills in the early grades may fail to graduate or drop out of school, and are less likely to access postsecondary education (U.S. Department of Education, 2005). As a result, these students may be economically disadvantaged because they lack the proficiency in science, technology, math, and reading expected for employment in well-paying jobs (U.S. Department of Education, 2005). Given the serious problems associated with academic deficits, one would expect that academic interventions for students with ADHD would be the focus of intense research. Unfortunately, this is not the case. A recent review found only 41 studies of academic interventions for students with ADHD (Trout, Lienemann, Reid, & Epstein, 2007), and in many of these studies academics was not the primary focus. To make matters worse, the existing research was described as a "hodgepodge of studies with no systematic replication and extension" (p. 222). As a result, we are not well informed as to how best to improve academic outcomes for students with ADHD (Loe & Feldman, 2007).

Though our knowledge base is not deep, there have been some encouraging developments and today academics are receiving increased attention. In this chapter we discuss how teachers can help students to improve their academic performance. First, we discuss two core problem areas—working memory and executive function deficits—and how they can adversely affect academic performance. Second, we discuss how teachers can address the problems of working memory and executive functions. We use an existing, validated instructional model to provide a framework and provide examples from research. Third, we present effective accommodations that can help to create an instructional environment that is more conducive to students with ADHD. Finally, we discuss peer tutoring, an effective instructional intervention for students with ADHD.

CORE PROBLEM AREAS

Students with ADHD often have deficits in working memory and executive functions (Martinussen, Hayden, Hogg-Johnson, & Tannock, 2005). This is significant because both working memory and executive functions are highly correlated with academic outcomes in students with ADHD (Alloway, Gathercole, & Elliott, 2010; Biederman et al., 2000; Clark, Prior, & Kinsella, 2002) and in the general population (Alloway, Gathercole, Kirkwood, & Elliot, 2009; Meltzer, 2007). Students with good working memory who can effectively use executive functions tend to be higher academic achievers. Problems in these areas are also thought to be related to the core problem areas associated with ADHD (i.e., inattention, impulsivity, and hyperactivity; Barkley, 2006). In this section we discuss working memory and executive functions and how they affect academics. Note that although we discuss each separately, in practice teachers need to consider both areas because problems in either area can affect the other.

Working Memory

Working memory refers to "a limited capacity system allowing the temporary storage and manipulation of information necessary for such complex cognitive tasks as comprehension, learning, and reasoning" (Baddeley, 2000, p. 418). The information can be either verbal (e.g., words, the steps in long division) or visuospatial (e.g., the layout of a football field, the relative position of two cities on a map). Working memory functions as a mental workspace where we can *temporarily* store limited amounts of information for use (e.g., to perform mental arithmetic; Alloway, 2006). The temporary nature of working memory is a critical factor for teachers to understand. Information in working memory is maintained only for a matter of seconds and if information is lost it is not retrievable. Working memory is not synonymous with short-term memory, although there is some overlap. The key difference is that working memory involves *processing or using* information to accomplish a task. It helps us to allocate and direct attention (e.g., shift between two aspects of a task such as the steps in long division and the product of multiplying two numbers; Engle, 2002). It also helps us to resist distractions (Conway, Cowan, & Bunting, 2001). The capacity to resist distraction is especially important during tasks that require prolonged attention. Here are two exercises that demonstrate the difference between short-term memory and working memory.

1. **Study the nonsense word below for few seconds, then cover it.**

OBECALP

   Task 1. Say the letters in order.

   Task 2. Take another quick look at the nonsense word, then cover it again. Now try to reverse the letters and pronounce the resulting word. For example, the word *flog* would be *golf.*

2. **Study the list of numbers below for a few seconds then cover them.**

4 7 2 5 4 9 6 4 8 7

   Task 3. Remember the order of numbers in the list. Think for a second about where you went on your last vacation and answer the following questions. Who did you go with? What was your most memorable experience? Did you purchase any souvenirs? How did you travel? Now remember the number of days you spent on the vacation. Multiply the number of days you spent on vacation by the last digit in your social security number. Now add the first number in the list and the sixth number in the list. Finally, multiply the sum of the first number and the sixth number by the seventh number in the list.

Hopefully you noticed that there was a considerable difference between the three tasks. Task 1 is a short-term memory task. All that is required is to store and retrieve the letters in order. There was no requirement that the information be processed or manipulated in any way. Task 2, on the other hand, required working memory and should have been more difficult because the demands are greater. First, you were required to remember the order of the letters. Next you had to reverse the order, which required you to systematically take the last letter, put it in first position, and maintain it in memory while retrieving the next-to-last letter and placing it second, and so on. Thus you had to remember the original order of letters while constructing the reverse order. Then you needed to maintain the reversed order of letters while you called up information needed to pronounce the new word (e.g., letter sounds, rules for syllabication). Finally you had to apply the information on how to pronounce the word. Task 3 is even more difficult. The amount of information is greater (nine digits) and is near the limit of what most people can easily maintain in working memory. The processing is also difficult. However, what distinguishes it is that a great deal of information and processing were irrelevant to the goal of the task (e.g., thinking about the vacation). It's quite likely that the irrelevant information storage and processing caused many people to forget the order of numbers in the list and therefore fail the task. At the least this interference probably caused the task to be much more stressful.

The tasks illustrate three important aspects of working memory that teachers should understand. First, working memory is limited. We can store only a small amount of information in working memory at any one time. If we are at maximum capacity and need to add another piece of information we can't temporarily expand capacity. Instead something must be dropped from storage. Second, working memory is temporary; once information is gone it is lost forever. For example, if while trying to reverse the order of OBECALP you had finished reversing the first three letters but were then interrupted, you would most likely have lost the information and would have to start again from the beginning. Third, if working memory becomes overloaded (i.e., the amount of information that must be stored is large and manipulations are complex), it can lead to task failure or other problems (e.g., failure to monitor performance or to detect errors in performance). The final task was intended to do just that by making more demands on storage and processing and introducing a number of extraneous bits of information and processing.

Working Memory Problems in the Classroom

Problems with working memory have direct implications for the classroom. Students with working memory deficits have difficulty with tasks that require holding large amounts of information in mind (Gathercole, Lamont, & Alloway, 2006). This in turn affects academically important skills such as listening and reading comprehension, mental computation, and written composition (Gathercole et al., 2006; Lorch, Berthiaume, Milich, & van den Broek, 2007). For example, to understand a text passage students must hold pieces of information in mind and establish links between the different ideas or content presented (e.g., main ideas and supporting details). Students with ADHD often report forgetting what they read at the top of the page when they get to the middle of the page, and forgetting what they read in the middle of the page by the end of the page (Barkley, 2006). As a result, students may be unable to answer even simple questions about a text. The same problems are evident in listening comprehension (Lorch et al., 2007). Students with working memory problems often have problems remembering and following directions. For example, if the teacher directs the students to get out their math books, turn to page 43, and do the odd-numbered long divisions problems in the right-hand column, the student with ADHD may get out the math book and turn to page 43, but fail to maintain the information on what problems to do. As a result the student might ask the teacher what to do, or sit and do nothing because critical information that would help him or her to accomplish the task was forgotten (Gathercole et al., 2006). Note that from the teacher's perspective this may appear to be the result of inattention (i.e., the student didn't pay attention to the directions) or laziness when in reality it was a working memory problem.

Complex tasks that require sequential steps (e.g., writing an essay or performing a science lab experiment) can be particularly troublesome because they involve significant demands both on storing and processing information. Note that even apparently simple tasks can pose serious demands on working memory. Gathercole et al. (2006) described the difficulties students with poor working memories encountered when asked to copy a sentence. Though seemingly simple, the task required students to remember the order of words in the sentence, the word to be copied, its spelling, and their place in the word while writing it, and to also generate the actual text. As a result, students made numerous errors. They would omit words, repeat a word, or substitute words that were not in the sentence. They might also be able to start the task successfully and write down the first few words, but be unable to remember the remainder. Note that at first glance these errors might appear to be careless errors or sloppy work. Tasks that require a student to rapidly shift focus between numerous aspects of a task can be extremely difficult. For example, writing a story requires attending to the mechanics of spelling and grammar, including necessary story elements (e.g., characters and setting), and using appropriate and interesting vocabulary. This places huge demands on working memory. Other tasks such as math problem solving place similar demands. Classroom teachers need to be sensitive to working memory demands because if working memory capacity is exceeded little or no learning will occur. Additionally, when demands on working memory increase, students with ADHD tend to exhibit increased levels of inattentive behavior (Kofler et al., 2009).

In addition to purely academic demands, teachers should also be aware that anxiety can have an effect on working memory (Owens, Stevenson, Norgate, & Hadwin, 2008). High levels of anxiety (e.g., worries about failure or negative evaluations) and the task-irrelevant thoughts that accompany high levels of anxiety can lead to diminished working memory capacity. In essence, high anxiety acts to drain cognitive resources. This in turn reduces students' ability to accomplish tasks in an efficient or effective manner. For example, if a student's working memory is filled with thoughts such as "I'll never get this done," "I can't do this," "I'm so bad at this," there is that much less space for task-related information that would actually help the student perform the task.

Executive Functions

Executive functions (EFs) are cognitive processes necessary for complex goal-directed behavior; EFs include metacognitive knowledge regarding strategies and tasks (e.g., knowledge of how a strategy can help or that different tasks require different strategies) and self-regulatory processes such as planning and self-monitoring (Meltzer, 2007). Students with ADHD often have EF deficits (Biederman et al., 2000). This is a serious concern because EFs involve planning, organizing, maintaining effort, and monitoring activities (Meltzer, 2007), all of which are necessary for academic success; and EF deficits negatively affect academic performance (Clark, Prior, & Kinsella, 2002). Thus, there is good reason to suspect that EF deficits play a significant role in the academic problems of students with ADHD. Three types of EFs pose serious problems for students with ADHD: (1) adopting a planful, strategic approach to academic tasks, (2) goal setting, and (3) persistence or maintaining effort on a task. In the following sections we describe the problems experienced in these areas.

Planning and Strategies

Students with ADHD seldom adopt a planful approach to tasks. They will often impulsively begin a task even when they have been directly instructed to plan the task before starting (e.g., Jacobson & Reid, 2010). They seldom analyze a task to determine the actions needed to accomplish it, and also may have difficulty effectively combining the actions needed to accomplish a task; thus constructing a plan or a strategy may be difficult (Barkley, 2006). Even when they do develop a plan they may be unaware of its shortcomings and may not actually follow the plan they have developed. For example, Kliegel, Ropeter, and Mackinlay (2006) asked 20 students with ADHD to develop and implement a plan to complete a computer game. All of the students claimed to have developed a plan; however, only three students were able to develop an effective plan, and only six students actually followed the plans they developed. Thus students with ADHD not only failed to develop effective plans but also failed to use the plans that they developed. Students with ADHD may struggle even when an optimal plan is obvious. When Kofman, Larson, and Mostofsky (2008) gave students with ADHD a copying task consisting of high- and low-point items, they found that students had great problems formulating an effective plan for maximizing points. Students could have scored the most points simply by copying only the high-point items, but most students with ADHD were unable to independently derive even this simple plan. Lack of a planful approach to academic tasks can result in erratic performance on tasks and work that is disorganized or appears sloppy.

Students with ADHD are also less likely to spontaneously use strategies (Hamlett et al., 1987). For example, when students with ADHD were asked to study some cards for a few moments and then tested to see how well they recalled the location of matching cards, they did not utilize strategies (e.g., chunking, verbal rehearsal) to help them remember locations. Students with ADHD also tend to adopt strategies that are easy but that also are less effective (O'Neill & Douglas, 1991). For example, when asked to remember and summarize a story, most students with ADHD tended to choose skimming as their strategy as opposed to a more effortful but effective approach such as rereading or taking notes (O'Neill & Douglas, 1996). When tasks call for pronounced and continued strategic processing, the deficit in strategy use for ADHD students becomes even more obvious (O'Neill & Douglas, 1996). For example, when asked to memorize word lists, students with ADHD often chose single-word repetition rather than more effortful and effective strategies such as grouping similar words into sets and repeating the sets. Even when provided with an effective strategy, students with ADHD may fail to employ it consistently (Kofman et al., 2008). Problems with strategy use (i.e., lack of a strategy or use of inefficient or ineffective strategies) can result in students performing below their potential.

Goal Setting

Students with ADHD may be unaware of the goal associated with an academic task or have difficulty maintaining a goal in working memory (Barkley, 2006). Moreover, some students with ADHD may adopt maladaptive performance-avoidance goals (in which the goal is to avoid appearing incompetent) that can serve to inhibit performance (Barron, Evans, Baranik, Serpell, & Buvinger, 2006). This is a serious problem because goals help to guide behaviors, provide feedback on progress, and enhance motivation (Schunk, 1990). Additionally, research suggests that goal setting can improve the academic productivity of students with ADHD (Konrad, Fowler, Walker, Test, & Wood, 2007). Without a specific and appropriate goal(s) in place, it will be difficult for students with ADHD to structure their behavior to effectively accomplish tasks. In the classroom, lack of goal knowledge may be reflected in an aimless (literally) approach to a task or in avoidance behavior (in the case of performance avoidance goals).

Persistence

Students with ADHD often struggle to maintain effort, especially if a task is repetitive or boring (Barkley, 2006). Compared to their peers without ADHD, they are more likely to quit a task. For example, when students with ADHD were asked to do simple word-finding puzzles, some of which were solvable and some of which were not, the students with ADHD gave up much more often than those without ADHD regardless of the difficulty of the puzzle (Milich & Greenwell, 1991; Milich & Okazaki, 1991). Even a small challenge may cause a child with ADHD to quit. In part this may be due to problems with regulation of emotion caused by frustration (Walcott & Landau, 2004). Students with ADHD report less "mood repair" when they experience frustration (i.e., they did not attempt to overcome their feelings of frustration), which makes it more likely for them to give up on a task when they began to feel frustrated (Scime & Norvilitis, 2006).

One source of frustration is lack of performance monitoring (Barkley, 2006). Students with ADHD do not effectively monitor their performance on tasks. They are often unaware of how well or how poorly they are performing a task or of their progress (or lack of progress) on a task. This in turn can lead to frustration that can negatively affect persistence. Another related problem is *positive illusory bias*. This refers to the tendency of students with ADHD to rate their performance much higher than is actually warranted (Hoza et al., 2004). This in turn can lead to unrealistic appraisals of their performance or a distorted perception of ability. It's possible that positive illusory bias serves a self-protective function (Waschbusch, Craig, Pelham, & King, 2007). However, it can be a serious problem for teachers because a student who does not understand or recognize that there is a problem is not likely to be willing or motivated to address the problem (Hoza et al., 2004). Additionally, positive illusory bias may lead to other maladaptive self-protection behaviors such as self-handicapping in which a student engages in self-sabotage (e.g., watched movies on the Internet till 2:00 A.M. the night before an exam) to provide him- or herself with an excuse for poor performance (Waschbusch et al., 2007).

EFFECTIVE INSTRUCTION FOR STUDENTS WITH ADHD

As we noted earlier, problems with adopting a planful strategic approach along with problems with EFs (which make it difficult to self-regulate behavior) are at the heart of many academic problems experienced by students with ADHD. These problems put students with ADHD at a tremendous disadvantage because adopting a planful strategic approach to a task is one of the hallmarks of a successful learner. One promising approach to the problem of the lack of a planful strategic approach is very straightforward: teach students how to plan and use strategies and to better organize their behavior. Teachers should treat planning and strategy use as skills that can be taught. There are several reasons why this approach holds promise.

First, strategy instruction has been demonstrated to be effective with students with LD (Swanson & Sachse-Lee, 2000). These students share common characteristics with students with ADHD (e.g., difficulty focusing attention, problems with persistence) and many students with LD also have comorbid ADHD.

Second, strategy instruction includes procedures that directly address problems with working memory and EF deficits. For example, strategy instruction incorporates explicit goal setting and self-regulation procedures (self-regulation procedures are discussed in detail in Chapter 11) that are known to be effective with students with ADHD (Reid, Trout, & Schartz, 2005). Note also that the procedures used in strategy instruction often are helpful for all students, not just those with ADHD.

Third, there is a small but growing body of research that has shown that strategy instruction can dramatically improve the academic performance of students with ADHD. Several studies have used strategy instruction successfully with students with ADHD (e.g., Jacobson & Reid, 2010; Lienemann & Reid, 2008; Mason, Kubina, & Taft, 2009; Reid & Lienemann, 2006b; Rogevich & Perin, 2008). In a number of cases student's performance was actually normalized (i.e., at or above the average for students in their grade).

On the surface teaching a student a strategy might appear simple: have the student memorize the steps in the strategy and then require the student to use the strategy. This approach is unlikely to be successful because effective strategy instruction goes well beyond rote memorization (Harris & Pressley, 1991). As we noted previously, students with ADHD often have problems using strategies. This should not be too surprising because problems with impulsivity and inattention are core symptoms of ADHD. Thus, it is very difficult for students with ADHD to approach a task in a strategic manner. Even when they are aware of effective strategies, they tend to immediately leap into a task with little or no consideration for how best to accomplish the task. As a result, their efforts may be disorganized and ineffective. Even more troubling is that when students with ADHD are provided with an effective strategy and prompted to use it, they may simply stop using the strategy in the midst of a task (Kofman et al., 2008).

Effective strategy instruction requires a process that is sensitive to the problems students with ADHD are likely to experience when learning and using strategies. Additionally, effective strategy instruction requires teachers to address the affective (e.g., anxiety, negative emotions), behavioral (e.g., difficulty maintaining focus), and cognitive (e.g., lack of background knowledge) needs of the learner (Lienemann & Reid, 2008). Attention to these needs is important for any student, but it is *critical* for students with ADHD who are likely to experience problems in some or all of these areas. This is why teachers must take a strategic, planful approach to instruction with students with ADHD using a model such as self-regulated strategy development (SRSD) to guide their instruction. In this section we describe how teachers can use procedures commonly incorporated in strategy instruction with students with ADHD. We first discuss the nature of strategies and why they can be helpful for students with ADHD. Then we present specific procedures using a well-validated strategy instruction model—SRSD—as a framework. We chose SRSD because it is a widely used strategy instruction model that has been employed effectively in several studies with students with ADHD.

Strategies: What and Why

A strategy can be defined as a series of ordered steps that allows one to accomplish a task (Reid & Lienemann, 2006a). Strategies are beneficial in that they help to structure and focus effort. In practice unstructured effort is a problem for students with ADHD. They may want to perform a task, but fail because they are unable to effectively focus their efforts. For example, after being asked to write an essay, one young student with ADHD worked for nearly 20 minutes trying to complete the task. He grew increasingly frustrated. Finally, after having produced only a few disconnected sentences, he put down his pencil and said sadly, "I want to, but I don't know how." The value of a strategy for students with ADHD is that it shows them how. An effective strategy provides a road map for how to effectively accomplish a task. The steps in a strategy literally guide a student through what is needed to accomplish a task. Having an effective strategy to use to attack a task may actually help students with EFs (Reid & Harris, 1993). For example, if a student knows what steps to follow to compute the solution to a multiplication problem he or she may be able to monitor progress through the process or detect procedural errors. In contrast, if a student has only a hazy idea of what process to follow, it's unlikely that any monitoring or error detection will occur because the student would not know what to monitor or how to detect a procedural error (because he or she had no procedure to follow).

A strategies-based approach is also useful for students with ADHD because it breaks up complex, amorphous tasks into a series of simpler and more do-able tasks. For example, for many students "doing a book report" might seem to be an extremely difficult, ill-defined, or even threatening task. The task becomes much more approachable if it is broken down into its components, such as: (1) Go to the library and pick out a book, (2) Read the book, (3) While you read jot down notes on interesting parts of the book, (4) Take your notes and make an outline, (5) Use your outline to write your rough draft, (6) Revise the rough draft to make your final report. Note that any of the steps could be further broken down if needed. For example, step 3 could be broken down into (a) Write down the main events in the story, the main characters, setting, and time the story took place; (b) Write down three reasons you liked (or didn't like) the story; (c) For each reason provide an explanation. Breaking down the task also reduces the amount of information students need to attend to at any one time. This in turn reduces the load on working memory (Alloway, 2006).

Instructional Procedures

The SRSD model is a six-stage approach to instruction. The stages may be combined, reordered, or even omitted if need be. The stages are also recursive, that is, a stage introduced in one lesson will commonly be revisited in subsequent lessons. Each stage has important aspects that are relevant to students with ADHD. In this section we present the SRSD stages in the order that they are commonly used. We explain what occurs at each stage and provide specific examples of problems that could affect students with ADHD. For more details on using the SRSD model, see Reid and Lienemann (2006a) or visit *www.unl.edu/csi/index.shtml* for a website devoted to strategy instruction.

Develop and Activate Background Knowledge

This is typically the first stage of instruction. Here the teacher determines whether the student has the necessary preskills to use a strategy. For example, before teaching a student a long division strategy, the teacher might assess the student's multiplication and subtraction skills. If, for example, the student had serious deficits in multiplication, he or she would find performing long division very difficult. To address this problem the teacher might provide additional instruction in multiplication, and delay instruction in long division, or help the student compensate for a multiplication deficit by providing a times table. Preskill assessment is extremely important for students with ADHD because many students will have serious deficits in core academic areas, such as reading, math, and written expression (Frazier et al., 2007; Mayes, Calhoun, & Crowell, 2000). For example, elementary students with ADHD often lack knowledge of the basic elements required for narrative texts (e.g., character, setting, plot) that results in poor-quality stories (Reid & Lienemann, 2006b). For this reason teachers might want to provide instruction in the elements of a story very early on.

Discuss the Strategy

In this stage the instructor (1) introduces the strategy to the student, (2) reviews the student's current performance, and (3) enlists the student's willing cooperation. Note that although we discuss the steps separately in practice, there may be considerable overlap (e.g., when discussing current performance instructors may also work toward enlisting willing cooperation). Introducing the strategy is straightforward. For example, to introduce the RAP strategy (Schumaker, Denton, & Deshler, 1984) the instructor tells the student about the strategy (e.g., "This is the RAP strategy. It can help you to remember what you read.") and presents the steps in the strategy. For instance, each letter in RAP stands for a step in the strategy: Read a paragraph, Ask yourself what is the main idea and two important details, Put the information in your own words. The instructor also discusses what the student will do at each step. At this stage the instructor will often provide prompts or other supports (see Figure 10.1). The prompt card serves to remind the student of the steps in the strategy. External prompts and cues are helpful for students with ADHD because they reduce demands on working memory (Gathercole et al., 2006). Later, the prompts can be faded and eventually phased out.

Next the instructor discusses the student's current level of performance. The instructor establishes that there is a problem with the student's performance. For example, the teacher might go over the student's grades on the weekly social studies tests, and note that the student got only 50% of the answers correct. In practice, using graphs to present performance levels can be particularly useful because the visual representation can be convincing. For instance, Lienmann and Reid (2008) provided students with a graph showing how many essay parts (out of a total of eight possible) that they included on their essays. Note that establishing current performance levels is especially important if there is a positive illusory bias. At this point instructors often work with the student to set a performance goal. For example, the students in Lienemann and Reid's (2008) study had a goal of writing an essay containing all eight elements. Explicit goal setting is extremely important for two reasons.

The Reading RAP!
Read each paragraph carefully
Ask myself, "What was the main idea and two details?"
Put it into my own words

The Reading RAP!
Read
Ask
Put

The Reading RAP!
R
A
P

FIGURE 10.1. Cue card for RAP strategy with fading.

First, many students may not realize the goal of academic tasks (e.g., the purpose of reading a chapter is to understand and remember the content). Understanding the goal of a task helps to guide behavior. Second, students with ADHD often have difficulty maintaining goals in working memory (Barkley, 2006); thus they literally may forget the ultimate purpose of a task. For these reasons the instructor should establish an explicit goal(s), regularly discuss the goal with the student, stress why the goal is important, and note progress toward the goal. The idea is to make the goal salient so that when students attempt a task they will remember the ultimate goal of the task. Teachers may also find that goals can be extremely motivating for students and may help to maintain high performance levels (Lienemann & Reid, 2008).

The final task of this stage is to enlist students' willing cooperation to learn and use the strategy. Instructors should literally "sell" the strategy to students as a tool that will help them to better perform a task. Teachers should be energetic and positive about the strategy; however, they should also be realistic (e.g., teachers shouldn't promise that using the strategy will put a student on the honor roll overnight). One effective way to sell a strategy is simply to tell students that it has helped many students just like themselves. Getting students to "buy in" to using a strategy is critical. If students are to use the study independently they must believe in and be committed to using the strategy. Instructors may even write up a "contract" in which the student agrees to learn to use the strategy.

There is one other important component to this step. Instructors should stress a positive, "can-do" attitude. They should stress that if the students use the strategy and give their best effort they will be successful at the task. This is important to help to prevent or alleviate any problems caused by anxiety regarding a task. This is a very real concern because many students with ADHD have experienced failure or difficulties with academic tasks. Remember that high levels of anxiety can detrimentally affect working memory. If a student's working memory is filled with anxious thoughts (e.g., "I can't do this!"), there is no room for constructive thought (e.g., the steps in the strategy). It's very important for teachers to consider the affective/emotional aspects of instruction. If a student is extremely anxious about a task, doubts his or her ability, or is focused on failure, it will affect his or her performance. This may be every bit as important as preskill development.

Model the Strategy

Using a strategy effectively might appear to be straightforward—simply go through each step in turn. In practice, however, it's a bit more complicated. For students to be able to use a strategy effectively they should have metacognitive knowledge regarding the strategy. For example, students should know why they are doing each step in the strategy, and what they should be thinking about when they do the step (Reid & Lienemann, 2006a). Lack of metacognitive knowledge of strategy use among students with ADHD is well documented (e.g., O'Neill & Douglas, 1991, 1996). The effects of lack of metacognitive knowledge are also documented. For example,

Cornoldi and colleagues (Cornoldi, Barbieri, Gaiani, & Zocchi, 1999) compared the performance of students with ADHD to control students using a memory task. The memory task consisted of a grid of small pictures of common objects. On each grid, half the objects could be categorized, and the other half could not. When students with ADHD were shown that some items belonged to the same category, taught that knowing the category would make it easier to remember those items, and provided with a demonstration of how to effectively categorize items, they performed as well as control students on the memory task.

Modeling can help to provide metacognitive knowledge by exposing the student to the thought processes of a skilled learner as he or she uses the strategy or performs a task. One way to provide this knowledge is through modeling a task using the think-aloud procedure (Reid & Lienemann, 2006a). In this procedure the instructor performs a task or uses a strategy and simultaneously verbalizes his or her thought processes. Note that an effective model involves much more than simply "skill stepping" (i.e., going through each step in a strategy). The value in the think-aloud procedure is the extent to which the instructor can provide the metacognitive knowledge associated with each step in the strategy (e.g., the how's and why's of the strategy). Figure 10.2 shows an example of skill stepping and modeling for a simple math problem.

Skills step	Modeling
First I'll add the 1's column.	What is it I have to do? Okay, this is a two-digit addition problem; I know it's addition because of the "+" sign. That tells me how to add. I know how to do this! I need to remember to follow the steps in my strategy and remember my basic facts.
Now I'll write the 5 and carry the 1.	First I need to start in the 1's column and add those. If I don't start at the 1's column I'll get the wrong answer! The 1's are on the right-hand side. I'll make a little mark to help me remember.
Now I'll add the numbers in the 10's column.	Okay, I'm ready to add the first two numbers. Did I get a two-digit number? Because if I do I need to carry the 10's digit to the next column, to the 10's column. Yep, "15" has two digits. I need to remember to write the numbers down correctly too. I only write one digit down under the line. The one I write down is the "5" 'cause that's in the 1's column. I need to be careful to write the "5" down under the 1's column. If I don't I can get my numbers messed up and get the wrong answer. Now what do I do with the "1." Oh, yes, I have to carry that number. I'll write it down above the 10's column of the problem. That way I'll remember that I've carried.
Finally, I'll write the answer	Now, what do I do next? I know, I need to add all the 10's digits that I have, the two in the original problem, and the one that I carried. I'm almost done, now all I need to do is write down the answer. I need to remember to keep my numbers lined up. I'll write them carefully. I knew I could do it. I took my time, used my strategy, and tried hard and I got the right answer.

FIGURE 10.2. Skill steps and modeling for adding 26 + 19. From Reid and Lienemann (2006). Copyright 2006 by The Guilford Press. Reprinted by permission.

Memorize the Strategy

It is very important for students to be able to recall the steps in a strategy quickly and accurately. After all, as one student noted, "If you can't remember it you can't use it" (Karen Harris, personal communication). The student should also be able to relate exactly what he or she needs to do for each step in the process. Often strategies will use mnemonics to help students remember the steps (e.g., RAP). Memorizing the strategy begins early on. Instructors discuss the need to memorize the strategy with students, and often quiz students on the steps. Games that require students to match a step in the strategy with the action they would perform (e.g., R = Read the paragraph; A = Ask what is the main idea and two details; P = Put it in my own words) are also used commonly. It is critically important for students to be able to recall strategies' steps accurately and effortlessly. Students should be focused on using the strategy, not struggling to recall strategy steps. Struggling to recall strategy steps consumes working memory, and may also lead to frustration and anxiety (which also consumes working memory), all of which are likely to have debilitating effects on performance.

Support the Strategy

After a student has learned the steps, he or she is ready to begin to use the strategy. However, the student is not yet ready to use the strategy independently. Actually using the strategy places different demands on the student. It's analogous to knowing the parts of an airplane and being able to fly an airplane. It's perfectly possible to know all the parts yet be unable to pilot an airplane. At this stage the instructor should work very closely with the student to help the student master *the use* of the strategy. This is accomplished through a scaffolding process. Together the student and instructor work through a task using the strategy. The instructor provides help to the student when necessary, but only as needed. As the student becomes more competent and conversant with the use of the strategy, the instructor systematically withdraws assistance. This process continues until the student can use the strategy without assistance.

There are a number of ways that instructors can scaffold instruction. In the initial lessons, when students are just beginning to use a strategy, instructors might use content material that is at an easy level. For example, for a student who was beginning to employ a reading comprehension strategy, using text that was one or two grades below the student's reading level would help the student to better focus on using the strategy and would lower demands on working memory. After the student had developed fluency with the strategy the difficulty of the text could be increased. One very simple way to scaffold is to let the student do the easier steps of the strategy or task while the instructor performs and models the more difficult steps. Over time, the student gradually can assume responsibility for the more difficult steps. Another approach is for the instructor to (1) ask the student to name the strategy step that should be performed, then the instructor describes the step and models its use; (2) ask the student to name the step and describe the step, then the instructor models the step; and (3) ask the student to name, describe, and model the step him- or herself. Finally, prompts and cues to help the student remember the steps in a strategy typically are faded over time.

There are no hard-and-fast rules for how long the scaffolding process should last. As a rule of thumb we suggest that it's better to be safe than sorry. If there is any doubt, continue the process. Skimping at this stage is counterproductive. Removing supports too early can literally undo all the gains the student has made. In practice, it is often very obvious when a student has mastered a strategy. For example, one girl we worked with dropped her pencil in the middle of her work and said, "You know this stuff is easy!" This is not an uncommon occurrence in practice. The key to remember is to keep demands on working memory and EFs as low as possible initially, and then gradually increase demands as the student becomes more accomplished at using the strategy. This will avoid overloading working memory and/or frustration and anxiety, all of which can result in problems such as inattention or even disruptive behavior (e.g., resistance to using the strategy).

Independent Performance

At this stage the student is ready to use the strategy independently. The instructor's job is primarily to monitor the student's performance and correct strategy use. The key concern is whether the strategy is improving student's performance. For example, if the student learned the RAP strategy, the concern would be whether the student was better able to answer comprehension questions. Maintenance is also important, especially with students with ADHD. If student's performance begins to deteriorate over time, then the strategy may need to be retaught. It's also necessary to check to see whether the strategy is used correctly. It's common for students to alter strategies when they begin to use them independently. Students with ADHD may alter or omit steps, especially those that require the most effort (see Johnson, Reid, & Mason, in press). This in turn can have detrimental effects on performance. If this occurs, instructors may wish to schedule booster sessions to reteach the parts of the strategy. Note that some changes may be benign or even an improvement. It is not a concern if a student modifies a strategy and the modification doesn't affect performance.

INSTRUCTIONAL ACCOMMODATIONS

Just as we can make accommodations in the physical environment to help students with ADHD function more effectively, we can also make accommodations in the instructional environment. Even under the best of circumstances many students with ADHD are likely to experience at least some academic difficulties. However, we can structure the instructional environment in a manner that minimizes the difficulties students with ADHD will encounter and maximizes the chances that they will benefit from instruction. There are three main areas that are amenable to accommodations: curriculum (what is taught), instruction (how it is taught), and independent seatwork.

Curriculum

In practice, teachers have little control over the sequence or content of curriculum. What is taught and when it is taught are typically determined by the school system. Few teachers have the authority to develop novel curricular areas. However, teachers can embed curriculum in *personally relevant contexts*. When curriculum is placed in a context of topics or activities that students value and find relevant, they are more likely to be actively engaged in learning (Glasser, 1992). For example, in our experience, one creative teacher managed to "hook" a group of car-crazy but extremely disruptive and noncompliant adolescent males by incorporating automotive magazines into the curriculum and presenting content areas in this context. A geometry lesson on the area of a cylinder was presented in the context of engine displacement and math calculations (e.g., distance = rate x time) were discussed using drag racing. In the case of children with ADHD, who actively seek high stimulation and can be easily distracted, this is even more important. Therefore, whenever possible, curriculum should be couched in a context that interests students or that takes advantage of their background knowledge.

Research has shown that the compliance, attention span, and academic productivity of students with ADHD are much better when they perform activities they perceive as meaningful (e.g., Dunlap et al., 1991; Dunlap, White, Vera, Wilson, & Panacek, 1996). For example, one student's interest in helping with the family grocery shopping led to using newspaper advertisements as a part of reading and vocabulary work. Math work consisted of using the advertised prices to plan a weekly grocery purchase (Dunlap et al., 1996). A problem-solving approach was effective for another student who often had problems with math drill and practice. His behavior improved when he was given work that related to a real-life activity that required problem solving such as reading a menu and computing the cost of a meal (Kern et al., 1994). Incorporating an outside interest or hobby, in this case photography, proved effective for one student. Her handwriting assignments were changed from copying pages from a workbook to writing captions for her photographs (Dunlap & Kern, 1993).

Curricular materials can be modified to increase the degree of stimulation provided by the task, which in turn can increase the degree to which students are engaged in a task. Introducing novelty into the task can also be effective. Zentall (1993) suggested that tasks can be made more stimulating through:

- The addition of color, shape, or texture changes.
- Varying the format in which tasks are presented (e.g., lecture, seatwork, activity, paper and pencil).

- Interspersing high-interest and low-interest tasks.
- Using tasks that require a motor response as opposed to a more passive response.

Teachers also can make routine tasks more stimulating. For example, math drill and practice activities can be combined with a puzzle. The answers to the questions form a "secret message" that the student can decode. However, inducing stimulation is not a long-term solution. Teachers may see the immediate effects of stimulation, but these effects tend to wash out fairly quickly.

Computer-assisted instruction (CAI) has long been thought to be a good match for students with ADHD. CAI can provide instruction in which (1) the instructional pace is set by the learner; (2) the learner is continuously prompted to make academic responses; and (3) the learner is provided frequent, immediate feedback about the quality of performance (Pfiffner et al., 2006). Additionally, CAI can highlight essential material (e.g., via large print and color), can use multiple sensory modalities (e.g., visual and auditory), and may utilize game-type formats that can be highly stimulating and motivating for students with ADHD (Mautone, DuPaul, & Jitendra, 2005). Despite the potential, little research has been conducted on CAI for students with ADHD, and much of the early research was poorly designed and did not address academic outcomes (Xu, Reid, & Steckelberg, 2002). More recently, the results of well-controlled studies suggest that CAI can have marked effects on engaged time and reduce time spent off-task; CAI also has positive effects on academic outcomes in terms of increased productivity and accuracy of responses—however, academic effects are not as pronounced as those for engaged time (Mautone et al., 2005; Ota & DuPaul, 2002).

In the classroom, CAI may offer several practical advantages for teachers in the general education classroom who must work with large classes. CAI can provide increased opportunities for a student to practice skills without requiring extensive teacher involvement and preparation time. Additionally, many programs can be adjusted to match each student's instructional level, and some monitor the student's progress and make instructional-level adjustments when appropriate (Mautone et al., 2005). CAI may also be useful as a potential reinforcer (e.g., after completing a task the student can go on the computer for a set period of time). However, there are some limitations. Most CAI is restricted to drill and practice programs designed to increase fluency on a task that has already been taught (e.g., math facts), and the range of CAI is quite limited in terms of coverage of the curriculum. For example, there are many programs for practicing math facts, but there are few programs in other areas such as history. In sum, CAI can be a useful adjunct to existing curriculum, but is unlikely to be a mainstay.

Instruction

Instructional variables can also affect children with ADHD. How instruction is delivered may help or hinder a child with ADHD. Teachers can present lesson material in a manner that accommodates problems with attention, distractibility, and working memory. This increases the likelihood that a student with ADHD will learn and maintain lesson material. Maximizing engagement is also important. The amount and type of responses students make during instruction can directly affect the degree of engagement of children with ADHD. Increasing engagement increases the likelihood that the student will remember lesson material and also decreases the likelihood that behavior problems will occur.

Delivering Instruction

Some general guidelines for more effective instructional delivery include (Alloway, 2006; DuPaul & Stoner, 2003; Gathercole et al., 2006; Mastropieri & Scruggs, 2005; Pfiffner & Barkley, 1998; Reid, 1999):

• Present material at an appropriate level of difficulty/abstraction. Teachers must ensure that students can follow lesson content. This cannot happen if students lack important background information or skills. Remember that students with ADHD often have gaps in their knowledge. Discussing key concepts or providing advanced organizers can help with this problem. Vocabulary deficits are another potential problem. Make sure vocabulary is at an appropriate level or teach necessary vocabulary prior to the lesson.

• Present lessons in an enthusiastic style. Students are more likely to maintain attention when teachers convey through their actions and tone of voice that the material is interesting and important.

• Set explicit goals and emphasize critical information and/or main points. Teachers can't assume that students with ADHD will identify critical information. Make sure that students understand the learning goal of a lesson. For example, "Today we are going to watch a video about the Industrial Revolution. I want you to watch for three ways that the Industrial Revolution changed America." This tells students exactly what their goal should be while watching the video, and thus what to focus on. Stress important information students need to remember verbally and graphically. For example, a teacher might directly state, "It's really important to remember that the abolitionists wanted to abolish slavery." Then write "abolitionists = abolish slavery" on the board and underline it to help make it clear to students that this is important information. It also reduces demands on working memory because students do not have to remember this information.

• Use a step-by-step, focused presentation of new material, and incorporate visual guides or summaries when possible. It's important for teachers to present material in a highly organized fashion. It's unlikely that a student with ADHD will be able to independently create an organizational structure to help understand or maintain information. If teachers jump around from point to point or backtrack, even accomplished students can easily become confused or frustrated because they must quickly retrieve needed information (the previous point) and maintain it while processing new information. Flipping back and forth puts demands on working memory and requires students to quickly shift focus from one set of information to another, both of which are likely to be difficult for students with ADHD.

• Avoid lengthy lectures. Any activity that requires students with ADHD to sit passively for long periods of time is a potential problem. Break up instruction into smaller chunks and intersperse it with activities that allow students to actively respond. Provide frequent opportunities for this kind of response. For example, "Okay class, we've been talking about the Industrial Revolution. Let's list some of the ways it affected people. Turn to your neighbor and write down two ways you think people were affected." The teacher would then call on several students and list their responses on the board. Opportunities for active responses by student help to keep students engaged and focused on the lesson.

• Provide frequent reviews and reminders of key information. Briefly re-cover major points in a lesson (e.g., "So as we discussed, there were three critical pieces of legislation that led up to the Civil War. Who can tell me one?"). Reiterate and stress key information that students need (e.g., "Remember that the first thing you need to do when you add fractions is to find the common denominator.").

• Support working memory. Provide students with prompts or other aids that reduce demands on working memory. For example, when working with the class on the steps of long division, provide students with a step-by-step example that they can refer to. Teachers also should remind students to actually use the prompts if they are unsure.

• Provide cognitive modeling and demonstrations of new procedures. Modeling and demonstrations can provide students with metacognitive information (i.e., information that gets at the thought processes behind actions) that can help them to better understand the "how and why" behind steps in procedures. For example, "Okay, I have to add these two fractions together. First, I have to remember that I can't just add the top and bottom numbers together. That would give me the wrong answer. I have to get my least common denominator. Let's see. How do I get that? I'll check with my reminder card." Note that here the teacher also modeled how to get help with the process if the student was unsure.

• Note that holistic or discovery-based approaches probably would not be appropriate for many children with ADHD because of their need for structure and difficulty with self-regulation (Reid, 1999). In contrast, direct instruction techniques, which are fast paced, highly structured, and incorporate frequent student responses, could be an ideal match.

Engagement

Children with ADHD often have difficulty maintaining engagement during large-group instruction (Pfiffner et al., 2006). Attention may wander, children may "tune out" or lose interest and, as a result, turn their attention to inappropriate behaviors.

One possible means of helping students with ADHD maintain engagement is the use of high-participation formats. High-participation formats are designed to provide students with frequent opportunities to respond to questions based on lesson content rather than sitting passively. Frequent opportunities to actively respond help to keep students with ADHD engaged and improve their performance (Zentall & Meyer, 1987).

One effective technique to increase the number of opportunities students have to respond is the use of response cards (Heward et al., 1996). To use response cards, teachers first prepare a series of questions about lesson content for students. Students are given cards to indicate a response to teacher questions. There are many types of cards. For example, teachers could use simple Yes/No cards (for true or false questions), cards with an A, B, C, or D (for multiple choice questions), or cards specifically related to a content area (e.g., each card has the name of one famous Civil War battle). Then, during designated times in the lesson (or at intervals throughout the lesson), the teacher questions the class and each student uses his or her response cards to answer. Alternatively, erasable white boards may be used for subjects such as math computation or spelling. Note that this technique can be useful in structuring guided practice of content and also can help teachers monitor student understanding. For example, students could be given a long division problem and asked to do the first step, then show their work. Based on students' responses teachers could move to the next step or provide needed corrective feedback. The key is to create situations in which all students *actively* participate as opposed to the one-at-a-time method where all but one student must sit passively.

Note taking is another type of engagement that that can pose problems for students with ADHD, especially when they reach middle school and beyond. Taking notes puts a tremendous strain on working memory because students must attend to the lesson, process the information in the lesson, identify important information, formulate the text to be written, and finally produce the text. Any of these tasks in isolation can be difficult for students with ADHD. Even the apparently simple act of producing text could pose problems (e.g., handwriting may be laborious, difficult to read, or the student may have spelling problems) for many children with ADHD. The fact that all of the activities must be done continuously and "on the fly" while the teacher presents information makes the task even more difficult. In this case, the teacher might consider the following accommodations: providing the child a copy of the lecture notes; using skeletal outlines to help the student organize notes (Lazarus, 1996); taping lectures so that the child can replay the lecture later, stop the tape to write, and start again when ready; or having a peer note taker (e.g., the teacher can photocopy the peer's notes).

Independent Seatwork

Independent seatwork provides practice that is important for building fluency. Keeping students with ADHD on-task during independent seatwork activities may be a problem because often there is less teacher supervision and independent work requires students to self-regulate their behavior (e.g., maintain focus, persist at a task), which often poses problems for students with ADHD. Factors that may influence the behavior of children with ADHD during independent seatwork include task difficulty, task length, and the amount and type of feedback provided during task performance.

Task Difficulty

The cognitive demands imposed by a task are directly related to student behavior. It is critical to match the difficulty level of the work to the student's current level of performance. Students should have attained a high degree of accuracy on a task *before* moving on to independent practice activities, such as completing worksheets (Mastropieri & Scruggs, 2005). Before assigning independent seatwork, the teacher should assess student performance to ensure that the work is at the appropriate level of difficulty. One good rule of thumb is that the student should be 90% accurate before given independent work. If students do not possess the prerequisite skills for an assignment, or if the difficulty level is too high (i.e., students cannot do the work with a high level of accuracy), they will become frustrated. For students with ADHD, frustration in turn can result in behavior problems (Cooper et al., 1992). Teachers should be sensitive to the fact that in the case of students with disruptive behavior problems, even a slight mismatch between task difficulty and student performance can significantly affect behavior. For example, DePaepe and colleagues (1996) gave students seatwork at two difficulty levels—one where students were 75% accurate, the other where students were 90% accurate. Even though the difference in difficulty between the two tasks was only 15%, students exhibited much higher rates of disruptive behavior at the 75% level compared to the 90% level.

A second common problem is getting "stuck." This can happen to any student for various reasons. Students with ADHD are probably more likely than other students to experience "stuckness." For example the student may not understand directions, forget important information needed to perform the task, or simply forget what he or she was supposed to be doing. For a student with ADHD, the problem is not so much getting stuck as it is obtaining help appropriately if the teacher is unable to provide immediate assistance. The student may call out, leave his or her seat and interrupt the teacher, or otherwise disrupt the class. To prevent potential problem behaviors, teachers should teach students a procedure to obtain help appropriately. One method for helping students obtain assistance appropriately is the use of assistance cards (Paine et al., 1983). Assistance cards are simple to construct. Simply fold a piece of card stock into thirds. On one third, the teacher writes "Please help me" and on another "Please keep working." The card it then folded into a triangle and taped to the student's desk. When the student needs assistance, he or she flips the card to the side that says "Please help me." This cues the teacher that the student requires assistance. If the teacher is busy with another student, she or he would walk over and flip up the other side of the card (Please keep working) indicating that the child should continue if possible or wait quietly. In this manner, the student's request is acknowledged and he or she knows that the teacher will be back shortly to help. Another technique that might be useful is the "study buddy" in which students are paired with a peer who provides assistance when needed. In both techniques the teacher must be sure to teach the students how to use the technique. Teachers also should be sure to praise compliance (i.e., use of the card or study buddy) or administer a mild reprimand for inappropriate help-seeking behavior (e.g., calling out).

Task Length

The length of tasks (i.e., amount of work assigned) can also affect behavior. If a student with ADHD feels overwhelmed by an assignment, he or she may not even start the assignment or may be unable to maintain attention and thus fail to complete it. One possible solution to this problem is to use shortened assignments, interspersing different activities within seatwork periods, and providing breaks. For example, rather than completing an entire 30-problem math worksheet, the student with ADHD might be assigned 10 math problems. When those are completed, the student can then practice five spelling words; then take a 5-minute break on the computer. Note that it is best to give the student one task at a time rather than a packet (Abramowitz, Reid, & O'Toole, 1994). Additionally, teachers must ensure that breaks are highly structured, and that breaks are awarded only *after* work completion. Shortened assignments can also be combined with providing students a choice of activities. Choice making involves providing students with a "menu" listing several different tasks (e.g., copy 10 spelling words, do a language arts workbook page, read a selection and answer five comprehension questions). Students are allowed to pick which task they wish to perform. When they complete the first task, they choose another from the menu. All tasks are drawn from the normal class curriculum and should be at the appropriate level of difficulty. The effectiveness of choice making for reducing disruptive behaviors and improving work completion in the classroom is well documented (e.g., Dunlap et al., 1991, 1994, 1996; Powell & Nelson, 1997).

Feedback

Children with ADHD typically perform better when they receive frequent feedback on their performance (Barkley, 2006). The use of self-correcting materials (e.g., flash cards, folders, or answer tapes) can be beneficial (Cohen & de Bettencourt, 1988). Self-correcting materials provide the student with ongoing performance feedback and immediate response confirmation, reduce failure experience, and can increase attention to task (Cohen & de Bettencourt, 1988). Self-correcting materials may also be used in conjunction with self-recording or self-graphing (see Chapter 11 for examples). Self-correcting materials are easy to use and practical. Students are given a seatwork assignment and a correction folder (which contains the answers). Students work as usual, but after each response (or set of responses), they use the correction folder to check their work. When using self-correcting materials, teachers should remember to give frequent feedback to students on their task engagement. Another type of feedback relates to the passage of time. Students with ADHD have problems accurately gauging passage of time (Barkley, 2006) and thus may subjectively feel that they have worked on a task "forever" when in reality they have only spent a few minutes. Alternatively they may believe that they have plenty of time to complete a task when their time is nearly up. One method that can help with this problem is the use of timers. For example, Fraser, Belzner, and Conte (1992) worked with an elementary school student who had problems getting ready for group work. They used an egg timer set for 5 minutes to provide feedback. If the student successfully accomplished all the tasks necessary within 5 minutes he received a token reinforcer. This approach was very successful and the student actually requested to use the timer in other situations (e.g., completing math seatwork).

PEER TUTORING

Peer tutoring is a well-established intervention that is effective for a wide range of students (Stenhoff & Lignugaris-Kraft, 2007). It is used for independent practice to help students solidify knowledge and/or develop fluency. Peer tutoring provides opportunities for extra instruction, practice, repetition, or clarification. Peer tutoring provides an excellent instructional environment for students with ADHD, because it combines (1) ongoing one-to-one peer attention, (2) frequent active responding with highly structured and individualized academic content that is presented at a student's pace, (3) frequent prompting to attend to task, (4) consistent and immediate feedback on performance, and (5) the elimination of wait time (DuPaul & Stoner, 2003). It is simple to implement and appropriate for both general education and special education classrooms. A typical peer tutoring interaction consists of:

1. The tutor provides a prompt (e.g., "What is 8 x 7?").
2. The tutee responds.
3. The tutor provides feedback and error correction if needed.
   a. If the answer is correct the tutor confirms (e.g., "That's right!"), then moves to the next prompt.
   b. If the answer is incorrect the tutor provides the correct answer (e.g., "8×7 is 56."), then repeats the prompt ("What is 8×7?"). After the tutee responds correctly the tutor moves on to the next prompt.
4. The tutor provides the next prompt.

For students with ADHD peer tutoring can increase academic responding, attention to task, and academic productivity, while decreasing noncompliance and inappropriate motor activity (e.g., fidgeting or remaining in seat; DuPaul & Henningson, 1993; DuPaul, Ervin, Hook, & McGoey, 1998). Peer tutoring may also benefit the teacher by decreasing the need to monitor behavior during peer tutoring time, and providing time that could be spent in one-to-one instruction or small-group instruction with other students. Figure 10.3 shows steps in implementing peer tutoring.

Step 1: Define the content of instruction and materials. Decide what content area(s) to address and what materials will be used. Peer tutoring will probably be most effective if it is correlated with class content. Focus on the skills that the student needs to succeed in the classroom. Some example areas might be basic math facts, phonics, oral reading, and language (e.g., spelling or writing practice). Identify or create the materials the tutor will need for instruction (e.g., flash cards with sight words, lists of states and their capitals)

Step 2: Lesson formats. Peer tutoring functions best when teachers create *highly structured and carefully prescribed lessons*. Peer tutors should know exactly what to do and how to do it for all parts of the lesson. Teachers need to develop step-by-step lesson guides so that tutors will be able to deliver instruction correctly. This allows tutors to function independently without asking the teacher, "What do I do now?" Additionally it ensures that instruction will be done correctly. Initially teachers may need to do a little "fine tuning" but with experience teachers should be able to quickly develop effective formats.

Step 3: Establish a schedule. Decide when peer tutoring sessions will be conducted and how long they will last. There are no set rules for scheduling. It may depend in part on the existing classroom schedule or other factors, but there are some guidelines. One rule of thumb is to have three to five session per week. Session length should be between 15 and 30 minutes. It's probably best to schedule peer tutoring 4–5 days per week because factors such as normal interruptions (assemblies, field trips, snow days), transitions, and absenteeism will always cut down instructional time.

Step 3: Recruit tutors. Identify and recruit the students who will make good peer tutors. Teachers should look for two factors. First, the student should have a sufficient level of mastery of the content material. The tutor will need to direct a lesson; therefore the tutor has to be able to perform the task well. Second, the student must have an acceptable level of interpersonal skills. Tutors must be able to work closely and positively with the tutee. When recruiting students to be peer tutors, frame the tutoring positively. Students are going to help the teacher and their classmates out with an important job.

Step 4: Train the tutors. Train tutors to conduct lessons correctly. To make peer tutoring work, tutors must be able to perform instructional tasks correctly and efficiently. When training a tutor, use the actual lesson format that you have developed. Model a lesson for the tutor and then ask the student to assume the role of the tutor for practice. Assess mastery before actual peer tutoring sessions begin. Remember that there is more to tutoring than just content. Tutors will need to be taught to give clear directions, encourage and praise learners for their efforts, confirm correct responses, correct errors positively, and not overprompt. Tutors need to be informed about the purpose of peer tutoring and the responsibilities of being a peer tutor. Tutors must make a consistent time commitment, be punctual, keep lesson results confidential, and have a positive relationship with the learner. Tutors must also be taught the appropriate measurement procedures and systematic recording procedures to enable you to assess a tutee's progress. Here's an example student progress record form.

(cont.)

FIGURE 10.3. Steps in implementing peer tutoring. Based on Miller (2005) and Lehigh University Project Outreach (n.d.).

Ask: What is the capital of _____? (say state name)			
States	Capitals	Correct	Incorrect
California	Sacramento		
Washington	Olympia		
Arizona	Phoenix		
Oregon	Salem		

During the initial peer tutoring session teachers should closely monitor sessions and conduct additional training if needed. Some teachers schedule regular training time with tutors. This allows for continual refinement of the tutoring procedures and is an excellent feedback mechanism.

Step 5: Do It! Monitor the initial sessions closely. Set high expectations for tutors and tutees, and reinforce students whose performance meet or exceed those expectations. You should *explicitly encourage respect and mutual concern between tutor and tutee.* Teachers should aim to interact with each dyad at least once during peer tutoring sessions. This allows teachers to monitor, establishes that the teacher is interested, and allows teachers to praise students who are exhibiting desirable behaviors and correct behaviors that are inappropriate. Teachers need to show their enthusiasm, interest, and commitment to high expectations. Your active involvement sends this message. You may wish to conduct "debriefing" sessions after the first few peer tutoring sessions. After peer tutoring becomes well established you may spend the majority of the time with one or two dyads or may use the time for other instruction; however, it's still a good idea to reserve time to interact with the dyads.

Support peer tutoring. Manage and maintain the peer tutoring program. One of the biggest challenges will be keeping peer tutors motivated. There are a number of ways to help maintain motivation. Perhaps the best way is through teacher attention. The time spent with tutors discussing the project, comments on the job they are doing, or just time spent shooting the breeze are all powerful reinforcers. Another reinforcer for tutors is being able to see the progress that their tutee is making. The use of graphs and charts or other visual displays can highlight progress. Teachers can draw attention to tutors' (and tutees') accomplishments through informal discussions with parents, teachers, or the principal. These serve to remind tutors of the importance of the job they are doing. Try to establish a systematic schedule of reinforcing events such as tutor luncheons, tutor parties, letters of thanks from the principal, or material rewards such as stickers or candy.

FIGURE 10.3. *(cont.)*

Peer tutoring can also be done with an entire class. There are a number of different types of whole-class peer tutoring approaches including classwide peer tutoring (CWPT), peer-assisted learning strategies, classwide student tutor teams, and START (see Maheady, Mallette, & Harper, 2006, for descriptions). One method that has been used successfully with students with ADHD is CWPT, where an entire class or large groups are divided into competing teams with points awarded for daily performance (DuPaul et al., 1998). For CWPT, the use of daily points may provide useful performance feedback; the points might also be used along with a token economy. The use of performance charting or graphing may also improve performance or motivation (Locke & Fuchs, 1995).

SUMMING UP

Students with ADHD are at high risk for academic difficulties. To help students with ADHD function effectively in the classroom, teachers need to create an instructional environment that is sensitive to the core problems of students with ADHD: working memory and EF deficits. Remember that activities that many students can perform routinely (e.g., understanding and following directions, completing work) may be difficult for students with ADHD. Here are some points to remember.

✓ Reduce demands on working memory as much as possible. Do not put students with ADHD in situations that require them to hold and process a number of pieces of information. Instead provide supports such as prompts or visual organizers.

✓ Some problems with working memory (e.g., not following directions) may appear to be the result of attention problems. Even tasks that appear simple can be very demanding for students with working memory problems.

✓ Students with ADHD will seldom if ever independently adopt a planful strategic approach to tasks. However, they can be taught to do so.

✓ Students with ADHD may not be aware of the goal of an academic task (e.g., the purpose of reading is to understand what is read). They may also have maladaptive goals (e.g., avoiding embarrassment). Teachers should establish explicit goals for tasks and communicate them to students.

✓ Some students with ADHD believe that their performance is much better than it actually is. Teachers should help students establish a realistic understanding of their performance, and set appropriate goals for improvements.

✓ An instructional approach that uses the components of strategy instruction may be helpful for students with ADHD.

✓ Strive to embed content in personally relevant contexts if at all possible.

✓ Try to keep tasks stimulating through novelty and active responding.

✓ Keep instruction focused and highly organized. Avoid jumping around or backtracking that requires students to rapidly shift from one set of information to another.

✓ To help keep students engaged, use an enthusiastic instructional delivery that incorporates frequent active responding.

✓ Keep independent work tasks at an appropriate level of difficulty. Students should be able to perform independent seatwork with 90% accuracy.

✓ Use a series of short assignments as opposed to a single long assignment. Incorporate choice to the extent possible.

✓ Peer tutoring can be an effective technique for students with ADHD.

CHAPTER 11

Self-Regulation Strategies

By the time I think about what I'm going to do
I've already done it.
—Dennis the Menace

The term "self-regulation" refers to skill in controlling and regulating one's behavior such as monitoring progress, checking outcomes, and redirecting unsuccessful efforts (Berk, 2003). Self-regulation can also be directed at cognitions and affect. Historically, being able to self-regulate one's behavior has been considered highly desirable (Harris, Reid, & Graham, 2004) and individuals who exhibit self-regulation are held in high esteem. For example, Ben Franklin used self-regulation to develop 13 virtues that he thought were desirable (Zimmerman & Schunk, 1989). He kept a detailed journal in which he established goals to increase each virtue, monitored his successes and failures, recorded daily results, and established new goals. In the case of students with ADHD, self-regulation is critically important because problems with self-regulation are central to the problems associated with ADHD (Barkley, 2006).

As we noted in the previous chapter, current conceptualizations of ADHD suggest that students with ADHD have difficulties with EFs that would help them to self-regulate their behavior. As a result these students experience difficulties with inhibition of behavior, delay of gratification, maintaining focus (e.g., inhibiting interfering cognitions), persistence, producing the amount and quality of work they are capable of, maintaining on-task behaviors, planning, and directing goal-directed future-oriented behaviors. Problems with these areas put students with ADHD at a distinct disadvantage academically and socially. Let's consider the following hypothetical scenario to illustrate why self-regulation is highly desirable:

You're taking a graduate course and it's a tough one with a demanding professor. It's not a particularly interesting course, but it's required for your graduate program that you need to complete your certification program for your new position. It's been a long day and you are having trouble getting through the assigned reading for the next class. The reading is important because it is the basis for the major assignment in the course. It seems like you have been at it forever and that you'll never get the assignment done. Moreover, you're starting to get a headache. You'd like nothing better than to go outside on your patio and relax with a cool drink.

How could we deal with a situation like this? It's obviously important to complete the readings. Failing to complete the reading might result in problems with a future assignment that could result in failing to pass the course. This in turn could lead to losing your new job. Most of us would realize the potential consequences and would realize that we needed to do something to help maintain effort and focus on the task. In truth scenarios such as this one are not uncommon; most of us deal with situations akin to this one frequently. In this particular situation there are numerous techniques we could use to help. For example, we might try some combination of the following:

- Promise oneself a small treat (e.g., a decadent dessert) after we finish the reading assignment, and a trip to a spa after the entire course has been finished.
- Divide the assignment into four equal 20-page chunks, and allow oneself a brief break after every 20 pages of reading.
- Chart progress by making a graph and checking off each page completed.
- Tell oneself, "I can do this. If I just stick to it, and it will help me keep my new job."
- Arrange our study space to be more comfortable, and block out distractions that might get us off-task (e.g., close the blinds so we can't see the patio).

Unfortunately, when students with ADHD are faced with analogous situations, the response is likely to be the equivalent of the "cool drink on the patio."

For example, faced with a homework assignment, the impulse to engage in a more stimulating activity (e.g., watch a TV show) may overpower the need to complete the homework. That is, they may be unable to inhibit their immediate desire to escape the situation (i.e., homework) and to persevere at the task. Instead they will often choose immediate gratification (i.e., the TV show). For students with ADHD, possible negative future consequences (e.g., the teacher's reaction when the homework isn't completed, effects on grades, parents' anger) wouldn't enter into their thinking. Long-term goals (e.g., failing the course could affect graduation) also would not even be considered. The impulse to escape the situation is overpowering. Note that this is not "laziness"; instead it is a classic symptom of ADHD. Like Dennis the Menace, by the time they think about consequences it's already much too late. As a result of these problems with self-regulation, students with ADHD may struggle to complete academic work, which in turn can result in lowered grades or failure to complete a course of study and reduced opportunities for learning.

THE CASE FOR SELF-REGULATION STRATEGIES

Teachers need to help students with ADHD develop self-regulation strategies (Strayhorn, 2002) because these strategies are unlikely to develop independently. One approach to developing self-regulation strategies is straightforward: teach the student effective self-regulation strategies. Self-regulation strategies are a family of methods used by students to manage, monitor, and/or assess behavior or academic activities (Reid, Trout, & Schartz, 2005). Research demonstrates that self-regulation strategies can help students with ADHD improve their academic accuracy and productivity, can increase time on-task, and can also help to decrease disruptive behaviors (Reid et al., 2005). Moreover, self-regulation strategies have a long history of classroom use, are not time-consuming or difficult to implement, and are seen by classroom teachers as practical for use in the classroom (Reid, 1996).

Self-regulation strategies are particularly appropriate for students with ADHD because, for students with ADHD, problems often occur as a result of a performance deficit rather than a skill deficit (Barkley, 2006). That is to say, students often possess the skills to accomplish a task, but are unable to martial them effectively. Thus, for example, a student may know her math facts, but be unable to complete a math worksheet because she cannot maintain focus on her work. She may not be able to shield her attention from competing stimuli (e.g., looking out the window) or classroom distractions (e.g., other students talking). She may also be *unaware* that she is spending much of her time off-task. Students with ADHD often are unaware of their behavior. This is a serious problem because conscious appraisal of immediate past behavior is necessary for self-regulation to occur (Barkley, 1997c). Self-regulation strategies can help students with ADHD by providing them with feedback on their behavior. This feedback helps to enable a comparison between what the student *is* doing and what the student *should* be doing. This in turn serves as a cue to maintain appropriate behavior or to change inappropriate behavior (Barkley, 2006).

Additionally, self-regulation strategies provide two potential advantages over other interventions (Graham, Harris, & Reid, 1992). First, self-regulation strategies allow students to change their own behavior as opposed to the teacher or another adult intervening. The lesson here is one of empowerment—students learn that they can independently regulate their behavior. For students with ADHD, this may be a very important learning experience. Second, and equally important, self-regulation strategies offer distinct practical advantages over many other approaches. After the student has been taught a self-regulation strategy the teacher's involvement may be minimal because the student is literally running the intervention. Compared to other approaches, self-regulation strategies can result in considerable savings in teacher time, and makes more time available for learning. For example, self-regulation strategies do not require teachers to take the time to constantly reinforce behaviors or track points earned from token economies; instead teachers are free to perform other instructional activities.

In this chapter we discuss how teachers can teach five self-regulation strategies—self-monitoring, self-management, goal setting, self-reinforcement, and self-instruction—in the classroom with students with ADHD. For each strategy we provide a brief background, examples from research on how the strategy can be used, and the steps needed to actually implement the strategies in the classroom. For additional information on self-regulation strategies, see Reid and Lienemann (2006a). Note that although we discuss the strategies individually, in practice they can be combined with other self-regulation strategies and can also be used in combination with content-area strategies.

SELF-MONITORING

Self-monitoring occurs when an individual self-assesses whether or not a target behavior has occurred, and then self-records the occurrence, frequency, or duration of the target behavior (Nelson & Hayes, 1981). For example, in one of the earliest self-monitoring studies, researchers taught a student to periodically ask herself whether or not she was working or paying attention in class (the self-assessment component) and to then make a tally of the times she was working or paying attention (the self-recording component; Broden, Hall, & Mitts, 1971). In contrast to behavioral approaches, self-monitoring usually does not involve the use of external reinforcers; the act of self-recording is thought to act as a reinforcer (Mace, Belfiore, & Hutchinson, 2001). Note, however, that self-monitoring can be effectively combined with external reinforcers (e.g., Barkley, Copeland, & Sivage, 1980). For some students adding external reinforcers may be beneficial (Graham-Day, Gardner, & Hsin, 2010).

Self-monitoring has been used successfully with a variety of behaviors (e.g., weight reduction, smoking cessation, nail biting). For our purposes, we focus on two problem areas that most directly affect classroom teachers: on-task behavior and academic responding. There are two main types of self-monitoring interventions: self-monitoring of attention (SMA) and self-monitoring of performance (SMP). Both of these have been used successfully with students with ADHD (Reid et al., 2005). In SMA, students are taught to self-assess whether or not they are paying attention when cued (typically, cuing is performed through the use of taped tones presented at random intervals), and then to self-record the results on a tally sheet (Figure 11.1 shows an example of a SMA tally sheet). A number of studies have successfully used SMA with students with ADHD. For example, Mathes and Bender (1997) used SMA with elementary school boys who had high rates of disruptive behavior (e.g., talking out), often failed to complete assigned tasks, and were noncompliant. Effects were pronounced and immediate: after SMA was introduced all students more than doubled the amount of time on-task. Additionally, all students were receiving medication for ADHD; thus self-monitoring resulted in improvements over and above medication.

Was I Paying Attention?	
• In my seat	
• Listening to the teacher	
• Doing my work	
• Asking for help	
YES	NO

FIGURE 11.1. Example of a self-monitoring of attention tally sheet.

In SMP, students first self-assess some aspect of academic performance (e.g., the number of correct addition problems on a work sheet) and then self-record the results (Reid, 1993). Self-assessments can occur during a work session (sometimes using taped tones as cues), but are more commonly used after a work session. In SMP, self-recording typically involves the use of charting or graphing. Figure 11.2 shows an example of a SMP graph. This provides students with a concrete representation of their progress that can prove to be quite motivating for students with ADHD (Lienemann & Reid, 2008). There are many types of SMP. For example, students may self-assess their productivity (e.g., the number of math problems they attempted), accuracy (e.g., the number of math problems completed correctly), or strategy use (e.g., whether or not steps in a math strategy were performed). SMP has also been used successfully with students with ADHD. For example, Shimabukuro and colleagues had nine students with ADHD self-monitor their accuracy and percent of work completed on reading comprehension, writing, and math seatwork (Shimabukuro, Prater, Jenkins, & Edelen-Smith, 1999). After each seatwork session students would compute their percent accuracy and the percentage of work completed and graph the results. All students markedly improved both the accuracy of their work and the percent of work completed. Some students more than doubled their accuracy and rate of work completion.

Typically either SMA or SMP is used alone; however, combining the two types of self-monitoring also can be quite effective with students with ADHD (Rock, 2005). At present it is not clear if SMA or SMP is more effective for students with ADHD. We are aware of only one study that has compared SMA and SMP (Harris, Friedlander, Saddler, Frizelle, & Graham, 2005). This study found that both SMA and SMP increased the amount of on-task behavior, and there was no difference between the methods in terms of their effects on on-task behavior. Both methods also improved academic productivity (number of spelling words practiced); however, four of six students completed more work in the SMA condition. All students reported that both SMA and SMP were acceptable, but while the SMA condition

How many words did I write in my story?

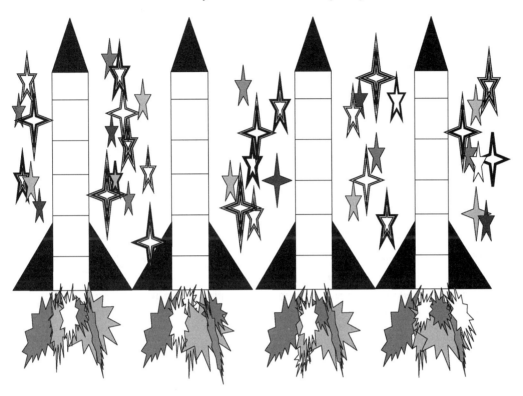

FIGURE 11.2. Example of a self-monitoring of performance graph. From Reid and Lienemann (2006a). Copyright 2006 by The Guilford Press. Reprinted by permission.

was more effective at increasing productivity, four of six students actually preferred the SMP condition.

Implementing Self-Monitoring

Teaching a student to use self-monitoring is straightforward and the actual training in self-monitoring procedures takes very little time. Reid (1993) outlined the following steps:

1. Select a Target Variable

The first step it to decide what behavior will be self-monitored: attention or performance. The behavior targeted for change and the behavior that is self-monitored are often the same; however, they are not *always* the same. For example, a student might self-monitor attention even though the teacher was actually concerned with increasing the amount of seatwork that was completed. A good target behavior is specific, observable, appropriate, and a personal match (Reid, 1993).

SPECIFIC

The teacher must *exactly* define the behavior to be monitored. Because the self-monitoring process begins with self-assessment, students must be able to easily and accurately determine whether or not a target behavior has occurred. Target behaviors such as "better reading" or "being good" are much too vague to be useful; instead use behaviors such as "number of math problems correct" or "listening to the teacher and doing my work" which are easily understandable and readily assessed by the student. Note that the target behavior can, however, consist of a number of behaviors (e.g., being in my seat, having my work,) so long as they are all well specified. For example, in Figure 11.1 the behaviors that constitute "paying attention" are spelled out.

OBSERVABLE

Students must be *aware* of the occurrence of a target behavior; otherwise they will be unable to self-assess whether the behavior has occurred. This could be a problem for students with ADHD who may engage in a behavior impulsively and/or unconsciously. They may be unaware of the occurrence of the behavior. For example, students who impulsively talk out of turn may be unaware of the behavior. The lack of awareness would preclude effective self-monitoring. In the case of students who talked out of turn the teacher might instead ask them to self-monitor the number of times they raise their hand to speak, as this might be more observable for the student.

APPROPRIATE

When selecting a target behavior, teachers should consider two factors: setting and task. It is important to be sensitive to the environment where self-monitoring will take place and try to imagine possible problems that could arise. For example, if taped tones were used to cue a student to self-assess during a group activity, a student might feel as though he or she were being singled out. The fit between self-monitoring procedures and academic tasks should also be closely examined. In some cases, self-monitoring procedures can be intrusive and can detract from performance (Reid, 1996). For example, using a procedure that required students to self-assess and self-record frequently would probably be inappropriate during a small-group reading lesson because it would distract from the lesson. Unfortunately, there are no established rules to help teachers select the best target behavior for any given combination of environment and task. One practical method might be to simply allow students to try self-monitoring different behaviors and let them choose the behavior they felt was most appropriate or effective for them to self-monitor. When given a choice between several alternatives, students are capable of selecting the most effective target behavior (Maag, Reid, & DiGangi, 1993).

PERSONAL

Self-monitoring may not appropriate for students who are very young or are imma-ture because students must be able to understand the connection between self-monitoring procedures and the target behavior (Graham et al., 1992). If this connec-tion is not made in the mind of the student there will be no effect on behavior. For example, imagine a student who self-monitored the number of spelling words she completed and graphed the results. For self-monitoring to be effective the student must be able to relate the graph to the work completed (i.e., be able to understand that the graph represented the amount of work completed). Unless the student can make the connection between the work done and the graphic portrayal of results, there's likely to be no change in the number of spelling words practiced. Teachers should also be sensitive to age level, which can affect the perceived value or salience of target behaviors. For example, a student may see value in "paying attention," but not in "how many practices completed" (or vice versa). The effects of age level on self-monitoring are not well understood; however, there is some evidence of differ-ential effectiveness of target variables across age levels effects (Maag et al., 1993).

2. Collect Baseline Data

Next, baseline data should be gathered and recorded. Data should be collected at the time and place where the self-monitoring intervention will take place. For example, if the intervention was to be directed at out-of-seat behavior during second period math class, the teacher would simply count the number of times the student was out of his or her seat during the period. In the case of interventions directed to academic accuracy or productivity, baseline data collection could be as simple as collecting work samples. Collecting baseline data is important because it provides an objec-tive benchmark to evaluate the success of the intervention. Note also that collecting objective data on the extent of the problem may obviate the need for an intervention. Teachers sometimes find that the problem was not nearly as serious as they believed. Alternatively, they may discover that they have targeted the wrong behavior.

3. Obtain Willing Cooperation

The "self" is the active ingredient in self-monitoring. This means that the teacher will need active and willing cooperation on the part of the student. Teachers should schedule a conference with the student and address the problem area(s) frankly. Discuss the benefits of self-monitoring with the student (e.g., staying in your seat means you don't lose recess; doing all your arithmetic problems means you'll do bet-ter on the test). Be optimistic, but also be realistic; don't make exaggerated claims. Instead, describe self-monitoring as "something that helped a lot of students like you with the same kind problem." If students are unsure, try using a contingency contract. If the student commits to trying self-monitoring for a specified period of time, he or she will receive a reinforcer. We have found that in practice students with ADHD often enjoy using self-monitoring and that it can be highly motivating. After you have enlisted cooperation, explain when and where self-monitoring will be used (e.g., during second period math class seatwork time).

4. Instruct Self-Monitoring Procedures

In this stage the student is taught how to self-monitor. The teacher and student together go through each self-monitoring step. For example, for SMA the student would listen for the beep, ask "Was I paying attention?," and mark the tally sheet. Note that the time spent on any one step may vary widely depending on the student and the choice of target variables. Students should master each step in turn before proceeding to the next. This process is not time-consuming; students typically can learn to self-monitor quickly and easily with total training time typically well under 1 hour. There are three critical tasks at this stage:

DEFINING THE TARGET BEHAVIOR

Explain to the student exactly what constitutes the target behavior. For most types of self-monitoring this is quite simple. For example, in SMP defining the target variable may involve little more than telling the student to count correct answers. For other types of self-monitoring, defining the target variable may be more complex. For example, in SMA interventions the student must understand what it means to "pay attention." Here the teacher and the student can develop a list of specific behaviors that constituted "paying attention" such as looking at the teacher or your work, writing answers, listening to the teacher, or asking a question. Remember that students must understand the target behavior before proceeding.

DISCRIMINATION OF TARGET BEHAVIOR

The student should be able to discriminate between the target behavior and other behaviors. One simple way to teach discrimination is for the teacher to model examples and nonexamples of the target behavior and ask the student to determine if they are examples of the target behavior. For instance, if the target behavior was paying attention, the teacher might fiddle with a pencil (nonexample) or write on a worksheet (example). This provides reinforcement of the knowledge of the target variable gained in the previous stage and also provides evaluative feedback for the teacher. Note that for some types of self-monitoring this might not be necessary (e.g., self-monitoring the number of practice items completed).

EXPLANATION OF SELF-MONITORING PROCEDURES

In this stage the teacher first directly explains the procedures involved in self-assessing and self-recording. Next, the teacher models proper performance while verbalizing the steps. The student is then asked to verbalize the steps as the teacher performs them. Following this, the student is asked to model and verbalize the procedures. It is extremely important that the student be able to perform the self-monitoring procedures effortlessly (Mace & Kratochwill, 1988). Self-monitoring procedures should be minimally distracting for the student. If the procedures are difficult for the student to remember or perform they are probably inappropriate for the student. After the student is able to demonstrate the procedures correctly, the teacher should provide a brief period of guided practice. This offers structured experience for the student and also allows the teacher to assess mastery. Again, in practice this entire procedure can be done very quickly.

Independent Performance

Now the student is ready to use self-monitoring. The first time the student self-monitors it is a good idea to prompt the student to use the procedures and/or to check for knowledge of the target variable. During the initial sessions the teacher should monitor the student to ensure that the self-monitoring procedures are used consistently and correctly. Remember that self-monitoring procedures must be used properly and consistently if self-monitoring is to be effective. If any problems are evident, reteach the procedures. If a student appears to be having problems additional training may be indicated. For less serious problems simply providing students with prompts, such as reminders of what constitutes the target behavior or cues to self-assess or self-record may be all that is required. However, if students consistently experience problems it may be best to rethink whether self-monitoring is appropriate.

Evaluation

After the student has begun to self-monitor independently, the teacher should continue to collect data in order to assess the effectiveness of the intervention. Typically, improvement occurs rapidly. The teacher should also assess for maintenance. In practice, students have been able to maintain increased performance levels for considerable periods of time in the classroom (e.g., Harris, 1986). However, if the student's performance begins to deteriorate, additional "booster sessions" in self-monitoring procedures may be necessary.

SELF-MANAGEMENT

Self-management (SMGT) (also called self-evaluation) is closely related to self-monitoring in that both require students to self-assess some aspect of their behavior and self-record at regular intervals. SMGT typically involves the use of self-monitoring in that it requires students to self-assess and self-record their rating of a behavior at set intervals (Shapiro & Cole, 1994). For example, students might rate their behavior on a scale of 1 (did not follow directions or finish work) to 5 (followed all directions and finished all work) at 15-minute intervals during a period and to record the results. Figure 11.3 shows an example of an SMGT rating sheet. SMGT differs from self-monitoring in that student self-assessments are compared to an external standard or criterion and students typically (but not always) receive reinforcement based on the accuracy of their self-assessments (Mace et al., 2001). Thus reinforcement depends on accurate self-assessment of behavior. Note that SMGT may often use goal setting (discussed later in this chapter).

SMGT has been used frequently and very effectively with children with ADHD (e.g., Shapiro, DuPaul, & Bradley-Klug, 1998). For example, in two studies Gureasko-Moore and colleagues used SMGT, self-monitoring, and goal setting to increase the classroom preparation (e.g., coming to class with needed materials) and homework completion of students with ADHD (Gureasko-Moore, DuPaul, & White, 2006, 2007). Students were taught to self-monitor using a checklist (Figure 11.4). Students also were taught to calculate the number of behaviors on the checklist that they performed in order to record them in a log. Students set goals for performance of checklist behaviors and recorded progress in the log. Students also used the log to self-evaluate the extent to which they were accomplishing their goals and their satisfaction with their progress. After the students completed their logs, they met with the teacher, who commented on their logs and commended students who met goals and performed classroom preparation behaviors. After SMGT training students were able to perform all the organizational behaviors successfully 100% of the time.

The steps in implementing SMGT are straightforward (Shapiro et al., 1998). Note that the same concerns regarding well-specified target behavior and teaching procedures discussed in the self-monitoring section also apply to SMGT. In the baseline stage, the teacher identifies the behavior(s) to be targeted (e.g., staying in seat, finishing homework, following classroom rules) and establishes the time and setting when the intervention will be used (e.g., during third period reading class). Next the teacher makes subjective ratings of the student's performance using a graduated scale (e.g., 1 = very bad, 5 = fair, and 10 = excellent; or 1 = poor, 5 = very good) at intervals during the period (e.g., every 15 minutes). These ratings are graphed, but are not immediately shared with the student. Next, in the teacher management stage, the teacher meets with the student and informs the student of the ratings. The teacher informs the student that he or she will be rated at regular intervals and that the ratings are worth points (which can be redeemed for reinforcement). They also share the baseline stage data with the students. During the time SMGT is in effect, the teacher verbally informs the student of the rating the teacher made of the student's performance. Once again ratings are graphed and shared with the student. This phase continues until the student receives acceptable ratings for several consecutive days.

The next phase involves matching the student and teacher ratings. The purpose of this phase is to help the student accurately judge his or her own behavior. After

How Did I Do Today?

Did I Follow Directions?   Did I Listen Quietly?

Did I Complete My Work?   Did I Respect Others?

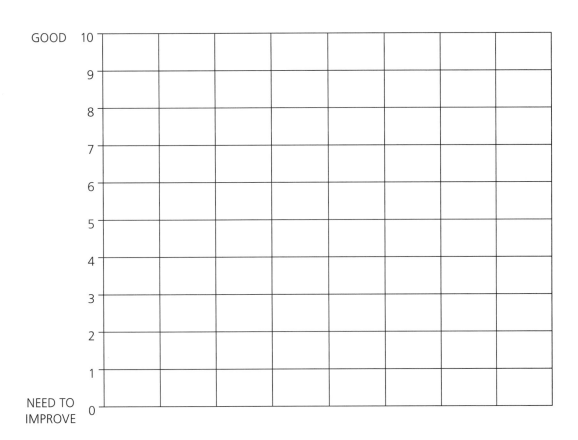

FIGURE 11.3. Example of a self-management graph.

Am I ready for class?	**Yes**	**No**
Was I at my desk?		
Did I stop talking when the teacher started class?		
Did I focus on the teacher during the lesson?		
Did I bring my pen/pencil?		
Did I bring my book?		
Did I bring my notebook?		
Did I bring my homework?		
Did I sit up straight and face the teacher during the lesson?		

FIGURE 11.4. Example of a self-monitoring checklist. Based on Gureasko-Moore, DuPaul, and White (2007).

every rating period the teacher and student compare ratings. If the student and teacher ratings are close (e.g., within 1 point) the student receives points for accurately self-assessing his or her behavior. The teacher and student also briefly discuss why the discrepancy occurred. If the teacher and student match exactly the student receives points equal to the rating (e.g., if the student rating was a 5, 5 points would be awarded) plus a bonus point. Ratings that differ greatly (e.g., by 2 or more points) receive no points for that rating period.

In the next phase, fading, the number of times the teacher and students evaluations are compared is gradually decreased, and the time periods in which the student rates his or her behavior are gradually increased. For example, if the teacher and student had four opportunities to match ratings, the teacher would first match four times, then three, and so on until matching was completely faded. In periods when no match occurs, points are awarded based on the student's rating. At the same time the length of the rating period is gradually increased (e.g., from 15 minutes to 20 minutes). Fading should take place gradually and only after the student's behavior has remained stable for a period of time. After the student has stable and improved behavior, the student moves to complete self-management. In this final phase, the student gradually shifts to oral assessments (as opposed to written) of behavior given to the teacher at the end of a class period, and external reinforcement is also gradually removed.

GOAL SETTING

Goal setting is a critical component of self-regulation (Bandura, 1986). Goals serve three important functions for learners (Schunk, 1990):

1. Goals structure effort by providing a target for our efforts (e.g., "I want to lose 10 pounds."). This in turn provides information on how to accomplish the goal (e.g., "I need to decrease my calories and increase my exercise.").
2. Goals provide information on progress. To continue the previous example, we would monitor our weight to see if we are making progress meeting the goal.
3. Finally, goals can motivate performance ("I lost 3 pounds this week. Yipee!").

Progress toward a goal and achieving a goal is reinforcing. Put simply, it feels good to reach a goal. Problems with goal-related behaviors are common among students with ADHD (Barkley, 2006). They may be unaware of the goal associated with a task and may also have difficulty maintaining goals in working memory. They also may set maladaptive goals that can serve to inhibit performance. For example, some students with ADHD have performance-avoidance goals (i.e., avoid appearing incompetent) (Barron et al., 2006). In this case students are not concerned with accomplishing tasks, but with avoiding being seen as lacking ability.

Goal setting has been used successfully for a variety of problems with students with ADHD. For example, Trammel, Schloss, and Alper (1994) taught middle and high school students to self-monitor their homework completion. This resulted in an increase in the rate of homework completion. They then taught students to set goals for homework completion and graph the results. Goal setting resulted in an additional improvement in homework completion rate. Barry and Messer (2003) used self-management and goal setting combined with reinforcement for goal attainment to reduce the levels of disruptive behavior for sixth-grade students with ADHD in the general education classroom. Goal setting is also useful in the instructional process. For instance, Lienemann and Reid (2008) used goal setting as a part of instruction in an essay writing strategy. The instructor and student first discussed the importance of writing essays that had all the necessary parts. They then examined the number of parts in past essays written by the student and graphed the results. They next set the goal of writing an essay with all the parts. After each essay the student wrote, the student counted up the number of essay parts and then recorded them on a graph. The authors concluded that reaching a goal was motivating for students. Note that goal setting typically involves a self-evaluative process where students compare current performance with a goal (Schunk, 2001). It is this evaluative process that is the source of motivation.

Teaching goal setting is a straightforward process. First, the teacher and student meet and discuss performance in an area (e.g., spelling test results). Together the teacher and student decide on an appropriate goal, determine a timeline for meeting the goal, and establish how progress toward the goal can be monitored. Choosing appropriate goals is important. For a goal to be effective it should be (Bandura, 1988):

- *Specific.* A good goal is well defined. Goals that are vague (e.g., try your hardest) are not as effective as those that are well specified (e.g., get 80% correct on the math test).
- *Proximal.* The best goals are ones that can be reached in the near term (e.g., copy my spelling words three times by the end of class). Proximal goals are more effective than distal goals that can only be completed in the far future (e.g., learn 100 new spelling words by the end of the year). The time taken to accomplish the goal may reduce or eliminate reinforcement or motivation. This factor will likely be important for students with ADHD who need frequent reinforcement. Note, however, that it is possible to use a series of proximal goals to accomplish a long-term goal.
- *Moderately difficult.* The most effective goals are those that are moderately challenging, that is, those that are neither too easy nor too difficult. Goals that are easily attained do not serve to enhance or maintain effort (Johnson & Graham, 1990).

Note that for goal setting to be effective goals *must be valued.* If a goal has little or no importance to the student, then it is unlikely to improve performance or maintain motivation or effort. Thus teachers may need to point out the benefits of accomplishing a goal (e.g., getting homework completed will mean not missing recess). Because the actual goal(s) selected are so important, it's best for the teacher to help with setting goals to ensure that goals are realistic and attainable. Otherwise students may set goals that are either much too high or much too easy.

Teachers should also ensure that students are aware of progress toward their goals. This provides student with self-evaluative feedback that increases motivation. One good way to help students see progress toward goals is to combine goal setting and self-monitoring where students self-record and graph their performance. Graphing provides powerful visual feedback. Additionally, teachers should stress that students' progress toward a goal is the result of their efforts rather than simply luck or factors outside their control (Schunk, 2001). Figure 11.5 shows an example of a goal-setting graph. Note that students may focus on a distal goal (e.g., get an "A" in math). This is perfectly understandable. In this type of situation, the teachers should establish more proximal (and readily attainable) goals (e.g., get a "C" on this week's math test). Note also that the teacher needs to establish procedures to help the student attain the goal. For example, the teacher might suggest daily 10-minute practice sessions on multiplication facts and have the student self-monitor the number of facts he or she got correct.

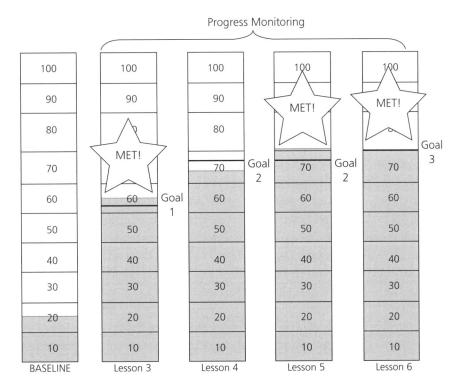

FIGURE 11.5. Example of a goal-setting graph. From Hagaman, Luschen, and Reid (2010). Copyright 2010 by the Council for Exceptional Children. Reprinted by permission.

SELF-REINFORCEMENT

Self-reinforcement occurs when a student selects a reinforcer and self-awards it when a predetermined criterion is reached or exceeded (e.g., when I read 20 pages, I get a break; Graham et al., 1992). Zimmerman and Schunk (1989) note that this process is analogous to the natural developmental process where a child learns that meeting expectations often results in positive reinforcement and conversely failure to reach expectations results in no response or a negative response. As a result, children learn to self-reinforce their own behavior. Learning to self-reinforce appropriately may be important for many students with ADHD. Students with ADHD may require frequent reinforcement to maintain or change behavior; self-reinforcement can be an efficient and effective means of providing needed reinforcement.

Although self-reinforcement has not been employed as frequently as other self-regulation strategies, it has been used effectively with students with ADHD. For example, Ajibola and Clement (1995) used a combination of self-monitoring, goal setting, and self-reinforcement with six students with ADHD in a tutoring class. The students set goals for the number of reading problems they hoped to complete and self-monitored the number of reading problems they actually completed. Each time they answered a reading comprehension question correctly, they awarded themselves one point. At the end of the tutoring session each day they received a stamp in a "payment book" for reaching their goal. When students earned four stamps they could redeem them for tangible reinforcers. This intervention led to significant improvement in academic performance.

Self-reinforcement is implemented using a four-step process. First, the teacher sets the standard that must be met for receiving rewards. This may be done in collaboration with a student if feasible. Standards should be clear and objective. For example, "getting better at math" would not be a good standard; "getting 80% correct on my math worksheets" would be more appropriate. Note that the standards should be set low enough that the student can receive at least some reinforcement relatively quickly. Second, the teacher and student should select a reinforcer. We recommend involving the student in this process for practical reasons: students know what is rewarding to them. Third, determine how students will evaluate whether or not they have met the standard for reinforcement. For example, the student may self-correct or bring the work to you to check. Finally, if the student met or exceeded the criterion they may award themselves the reinforcer. Note that awarding reinforcements does not need to be totally independent. For example, the student could be taught to check with the teacher before self-awarding reinforcement. Self-reinforcement is often combined with goal setting since they have so much in common (e.g., setting a criterion for performance, reinforcement based on achieving criterion level).

SELF-INSTRUCTIONS

Self-instruction strategies involve the use of self-statements to direct or self-regulate behavior, affect, or cognitions (Graham et al., 1992). They take advantage of the fact that language is often used to self-regulate behavior, and that this is a part of the normal developmental process (Harris, 1990). Self-instruction interventions involve the use of *induced* self-statements to direct or self-regulate behavior (Graham et al., 1992). Self-instruction strategies quite literally teach students to talk themselves through a task or activity. Self-instructions can be used for many different purposes. Figure 11.6 shows some basic functions of self-instructions (Graham et al., 1992). Self-instruction strategies may be particularly useful for students with ADHD because the difficulty using language to moderate behavior is seen as one of the key EF deficits in students with ADHD (Barkley, 2006).

Self-instruction strategies have been dismissed as ineffective by some researchers (e.g., Braswell, 1998) based on the results of reviews of literature by Abikoff (1985, 1991). However, as Harris et al. (2005) noted, the claim that self-instruction strategies are ineffective is based largely on research that taught self-instruction strategies in an experimental setting (e.g., a hospital) that were aimed at complex global social and problem-solving behaviors. These strategies were then expected to generalize to home and school settings. In contrast, when self-instruction strategies are taught in the environment in which they will be used and aimed at more specific problem behaviors they can be quite effective, as more recent analyses indicate (Robinson, Smith, Miller, & Brownell, 1999). For example, Hogan and Prater (1993) used self-instructions and self-monitoring to help reduce the number of outbursts with a student with extremely disruptive behaviors, attentional problems, and distractibility. The student was taught that when he became frustrated he should Stop, Count, and Think before he reacted. The student was given a checklist showing the self-instruction steps and taught to go through the checklist and use the self-instructions

Type of self-instruction	Example
Problem definition: defining the nature and demands of a task	"Okay. What do I need to do now?" "What's my next step?"
Focusing attention/planning: attending to task and generating plans	"I need to take my time and concentrate." "What's the best way to do this problem?"
Strategy related: engaging and using a strategy	"I need to remember to use my strategy." "Okay, what I need to do is remember my four B's strategy."
Self-evaluation: error detection and correction	"I need to check and see how I am doing?" "Does this answer make sense?" "Oops, this isn't right. I need to fix it."
Coping: dealing with difficulties/ failures	"I can do this if I keep at it." "This isn't rocket science, I know I can do it." "Take a deep breath and relax."
Self-reinforcement: rewarding oneself	"I did it! Great job!" "I worked hard and I got it right!"

FIGURE 11.6. Self-instruction examples. From Reid and Lienemann (2006a). Copyright 2006 by The Guilford Press. Reprinted by permission.

for each step when he felt he might become disruptive. The use of self-instructions nearly eliminated the outbursts in both a resource room and the general education classroom.

Teaching students to use self-instructions is straightforward (Graham et al., 1992). First, the teacher and student discuss the importance of verbalizations, and how what we say to ourselves can help or hurt us. This is very important because students with ADHD may exhibit high rates of very negative self-statement (e.g., "I'm stupid." "I'll never get this."). The focus of the discussion is on how to use words to help yourself. Second, the teacher and student collaboratively develop meaningful, individualized task-appropriate self-statements together. At this point we would stress that teachers must remember that self-instructions are not simply parroting back statements created by the teacher. Self-instruction training is a *dialogue* not a monologue. For self-instruction to be successful, self-statements must be meaningful to the student, and the most meaningful statements often are those that the student develops. Note, however, if a student likes a teacher's example it's perfectly appropriate for him or her to use it. Third, the teacher and student model the use of self-statements and discuss how and when they would use them. Finally, the teacher provides opportunities for collaborative practice in the use of self-instructions to perform the task. This would include modeling the self-statements and discussing how and when to use the self-statements. The ultimate goal is for students to progress from the use of modeled, overt self-statements (i.e., talking aloud to oneself) to covert, internalized speech (Harris, 1990).

CAUTIONS AND LIMITATIONS

In this chapter we have argued for the use of self-regulation strategies with students with ADHD and provided a number of examples where these strategies have been used successfully with students with ADHD in the classroom. However, we would caution that while these strategies are powerful and potentially very useful there are limitations and concerns that teacher should be aware of.

- *Self-regulation strategies don't create new behaviors.* Self-regulation strategies allow students to use behaviors that they already possess, they don't create new ones. What self-regulation strategies can do is increase the frequency of behaviors (e.g., persisting on a task) or help a student guide him- or herself through a task. For example, teaching a student to self-monitor the number of correct math problems on daily work sheets would be appropriate if the student knew his or her math facts and had a problem maintaining focus or with careless errors. However, self-monitoring alone would not teach the student math facts.

- *Self-regulation strategies are not for students who are out of control.* Self-regulation strategies are not appropriate for students who exhibit extreme behaviors (e.g., physical violence) on a frequent basis. For these types of problems behavioral interventions are more appropriate.

- *Don't expect generalization.* The most effective self-regulation interventions are those that are targeted at a specific behavior in a specific setting. Remember that even if a student shows tremendous improvements in one setting it is not likely that the improvements will generalize to other settings or behaviors. For example, if a student learns to self-manage homework and the rate of homework completion and quality improve markedly, it's unlikely that the student would spontaneously apply the strategy to organizing materials for the classroom. However, if a technique is effective, the teacher can work with the student to help him or her use the technique in a different setting or for a new task. Thus, in our previous example, the teacher could work with the student to develop self-management to help organize class materials. Note that students often find self-regulation strategies helpful, and are amenable to using them for other purposes; it's just that it's unlikely that students will do this independently.

- *Remember the environment.* Self-regulation does not take place in a vacuum. The environment is a significant factor in self-regulation that can enhance or enable self-regulation or make it unlikely that it will be feasible (Mace et al., 2001). Providing students with a structured environment and a predictable, stable routine is an important prerequisite for self-regulation that can increase the likelihood of effective self-regulation. In contrast, when a classroom environment is disordered or chaotic, successful self-regulation is unlikely to occur. Students also may self-regulate their environment to help themselves complete tasks (e.g., finding a place to study that is quiet and free of outside distractions). Remember that even in the *best possible* environment students with ADHD may have some problem with self-regulation. Additionally, there are many simple environmental changes that can enhance self-regulation, such as providing students with folders to serve as organizers for assignments, taping prompts to lockers ("Did you remember to bring your book?"), or using prompt cards (which list the steps for a task and serves to cue performance). Teachers need to remember to attend to both self-regulation strategies and creating supportive environments.

SUMMING UP

Difficulties with self-regulation are the root of many problems experienced by students with ADHD. For example, they might be able to complete the homework, but then lose it or forget to hand it in. Providing self-regulation strategies can help students with ADHD deal more effectively with many problems they experience. Here are some points to remember:

- ✓ Self-regulation strategies can be effective with students with ADHD especially if their problems are due to performance problems as opposed to skill deficits.
- ✓ A self-regulation strategy can be used in isolation, but self-regulation

strategies are frequently combined (e.g., using self-monitoring and goal setting together).

✓ Self-monitoring involves students self-assessing and self-recording the results. One major advantage of self-monitoring is that it can provide ongoing performance feedback.

✓ Self-management involves evaluative feedback that compares a teacher's ratings of performance with the student's self-ratings. This technique may be useful if a student's perception of his or her performance (i.e., positive illusory bias) is very inaccurate.

✓ Goal setting is particularly appropriate for students with ADHD because they often experience difficulties maintaining goals in working memory. However, teachers need to ensure that students have the means to achieve their goals.

✓ Self-reinforcement may be useful to help provide additional reinforcement for students with ADHD.

✓ Using language to help guide and structure behavior is difficult for students with ADHD. Self-instructions that use induced self-statements can be beneficial in helping students to use language to help themselves accomplish tasks or reduce inappropriate behaviors.

✓ There are limitations to self-regulation strategies. Self-regulation strategies don't create new behaviors. They are not appropriate for students who are out of control. They are not likely to generalize across settings.

✓ Environment is a critical factor in successful self-regulation. A stable classroom environment is a prerequisite for effective self-regulation.

CHAPTER 12

Survival Skills

For want of a nail the shoe was lost.
For want of a shoe the horse was lost.
For want of a horse the rider was lost.
For want of a rider the battle was lost.
For want of a battle the kingdom was lost.
And all for the want of a horseshoe nail.
—OLD PROVERB

Small things matter. As the old proverb illustrates, sometimes one small problem can cause a chain of events that results in a much larger problem. No single problem in and of itself was critical, but because each small problem produced a larger problem, the end result was a disaster. Unfortunately, in the classroom, we may overlook small things or take them for granted. One "small thing" that is crucial to success in the classroom is survival skills. Survival skills refer to nonacademic behaviors that allow students to meet classroom demands (Zigmond, Kerr, & Schaeffer, 1988). Figure 12.1 shows examples of important survival skills. These skills are termed survival skills for a very good reason—they are social and organizational behaviors that are critical for success in the classroom. These are small things that we may take for granted; we simply expect them to happen normally. There are also survival skills problems. Students who exhibit these social and organizationally related problems will encounter difficulty in the classroom and may experience negative relations with the classroom teacher. Figure 12.2 shows examples of behaviors identified as survival skills problems.

Students with ADHD often lack survival skills and exhibit survival skills problem behaviors. As we've noted in previous chapters, many of the survival skills problems are behaviors that are common among students with ADHD. In fact some

- Finishes assignments on time.
- Comes to school on time.
- Attends class regularly.
- Accepts consequences for inappropriate behavior.
- Interested in improving academic performance.
- Behaves appropriately in a variety of settings.
- Makes plans for achieving goals.

FIGURE 12.1. High school survival skills. Based on Brown, Kerr, Zigmond, and Harris (1984).

(e.g., seldom completes tasks, difficulty with directions) are very close to symptoms on the DSM-IV diagnostic criteria. The problems may be small ones such as forgetting pencils, losing assignments, or talking to a neighbor at the wrong time. Problems may also be social. For example, a student may fail to recognize important social cues (e.g., the teacher is in a bad mood today) or make inappropriate comments. There may also be problems with oppositional behavior (e.g., back talk). None of these problems at low levels or in isolation would be cause for concern. Forgetting a pencil once in a while or making an inappropriate wise crack aren't likely to seriously affect academic performance or impair the student's relationship with the teacher. However, with students with ADHD the problem behaviors are likely to appear consistently and can negatively affect academics and teacher–student relationships. There may also be problems relating successfully to peers (e.g., the student may lack friends). Lack of an established peer group affect can affect the extent to which a child is engaged with school activities. For this reason, teaching social skills and organization skills can be a lifesaver for children with ADHD.

In this chapter we discuss survival skills for students with ADHD. First, we describe common social skills problem among children with ADHD, provide information on how social skills problems can be assessed, and give recommendation on what teachers can do to help with social skills problems. We then discuss how

- Consistently fails to completes tasks assigned by the teacher.
- Talks back to teachers.
- Is unable to follow written directions.
- Sleeps in class.
- Gives up quickly.
- Fails to bring necessary materials to class.

FIGURE 12.2. High school survival skill problems. Based on Brown, Kerr, Zigmond, and Harris (1984).

teachers can help students with organizational skills, and provide examples of strategies to help students improve organization and class participation.

SOCIAL PROBLEMS OF STUDENTS WITH ADHD

Effective social functioning in the school is important for several reasons. First, problems with social behavior may serve to exacerbate stress. The school environment can be a stressful environment for students with ADHD. For example, students may be the subject of bullying or rejection (Exley, 2008). Adolescent students with ADHD have reported experiencing high levels of stress and having occasional emotional outbursts (Brook & Boaz, 2005). High stress levels are not conducive to effective classroom functioning. Second, socially appropriate behaviors help students make friends, which helps to establish a supportive peer group. Support from friends increases engagement in school (e.g., attendance, participation in class or school activities), which in turn is predictive of future academic achievement (Finn & Cox, 1992; Perdue, Manzeske, & Estell, 2009).

Social problems are common among students with ADHD. Problems often appear early in childhood and can persist into adulthood (Mannuzza & Klein, 2000). While we may tend to think of social difficulties in terms of relations with peers, students with ADHD also experience social problems in their relationships with teachers, parents, and other adults (Mikami, Jack, & Lerner, 2010). The magnitude of their social skills problem is large; studies have found that teachers and parents rate average students without ADHD as having better social skills than 84% of students with ADHD (Mikami et al., 2010). As a result of these problems, students with ADHD are more likely to be avoided or rejected by peers and to experience narrowly delimited social interactions (Cunningham & Siegel, 1987). They also tend to have significantly fewer friends than their peers or even be rejected entirely by their peers (Blachman & Hinshaw, 2002; Mikami et al., 2010). This is a serious concern because having even one friend can reduce the risk of later social adjustment difficulties (Bagwell, Newcomb, & Bukowski, 1998). Unfortunately, students with ADHD also have a positive illusory bias toward their social skills. They tend to significantly overestimate their social competence; thus students with ADHD are likely to be ignorant of their own social skills deficits (Evangelista, Owens, Golden, & Pelham, 2008).

Students with ADHD will often exhibit overactive, inattentive, and impulsive behaviors that interfere with effective social relations (Cunningham & Cunningham, 2006). For example, compared to peers, students with ADHD:

- Are more physically active and talkative during peer interactions (Madan-Swain & Zentall, 1990)
- Are likely to exhibit difficulty with conversational turn taking (Clark, Cheyne, Cunningham, & Siegel, 1988)

- Express fewer positive social statements (Madan-Swain & Zentall, 1990)
- Make more irrelevant comments in conversations and be less sensitive to peer's needs (Mikami et al., 2010)
- Demonstrate a controlling, uncooperative interaction style (Cunningham & Siegel, 1987)
- Exhibit more aggressive or hostile behaviors and be perceived as more aggressive than peers from as early as preschool (DuPaul et al., 2001)

Students with ADHD also have difficulties with understanding or interpreting the emotions of others and expressing their own emotions appropriately (Kats-Gold, Besser, & Priel, 2007; Kats-Gold & Priel, 2009). Thus they are prone to misread others' intent (e.g., they may interpret benign behaviors as hostile). There is some evidence that students with different types of ADHD exhibit different types of social problems. For example, students with the inattentive type may appear passive or withdrawn, while students with the combined type are more likely to exhibit aggression or to make off-topic statements (Mikami et al., 2010). The effect of gender on the social skills of students with ADHD is unclear. Some studies have found that girls are less likely to be rejected than boys, while others have reported no differences (Mikami et al., 2010). As a result of these problems, students with ADHD are more likely to be negatively perceived by peers, often after only a brief contact period (Ernhardt & Hinshaw, 1994; Hinshaw, 2002).

Teachers also need to realize that social relationships don't occur in a vacuum: the behavior of peers toward students with ADHD will also affect their social functioning (Mikami et al., 2010). The ADHD label itself can have a negative effect on how peers perceive students with ADHD, which can in turn affect peers' behavior toward students with ADHD. Studies show that the label of ADHD is likely to elicit negative peer judgments, and that peers report unwillingness to be friends with someone who is labeled ADHD (Mikami et al., 2010). One study (Harris, Milich, & McAninch, 1998) used target children who did not have ADHD. When peers were told that the target student had ADHD—even though this was not true—they behaved poorly toward the student, who in turn responded with negative behaviors. Ironically, the target student's behavior actually served to confirm peer's expectations.

Assessing Social Skills

A number of social skills assessment instruments may be used to assess the severity and nature of social skills problems. The type of assessment used will vary (Spence, 2003) depending on whether the purpose of the assessment is to (1) screen to identify students with social difficulties, (2) provide information about specific deficits and competencies to guide intervention, or (3) evaluate the effectiveness of intervention. There are several different types of assessment including interviews, rating scales, direct observations, and sociometry. Interviews involve questioning the student about aspects of social functioning (e.g., How many friends do you have?).

They can provide information on general functioning and social relationships useful for identifying potential problems area that might be targeted for intervention. Rating scales require teachers to rate students (or students to rate themselves) on a series of items relating to social skills (e.g., Makes friends easily). Rating scales can be useful in screening because they typically provide norms that allow teachers to compare students' social skills to those of their peers.

Direct behavioral observation involves observing students during naturally occurring situations where social skills would be exhibited (e.g., on the playground). This type of assessment is labor-intensive and requires training observers; however, it can provide useful information on specific social behaviors (e.g., participation in play activities). Sociometry is used to identify students who are isolated or neglected by peers (Spence, 2003). This method requires each student in an entire classroom to list peers who they most like and dislike, and who they would most prefer or not prefer to play or work with. There are two concerns relating to the use of sociometry (Merrell, 2001). First, sociometry does not measure social skills. Thus while it could provide information on the extent to which a student was not accepted, there would be no information on why. Second, to ethically conduct sociometry, it's necessary to get informed consent from parents for all students in a class to participate. In practice this may not be feasible. Figure 12.3 shows examples of social skill assessment instruments that might be used in school settings. For more information on social skills assessment for school populations, see *csefel.vanderbilt.edu/documents/rs_screening_assessment.pdf*.

Teaching Social Skills

Social skills training (SST) is recommended as an important part of treatment for students with ADHD and is regarded as a promising practice (Barkley, 2006). Note that SST is not intended to be used in isolation. SST is most effective when it is combined and integrated with parent training and ongoing behavioral supports for appropriate social behaviors (e.g., systematic reinforcement for the use of appropriate social behaviors) (Barkley, 2006). Combining SST and parent training increases the likelihood that students' efforts to employ newly learned skills will be recognized and supported (Spence, 2003). Note that medication may also be helpful in that it can reduce the amount of oppositional (e.g., argumentative responses) and/or aggressive behaviors that can impair social relationships; however, medication alone is not sufficient. It can neither create new skills nor help students recognize when to deploy skills they already possess (Mikami et al., 2010). Figure 12.4 shows examples of SST programs recommended by the National Association of School Psychologist (NASP; 2002) that have demonstrated effectiveness with students with social skills problems.

Components of SST programs vary, as do the nomenclature used to define the components, but most SST typically address the following broad skill areas (Gresham, Sugai, & Horner, 2001; NASP, 2002; Spence, 2003):

Social Adjustment Inventory for Children and Adolescents (SAICA)

The SAICA is a semistructured interview intended for children ages 6 to 18. It can be administered by a parent or teacher who knows the child well. Interviewers who use the SAICA are expected to have experience working with children. The SAICA contains a total of 77 items that cover a full range of observable and well-defined social interactions and outcomes, including potential activities and interactions characteristic of childhood. The SAICA takes about 30 minutes to complete (John, Gammon, Prusoff, & Warner, 1987).

Social Skills Improvement System Rating Scales (SSIS)

The SSIS is a norm-referenced rating scale intended for children ages 3 to 18. There are three versions of the SSIS: Teacher, Parent, and Child self-report. The SSIS is intended to identify specific social skill and performance deficits that can be directly addressed with skill-building interventions. Social skills areas assessed include Communication (e.g., takes turns in conversations, makes eye contact when talking), assertion (e.g., asks for help from adults), Responsibility (e.g., takes responsibility for own actions), Empathy (e.g., feels bad when others are sad), Engagement (e.g., makes friends easily), and Self-control (e.g., stays calm when teased). The SSIS can be completed in 20 minutes (Gresham & Elliot, 2007).

School Social Behavior Scales–2 (SSBS-2)

The SSBS-2 is a norm-referenced rating scale intended for children ages 5 to 18. The SSBS-2 consists of two scales. The Social Competence scale has 32 items that measure adaptive prosocial skills. It consists of three subscales: Peer Relations (e.g., cooperates with other students), Self-Management/Compliance (e.g., shows self-control), and Academic Behavior (e.g., completes assignments on time). The Antisocial Behavior scale consists of 32 items that address social problem behaviors. It consist of three subscales: Hostile/Irritable (e.g., whines and complains), Antisocial–Aggressive (e.g., gets into fights), and Defiant/Disruptive (e.g., is defiant to teacher or other school personnel). Total administration time is around 15 minutes (Merrell, 2002).

Matson Evaluation of Social Skills for Youngsters (MESSY)

The MESSY is a norm-referenced rating scale intended for children ages 4 to 18. It is intended to be used by certified teachers or mental health professionals The MESSY contains 64 items based on observable behaviors that are representative of social skills of children. The MESSY assesses both appropriate and inappropriate social skills to avoid focusing exclusively on the negative aspects of a child's behavior. Examples of appropriate social skills are "Helps a friend who is hurt" and "Walks up to people to start a conversation." Examples of inappropriate social skills are "Gives other children dirty looks" and "Wants to get even with someone who hurt him/her." The MESSY takes approximately 15 minutes to administer (Matson, Rotatori, & Helsel, 1983).

FIGURE 12.3. Instruments for assessing social skills.

"Stop and Think" Social Skills Program

The "Stop and Think" Social Skills Program focuses on interpersonal, problem-solving, and conflict resolution skills. The skills addressed help students to manage their own behavior and more successfully interact with others. Skills include listening, following directions, asking for help, ignoring distractions, accepting consequences, apologizing, dealing with teasing, handling peer pressure, and how to set goals. The program has demonstrated success in reducing student discipline referrals, school suspensions, and expulsions; fostering positive school climates and prosocial interactions; increasing students' on-task behavior; and improving academic performance.

Website: *www.projectachieve.info*

EQUIP Program

The EQUIP program has versions for students in grades 5 to 8 and also for adolescents and young adults. EQUIP program is a 10-week program that can be used in large- or small-group settings. The program covers training in moral judgment, anger management/ correction of thinking errors, and prosocial skills. Training includes the use of role play, group discussions, stories, and self-relaxation exercises. EQUIP has been used successfully with students who have behavioral and emotional disorders.

Website: *www.researchpress.com/scripts/product.asp?item=4848#5134*

PREPARE Curriculum

The PREPARE Curriculum is designed for middle and high school students. PREPARE consists of a series of 10 course-length interventions grouped into three areas: Reducing aggression includes anger management and situational perception training. Reducing stress includes stress management training, problem-solving training, and recruiting supportive models. Reducing prejudice includes empathy and cooperation training. The program also addresses transfer and maintenance of skills.

Website: *www.researchpress.com/scripts/product.asp?item=5063*

ACCEPTS Program

The ACCEPTS program is designed for grades kindergarten through 6. It teaches peer-to-peer skills, skills for relating to adults, and self-management skills. It was designed to be taught by classroom teachers and can be used in individual, small-group, or large-group formats. Skills included in the program are classroom skills (e.g., listening to the teacher, following class rules), basic interaction skills (making eye contact, using the right voice, taking turns), getting along skills (e.g., using polite words, sharing, touching the right way), making friends skills (e.g., smiling, complimenting), and coping skills (e.g., when someone teases you, when things don't go right).

Website: *www.proedinc.com/customer/productView. aspx?ID=625&SearchWord=ACCEPTS%20PROGRAM*

FIGURE 12.4. Social skills programs for students.

- Peer relations skills (e.g., making eye contact, inviting peers to play appropri-
  ately, conversational turn taking, waiting your turn)
- Self-regulation (e.g., self-monitoring behavior or emotions; inhibiting impulsive response)
- Compliance skills (e.g., listening to the teacher, following directions)
- Problem solving (e.g., recognizing problem situations, deciding on a course
  of action, seeking help appropriately)
- Conflict resolution (e.g., responding appropriately to teasing or losing a
  game)
- Perspective taking (e.g., recognizing how others might feel, recognizing
  social cues)

How socials skills are taught is also important. For example, simply giving a lecture
on what to do is not likely to have any effect whatsoever. Instruction in social skills
(Spence, 2003) should incorporate:

- Explicit instruction in skills (e.g., making eye contact) along with explanations of why the skills are important.
- Modeling of the skill by a competent peer in a realistic situation.
- Opportunities to rehearse behaviors through role play and practice activities.
- Structured opportunities to use skills outside of the training setting (e.g.,
  homework assignments to practice skills).
- Reinforcement from teachers, parents, and/or peers when skills are used
  appropriately.
- Sufficient duration and intensity to allow for the skills to be mastered. For
  many students training may require months as opposed to weeks and should
  be conducted on a daily basis.

Note that SST is not "one size fits all." Students can vary widely in the type of
social skills problems they exhibit. Additionally, it is important to recognize that
students may have difficulty with social skills for different reasons. This is especially true for students with ADHD. Students with ADHD may exhibit social skill
problems for two reasons. First, there is a skill deficit: they have not learned or are
unaware of the appropriate behavior (e.g., the student butts into peers' conversations because he or she has not learned to wait for an appropriate moment). Second,
there is a performance deficit: they have the appropriate behavior in their repertoire
but are unable to deploy it (e.g., the student knows to ask for a pencil but impulsively grabs it rather than asking to borrow it). Barkley (2006) has suggested that for
many students with ADHD the problems are largely due to performance deficits,
and therefore SST should focus on helping students with ADHD to use social skills
they already possess. Note, however, that there is also evidence that some students
with ADHD appear to exhibit skill deficits (Mikami et al., 2010).

In practice, teachers may not be able to institute a formal SST program with a student. In this case teachers might target one or two specific behaviors to improve. For example, if a student had problems sharing materials or asking to borrow needed materials during group work, the teacher might conduct a minilesson on how to perform appropriate behaviors (e.g., use calm voice, ask politely, thank for lending, and be sure to return promptly). Then the teacher would systematically praise the student with ADHD for using the appropriate behaviors. The teacher would also praise and reinforce the student's classmates for responding appropriately. There are also some strategies for appropriate nonverbal classroom behavior such as the SLANT strategy (Ellis, 1989). SLANT stands for "Sit up straight," "Lean forward," "Act like you're interested," "Nod," and "Track the teacher." This strategy helps students convey the message that they are engaged and actively paying attention. Note that simply giving the student with ADHD the steps of the strategy would not be effective. Instead the teacher would need to use the strategy instruction procedures described in Chapter 10.

We can't overstate the importance of helping students attain more normal social functioning. Otherwise students with ADHD may be caught in a vicious cycle in which their inappropriate social behaviors cause negative reactions on the part of their peers or teachers, which in turn leads to more inappropriate behaviors on the part of the students with ADHD (Mikami et al., 2010). We must also note that changing a student's social behavior and social status is not an easy task (Spence, 2003). For example, students can make socially appropriate overtures and be rebuffed because their past history of inappropriate behavior is still fresh in the minds of peers. In sum, teachers should realize that changing social behavior and improving the social status of a student with ADHD is a long-term process.

ORGANIZATIONAL SKILLS

O'Regan and Cooper's (2001) case study of "Ruby Tuesday," a 15-year-old student with ADHD, is an excellent example of how organizational problems can frustrate and confound both students and teachers. Ruby had an ongoing problem getting her homework assignments and other supplies (e.g., books, gym clothes, sneakers) from home to school. She had been warned about the problem repeatedly, but even reinforcement and punishment didn't seem to help. Finally when the parents and school personnel met to discuss the problem, Ruby broke down and sobbed, "It's just too much to do altogether" (p. 265). It seemed that Ruby's problem was that her school bag was not large enough to contain all the items she needed, and she did not want to take two bags to school. Unfortunately, what she did choose to take often appeared to be random as opposed to the items she would need that day. This problem was easily solved: Ruby received a new and larger school bag as a birthday gift. Ruby's case aptly illustrates how difficult even a simple organizational problem can appear to students with ADHD, and also the frustration they experience when trying to deal with organizational problems that to most students would be trivial. Note that there is an important lesson for teachers in this case: sometimes "carelessness" or "irresponsible" behavior is actually a problem with organization. For Ruby, reinforcement and punishment were ineffective because they didn't address the underlying organizational difficulty that was the cause of the problem.

As we noted earlier, problems with organization are typical for students with ADHD. In this section we discuss how ADHD affects organization skills and what teachers can do to address these problems. First we discuss the nature of the organizational problems and how they are commonly manifested. We then provide examples of strategies from research that teachers can use in their classrooms to helps student cope with organizational difficulties.

ADHD and Organizational Problems

As we noted earlier, even a cursory examination of the diagnostic criteria for ADHD shows that problems with organization are one of the ways in which ADHD is manifested. This is not surprising due to the problems with executive functions (EFs) among students with ADHD. EF problems quite often result in an outright lack of planning even when students are expressly prompted to plan. Additionally, even when students with ADHD try to plan and organize, their efforts are often ineffective. For example, Brown (2005) noted that individuals with ADHD often complain of difficulties with prioritizing among tasks, and appear to have little or no idea of how much time tasks require, or how many tasks they could reasonably accomplish in a given time. Additionally, while students with ADHD may be impulsive in many situations, in many instances they are likely to procrastinate or report that they have difficulty getting started at even routine tasks (Brown, 2005). Note also that problems with organization are not limited to the school environment; parents also report organizational problems at home (Zentall, Harper, & Stormont-Spurgin, 1993).

Research shows that, on average, students with ADHD are well behind students without ADHD and even students with learning disabilities in terms of their organizational skills (Shin, Kim, Cho, & Kim, 2003). There is also some evidence that suggests students with ADHD develop organization skills at a lower rate than students without ADHD (Shin, Kim, Cho, & Kim, 2003). Moreover, research also suggests that problems with EF and organizational skills are likely to persist into adulthood (Biederman et al., 2007). Thus students with ADHD are unlikely to grow out of their problems after adolescence. Problems with organization among students with ADHD are a serious concern for teachers. Many of the academic difficulties for students with ADHD are due to problems with organization (Pfiffner et al., 2006).

Improving Organizational Skills

The ability to organize is critical for success in the classroom for students at all levels (Krishnan, Feller, & Orkin, 2010). Students who come to class unprepared (e.g., without needed materials) or who fail to complete or turn in assignments are at increased risk for academic problems (e.g., failing to master course content, receiving a low grade in a class). We recommend that teachers treat organizational skills as a part of their curriculum beginning early on in elementary school. Teaching how to organize would likely be useful for most students; it could literally be a lifesaver for students with ADHD. We believe that an early start is important because the demands for organization and independent functioning increase markedly as students progress from elementary to middle and high school. Students with ADHD should learn organization skills early on so that they can become fluent in their use and appreciate how organizational skills can help them be more successful. In this section we provide examples of three approaches to help students become better organized: organizational prompts, self-regulation strategies, and organizational skills and strategies. Note that although we discuss each separately, in practice they can, and often should, be used together. For more on teaching organizational skills and strategies to student, see Meltzer's (2007) book on the topic.

Organizational Prompts

Organizational prompts are materials that cue a student to plan or organize his or her efforts. At the most basic level an organizational prompt might be as simple as a sign taped inside a locker. Figure 12.5 shows an example of a prompt that might be used to help remind a student to bring needed materials to class. Planner and homework folders are other examples of organizational prompts. Figure 12.6 shows an example and Figure 12.7 shows a completed example. There are numerous commercially available planners that could also be used. Note that simply providing material is not sufficient. Giving a student with ADHD a planner and telling him or

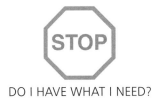

DO I HAVE WHAT I NEED?

BOOKS?
PENCIL?
BINDER?
HOMEWORK
ASSIGNMENTS?
PLANNER?

THINK!!
IS THERE ANYTHING SPECIAL TODAY?

FIGURE 12.5. Example of an organizational prompt.

Day	Assignment	Materials	Due

FIGURE 12.6. Simple planner.

Day	Assignment	Materials	Due
Monday	Problems 1–20 on page 57	Math book	Tuesday
Monday	Read Chapter 6 in social studies and do questions	Social Studies book	Wednesday
Tuesday	3-page report on lasers	Library books, web search	Friday
Wednesday			

FIGURE 12.7. Example of a completed simple planner.

her to use it is unlikely to have much effect. It's critical for students to use organizational prompts. It's also important for the teacher to explicitly show students why the materials were provided and how using the materials can help them. Teachers need to remember that while this may be obvious to us it is likely not obvious to students with ADHD.

For example, with the locker prompt, the teacher, Mrs. Jones, first might meet with Bruce to establish that there is a problem and then discuss the nature of the problem. Mrs. Jones would point out that several of Bruce's teachers were frustrated with him because he consistently came to class without needed materials. Several times he forgot to hand in assignments that he had completed, which resulted in lower grades because they were handed in late. He also got a low grade on an exam because he forgot to bring a pen and could not take notes on several occasions. Mrs. Jones would then discuss with the student why the problem occurs. The problem seems to be that Bruce has a hard time remembering to bring all the materials he needs to class. He makes it to his locker, but gets distracted or is in a rush and forgets to check to see that he has everything he needs. The teacher would then introduce the prompt. Together, Bruce and the teacher would discuss how to use the prompt card. The teacher will stress that every time Bruce goes to his locker he will see the prompt. This will remind him to go through the list of items. Mrs. Jones might even go with Bruce to his locker and model using the prompt card by systematically going through the list and verbally asking herself whether she needed each item on the list. After Bruce began using the prompt card independently, Mrs. Jones would be sure to check with Bruce's teachers to see if he was consistently coming to class prepared. Assuming that the prompt was helping Bruce to come prepared, Mrs. Jones would also be sure to reinforce (e.g., praise) Bruce for his performance.

Self-Regulation Strategies

Self-regulation strategies have been used successfully with students with ADHD to help them come to class prepared (e.g., Gureasko-Moore, DuPaul, & White, 2006, 2007), to help them complete and return homework (e.g., Axelrod, Zhe, Haugen, & Klein, 2009; Meyer & Kelley, 2007), and to help them with time management and planning (Solanto et al., 2010). Gureasko-Moore et al. (2006) provides an excellent example of how teachers can effectively use self-regulation strategies with students with ADHD. In this study the authors used an intervention with several self-regulation strategies to help three male high school students with ADHD improve their class preparation.

The first step in the intervention was to meet with each student individually and (1) establish that there was a problem with preparation, (2) stress exactly why coming to class was important (e.g., the student might miss important information), and (3) specify exactly what is needed to come to class prepared (e.g., bring paper and pencil, textbook, any assignments that are due). The instructor then helped the student identify all his problems with class preparation and list them in a logbook. Next the student and instructor collaboratively worked to set a weekly goal for preparation (e.g., the student would complete at least four of six preparation activities each day). The instructor then introduced the self-monitoring form, and the student wrote the goal down. Students were told that each day after the targeted class they were to use the self-monitoring form to self-assess their class preparedness by checking yes or no for each item. See Figure 12.8 for an example of a self-monitoring form.

Students were also instructed to write in their logbook the number of preparation behaviors that they performed and what they could do to be more effective at preparation. Students also were asked to rate the extent to which they were satisfied with the effort they expended at meeting their goals (e.g., 0 = no effort/total dissatisfaction to 5 = best effort/total satisfaction; p. 169). This served as self-reinforcement. After a 4-day training period, the students began using the procedures each day in the targeted classroom. Initially, the instructor met with students daily to monitor the extent to which students were using the procedures and for students to self-critique their performance. The instructor praised students for meeting goals and problem-solved with students when they failed to meet a goal. When students met weekly goals they set new goals. Meetings with the instructor were gradually faded from once a day, to every other day, to once a week. The results were impressive—after learning these procedures all student were almost always 100% prepared for class.

Organizational Skills and Strategies

Helping students to learn to plan, organize, monitor, prioritize, and evaluate efforts can help them to be more efficient and effective students. There are many organizational skills that would be helpful for students with ADHD. Among the most critical (Krishnan et al., 2010) are:

Date: _____

Classe: _____

Was I Prepared Today?

Did I come to class on time?	Yes	No
Did I bring my:		
Paper/binder	Yes	No
Pen or pencil	Yes	No
Text	Yes	No
Assignments	Yes	No
Planner	Yes	No

My goal for today is _____ out of 6.

FIGURE 12.8. Example of a self-monitoring chart for class preparation.

- *Goal setting:* being able to set realistic achievable goals. Goals provide structure for efforts, enable progress monitoring, and enhance motivation. The goal-setting process was discussed in Chapter 11.
- *Task analysis:* being able to take a task and break it down into its components. This allows students to take a complex task and convert it into a series of smaller and more manageable tasks.
- *Time management:* being able to take the components of a task (defined by a task analysis) and estimate the amount of time needed to complete each of them. This allows students to make an estimate of how long it will take them to complete a task and also to determine when they need to start a task in order to complete it ontime.

Note that there are also prerequisite skills for organizational skills (Krishnan et al., 2010). Some important preskills are:

- *Knowledge of time.* The student must be able to make a reasonably accurate estimate of the passage of time. This is a critical skill for time management. It is also potentially a serious problem for students with ADHD because an impaired sense of time is common among students with ADHD (Barkley, 2006).

- *Understanding of tasks.* The student must have sufficient knowledge of a task to analyze it, identify the components of the task, and then estimate the time required to perform each component of the task. This could be a problem for students with ADHD because they typically do not engage in planning activities prior to attempting tasks (e.g., Jacobson & Reid, 2010).

- *Prioritizing tasks.* The student must be able to distinguish between tasks that must be done (e.g., homework), and tasks that he or she wants to do (e.g., horseback riding). Students will usually be in a position in which they face competing demands on their time (e.g., schoolwork, household chores, softball practice, going to the mall with friends). Successful time management requires students to allow sufficient time for tasks that they must accomplish. In the case of students with ADHD this may be difficult because delaying gratification (e.g., completing homework before going on a long bike ride) is very difficult for them (Barkley, 2006).

There are also specific strategies to help students with organizational problems. One example is the WATCH strategy (Glomb & West, 1990) that is designed to help students complete assignments (see *www.unl.edu/csi/study.shtml* for other examples of organizational strategies). WATCH is a mnemonic for:

Write—Write down the assignment when it is given and write the due date.
Ask—Ask the teacher for clarification or help on the assignment if needed.
Task Analyze—Task-analyze the assignment and make a schedule for the tasks identified.
CHeck—Check the finished work for completeness, accuracy, and neatness.

Teachers would teach this strategy just as they would any other content-area strategy and would go through all the strategy instruction steps discussed in Chapter 10. Figure 12.9 shows an example of how a teacher might model the use of the strategy. Note that important parts of the strategy such as task analysis and time management are also modeled in some detail. Note also that in the Ask step, the teacher would model asking appropriately (e.g., don't interrupt to ask for clarification). Teachers should be careful not to overlook social aspects of strategy performance and should not assume that students with ADHD will know how to perform them correctly.

Teachers should remember that the skills and strategies taught will depend on the student's grade level and specific needs. Krishnan et al. (2010) have suggested that instruction in organizational strategies should begin in the elementary grades, and that there should be a developmental progression when teaching organizational strategies. In elementary school instruction should be focused on modeling strategies and helping students develop fluency with strategies. At the middle and high school levels, the focus is promoting and supporting independent strategy use. Here the teacher's focus shifts to cueing student's to consistently use strategies and to personalize them. This progression also appears to be appropriate for students with ADHD regardless of grade level. That is to say, teachers should not assume that simply because a student is in high school that she or he has learned organizational skills or developed effective strategies. Note also that demands for independent performance increase as students progress through elementary, middle, and high schools. Thus the need for well-developed organizational skills and effective strategies also increases.

SUMMING UP

Survival skills are those "small things," both social and academic, that potentially can have a disproportionate impact on a students' successful functioning in the classroom. They are easy to overlook in part because most students perform them as a matter of course. Unfortunately, survival skills are an area where many students with ADHD are likely to struggle. Some important points to remember are:

✓ Social skills are important. Students with a supportive peer group are more likely to be engaged in school.

✓ Social skills problems are common among students with ADHD.

✓ Students with ADHD are likely to overestimate their social competence.

✓ Social skills training programs are a recommended component of treatment for ADHD. These training programs should be integrated with other components of treatment (e.g., parent training).

✓ Improving social skills is a long-term process. It's very unlikely that a student will suddenly develop social competence after a few lessons. Additionally,

1. The first step in WATCH is "write down the assignment when it is given and write the due date." I will take out my planner as soon as I get a chance and write "Book report due November 30" on today's date. I would also add a note that says, "Pick and read reading-level book and one page double-spaced typed." This way I have everything important written down so I do not forget all the important information I need to complete the assignment. When I hear about an assignment, I need to remember to write down the important things:

    *   When it is due
    *   How it needs to be done (Does it need to be typed or written? How many pages does there need to be?)
    *   What do I need to do in the assignment?

    I do not need to write every single thing the teacher says when I am getting the assignment, but I do need the important parts.

2. The second step in WATCH is "Ask." I need to ask myself, "Is there anything that is confusing to me that I would like to ask the teacher about?" I think I am not sure about finding a book at my reading level. Since I found something that I need clarification about, do I ask my teacher if she is teaching math? No, that's probably not a good time. I think I'll ask her if she is not busy, like after class or when she is at her desk. If I think of something I want to ask her and it is not a good time to ask, I will write it down, maybe in my agenda or somewhere else I will know I will see it, and ask her later. When it is a good time, I will go up to my teacher and maybe say something like this: "Hi, Miss Swift. I was looking over the book report assignment and there's something I think I need help with. I'm not sure that I understand how to find a book at my reading level. Can you help me figure this out?" Once my teacher answers my question, I will repeat back her answer to make sure that I understand her correctly.

3. The third step in WATCH is "Task-analyze." This is when I'm going to look at my assignment and break it down into smaller parts. Okay, this seems like a really big project and I'm feeling overwhelmed. Maybe if I make this into smaller parts first, it will be a little easier to do. Okay, so the first thing I will do is ask, "What are the really big parts of this? Where is the beginning, middle, and end of my assignment? Well, the beginning is reading my book. Then I guess the middle would be writing my report. Finally, I type my report and hand it in.

    That's a good start, but maybe if I break it into smaller parts it will be even easier. Okay, so the beginning of my report is reading the book. First, I need to pick out my book. To make things easier I will get a book from our class library because I know a book with a red or yellow sticker is at my reading level. Then I will read it. Okay, I broke my beginning into two smaller parts.

    Now my middle. Okay, I will write my report. I know that when I write a report, I gather my information first. I know that I need to include "WHO was in the story." I need to write "WHAT is the name of the book and WHAT happened in the story." I also need to write "WHEN and WHERE the story took place." Looking back through my notes I see I need to write "WHY I liked the book or did not like the book" and "How I picked my book." I know that in reports I need an introduction and a conclusion. I will take all the information I found, and write a rough draft. So for my middle, I broke that into nine even smaller parts. That is much easier! But I still have to look at the end of the assignment.

    The end of my assignment is typing my report. First, I think I'll reread my rough draft to make sure I wrote everything I needed to write. I'll ask myself "Did I write all five W's and H, an introduction and conclusion?" If I did then I can type my report. Once I have typed it, I will print it off. I broke the end of my assignment into three extra parts. Now I have a really great idea of what I need to do.

(cont.)

FIGURE 12.9. Example of think-aloud segments for the WATCH strategy. Developed by Ms. Sarah Swift, University of Nebraska–Lincoln. Used by permission.

Now I can go through all of the parts of my report and figure out how much time I need to spend on each part. Okay, I know that I have until November 30th to finish my assignment. That gives me 29 days. I think I will look through all of the parts I found in my assignment and figure out how long each should take. First I need to pick out a book. I can look in my class library for a book with a red or yellow sticker. I will look for something with an interesting title or cover. Maybe I will ask my friends what they read and enjoyed. I can also ask my teacher so this step will probably take an hour or less.

Next I will read my book. I can read about two chapters a day and there are 14 chapters, it will take me one week to read my book. This means that by November 7 I should have finished my book. I think it might be a good idea to put that in my assignment notebook so I don't forget. I'll open it up to November 7 and write, "Finish book for book report." When I look over an assignment, I'll see important parts that I need to finish by certain days to make sure that I do not get behind.

I have six things I need to look for in my book that I will write about—who, what, when, where, why, and how. For each of those, I will probably have to look back in my book and write important information about each of them to stay organized. This will probably take an hour for each part—so that is 6 hours. If I do one of the five W's and H a day, I will be done with this part by November 13. That is another "landmark" so I will write "Write five W's and H" down in my assignment notebook on November 13. That means I have 17 days left to finish my assignment. Wow! When I make a time line like this, I can do my assignment pretty quickly!

The next step is to write my report. Since I already have the information I need for my middle with my five W's and H, this should go pretty quickly. I'm going to guess and say this part should take about 3 hours at the most.

My next step is to write an introduction and conclusion. Usually writing a paragraph takes about 30 minutes, so since I have two paragraphs that will take me an hour. With the 3 hours from my middle and the hour for my introduction and conclusion, writing the actual report should take 4 hours. I can probably do this over 2 days. I should be able to write my report by November 15, so I will write in my assignment notebook on November 15 "Rough draft of book report DONE." I still have 15 days left to finish my report!

The next step of my assignment is to review my rough draft to make sure I have everything written that needs to be in my report. This will take about 2 hours. I'll do this over 2 days, so that if I need to fix something, I will have plenty of time to finish it.

Once I have finished reviewing my rough draft, I can type my report. This will take me about 1 hour since I will be typing what is on my rough draft. WOW! This means that I can have my entire assignment done by November 18—12 whole days before it is due! That will give me plenty of time to make sure my report is done correctly, do other assignments and the fun things that I enjoy instead of worrying about finishing my book report!

The last step of WATCH—is CH, check for completeness, accuracy, and neatness. Since I will have my whole assignment typed out, I can go back to make sure I have everything done that I need. Do I have the five W's and H in my paper? Uh oh, I forgot to write HOW I chose the book. Thank goodness I checked my paper. I can go back and fix it. Once I have fixed that, I can continue checking for completeness. Is my paper one page, double-spaced? Yes it is! Is everything accurate or correct about what I wrote. Hm, looking over I notice that I wrote the author's name wrong. That's okay. I can fix that now. Okay, is everything else accurate? Yes it is! Now I can check for neatness. Is my paper clean? Is it wrinkled? Yes it is. Now I can hand in my assignment early or put it in a folder so it stays neat. Wow! I got everything done way before my assignment was due. WATCH really helped me do my assignment.

FIGURE 12.9. *(cont.)*

there is the problem that past behavior problems may affect peers' perceptions of present behavior and impair acceptance.

✓ Even the most rudimentary organization may be difficult for students with ADHD. This problem tends to persist over time.

✓ Providing supports for organization and teaching organizational skills and strategies should be a priority for teachers.

✓ Self-regulation strategies can be effective in helping improve students' organizational skills.

✓ Students with ADHD will likely need to be taught to set goals, perform a task analysis, and use time management skills.

References

Abikoff, H. (1985). Efficacy of cognitive training interventions in hyperactive children: A critical review. *Clinical Psychology Review, 5,* 479–512.

Abikoff, H. (1991). Cognitive training in ADHD children: Less to it than meets the eye. *Journal of Learning Disabilities, 24,* 205–209.

Abikoff, H., Courtney, M., Pelham, W., & Koplewicz, H. (1993). Teachers' ratings of disruptive behaviors: The influence of halo effects. *Journal of Abnormal Child Psychology, 21,* 519–533.

Abramowitz, A. J., & O'Leary, S. (1991). Behavioral interventions for the classroom: Implications for students with ADHD. *School Psychology Review, 20,* 220–234.

Abramowitz, A. J., Reid, M. J., & O'Toole, K. (1994). *The role of task timing in the treatment of ADHD.* Paper presented at the meeting of the Association for Advancement of Behavior Therapy, San Diego, CA.

Acevedo-Polakovich, I. D., Lorch, E. P., & Milich, R. (2007). Comparing television use and reading in children with ADHD and non-referred children across two age groups. *Media Psychology, 9,* 447–472.

Achenbach, T. M., & Rescorla, L. A. (2001). *Manual for the ASEBA School-Age Forms and Profiles.* Burlington: University of Vermont Research Center for Children, Youth, and Families.

Acker, M., & O'Leary, S. (1987). Effects of reprimands and praise on appropriate behavior in the classroom. *Journal of Abnormal Child Psychology, 15,* 549–557.

Ajibola, O., & Clement, P. W. (1995). Differential effects of methylphenidate and self-reinforcement on attention deficit hyperactivity disorder. *Behavior Modification, 19,* 211–233.

Alberto, P. A., & Troutman, A. C. (2006). *Applied behavior analysis for teachers* (7th ed.). Columbus, OH: Merrill.

Alloway, T. P. (2006). How does working memory work in the classroom? *Educational Research and Reviews, 1,* 134–139.

Alloway, T. P., Gathercole, S. E., & Elliott, J. (2010). Examining the link between working memory behaviour and academic attainment in children with ADHD. *Developmental Medicine and Child Neurology, 52,* 632–636.

Alloway, T. P., Gathercole, S. E., Kirkwood, H. J., & Elliott, J. E. (2009). The cognitive and behavioral characteristics of children with low working memory. *Child Development, 80,* 606–621.

American Academy of Child and Adolescent Psychiatry. (2007). Practice parameters for the assessment and treatment of children and adolescents with attention-deficit/hyperactivity disorder. *Journal of the American Academy of Child and Adolescent Psychiatry, 46,* 894–921.

American Academy of Child and Adolescent Psychiatry. (2009). Practice parameters on the use of psychotropic medication in children and adolescents. *Journal of the American Academy of Child and Adolescent Psychiatry, 48,* 961–973.

American Academy of Pediatrics. (2009). Policy statement—Guidance for the administration of medication in school. *Pediatrics, 124,* 1244–1251.

American Psychiatric Association. (1968). *Diagnostic and statistical manual of mental disorders* (2nd ed.). Washington, DC: Author.

American Psychiatric Association. (1980). *Diagnostic and statistical manual of mental disorders* (3rd ed.). Washington, DC: Author.

American Psychiatric Association. (1987). *Diagnostic and statistical manual of mental disorders* (3rd ed., text rev.). Washington, DC: Author.

American Psychiatric Association. (1994). *Diagnostic and statistical manual of mental disorders* (4th ed.). Washington, DC: Author.

American Psychiatric Association. (2000). *Diagnostic and statistical manual of mental disorders* (4th ed., text rev.). Washington, DC: Author.

Anastopoulos, A. D., Hennis Rhoads, L., & Farley, S. E. (2006). Counseling and training parents. In R. A. Barkley (Ed.), *Attention-deficit hyperactivity disorder: A handbook for diagnosis and treatment* (pp. 453–479). New York: Guilford Press.

Anastopoulos, A. D., & Shelton, T. L. (2001). *Assessing attention-deficit/hyperactivity disorder.* New York: Kluwer Academic/Plenum.

Angello, L. M., Volpe, R. J., DiPerna, J. C., Gureasko-Moore, S. P., Gureasko-Moore, D. P., Nebrig, M. R., et al. (2003). Assessment of attention-deficit/hyperactivity disorder: An evaluation of six published rating scales. *School Psychology Review, 32,* 241–262.

Angold, A., Costello, E. J., & Erkanli, A. (1999). Comorbidity. *Journal of Child Psychology and Psychiatry, 44,* 69–76.

Applegate, B., Lahey, B. B., Hart, E. L., Waldman, I., Biederman, J., Hynd, G. W., et al. (1997). Validity of the age of onset criterion for ADHD: A report from the DSM-IV field trials. *Journal of the American Academy of Child and Adolescent Psychiatry, 36,* 1211–1221.

Arcia, E., Frank, R., Sánchez-LaCay, A., & Fernández, M. C. (2000). Teacher understanding of ADHD as reflected in attributions and classroom strategies. *Journal of Attention Disorders, 4,* 91–101.

Armstrong, T. (1995). *The myth of the A.D.D. child.* New York: Penguin Books.

Arnold, L. E. (2002). Treatment alternatives for attention deficit hyperactivity disorder. In P. S. Jensen & J. R. Cooper (Eds.), *Attention deficit hyperactivity disorder: State of the science-best practices* (pp. 13.1–13.29). Kingston, NJ: Civic Research Institute.

Arnold, L. E., & DiSilvestro, R. A. (2005). Zinc in attention-deficit/hyperactivity disorder. *Journal of Child and Adolescent Psychopharmacology, 15,* 619–627.

Atkins, M. S., Graczyk, P. A., Frazier, S. L., & Abdul-Adil, J. (2003). Toward a new model for promoting urban children's mental health: Accessible, effective, and sustainable school-based mental health services. *School Psychology Review, 32,* 503–514.

Axelrod, M., Zhe, E., Haugen, K., & Klein, J. (2009). Self-management of on-task homework behavior: A promising strategy for adolescents with attention and behavior problems. *School Psychology Review, 38,* 325–333.

Baddeley, A. D. (2000). The episodic buffer: A new component of working memory? *Trends in Cognitive Science, 4,* 417–423.

Bagwell, C., Newcomb, A., & Bukowski, W. (1998). Preadolescent friendships and peer rejection as predictors of adult adjustment. *Child Development, 69,* 140–153.

Baker, L., & Cantwell, D. P. (1987). A prospective psychiatric follow-up of children with speech/language disorders. *Journal of the American Academy of Child and Adolescent Psychiatry, 26,* 545–553.

Bandura, A. (1986). *Social foundations of thought and action.* Englewood Cliffs, NJ: Prentice-Hall.

Bandura, A. (1988). Self-regulation of motivation and action through goal systems. In V. Hamilton, G. H. Browder, & N. H. Frijda (Eds.), *Cognitive perspectives on emotion and motivation* (pp. 37–61). Dordrecht, The Netherlands: Kluwer Academic.

Banerjee, T. D., Middleton, F., & Faraone, S. V. (2007). Environmental risk factors for attention-deficit hyperactivity disorder. *Acta Paediatrica, 96,* 1269–1274.

Barkley, R. A. (1988). Attention. In M. Tramontana & S. Hooper (Eds.), *Assessment issues in child neuropsychology* (pp. 218–243). New York: Brunner/Mazel.

Barkley, R. A. (1990). *Attention-deficit hyperactivity disorder: A handbook for diagnosis and treatment.* New York: Guilford Press.

Barkley, R. A. (1994). Impaired delayed responding: A unified theory of attention deficit hyperactivity disorder. In D. K. Routh (Ed.), *Disruptive behavior disorders: Essays in honor of Herbert Quay* (pp. 11–57). New York: Plenum Press.

Barkley, R. A. (1997a). Behavioral inhibition, sustained attention, and executive functions: Constructing a unified theory of ADHD. *Psychological Bulletin, 12,* 65–94.

Barkley, R. A. (1997b). *Defiant children: A clinician's manual for assessment and parent training* (2nd ed.). New York: Guilford Press.

Barkley, R. A. (1997c). *ADHD and the nature of self-control.* New York: Guilford Press.

Barkley, R. A. (2000). *Taking charge of ADHD* (rev. ed.). New York: Guilford Press.

Barkley, R. A. (2006). *Attention-deficit hyperactivity disorder: A handbook for diagnosis and treatment* (3rd ed.). New York: Guilford Press.

Barkley, R. A., & Biederman, J. (1997). Towards a broader definition of the age of onset criterion for attention deficit hyperactivity disorder. *Journal of the American Academy of Child and Adolescent Psychiatry, 36,* 1204–1210.

Barkley, R. A., Copeland, A. P., & Sivage, C. (1980). A self-control classroom for hyperactive children. *Journal of Autism and Developmental Disorders, 10,* 75–89.

Barkley, R. A., DuPaul, G. J., & McMurray, M. B. (1990). A comprehensive evaluation of attention deficit disorder with and without hyperactivity defined by research criteria. *Journal of Consulting and Clinical Psychology, 58,* 775–789.

Barkley, R. A., & Edwards, G. (2006). In R. A. Barkley (Ed.), *Attention deficit hyperactivity disorder: A handbook for diagnosis and treatment* (3rd ed.). New York: Guilford Press.

Barron, K. E., Evans, S. W., Baranik, L. E., Serpell, Z. N., & Buvinger, E. (2006). Achievement goals of students with ADHD. *Learning Disability Quarterly, 29,* 137–158.

Barry, L. M., & Messer, J. J. (2003). A practical application of self-management for students diagnosed with attention deficit/hyperactivity disorder. *Journal of Positive Behavior Interventions, 5,* 238–248.

Bauermeister, J., Shrout, P., Chavez, L., Rubio-Stipec, M., Ramirez, R., Padilla, L., et al. (2007). ADHD and gender: Are risks and sequela of ADHD the same for boys and girls? *Journal of Child Psychology and Psychiatry, 48,* 831–839.

Bender, W. N., & Mathes, M. Y. (1995). Students with ADHD in the inclusive classroom: A hierarchical approach to strategy selection. *Intervention in School and Clinic, 30,* 226–234.

Berk, L. E. (2003). *Child development.* Boston: Allyn & Bacon.

Bernfort, L., Norfeldt, S., & Persson, J. (2008). ADHD from a socio-economic perspective. *Acta Paediatrica, 97*, 239–245.

Biederman, J., Faraone, S. V., Keenan, K., Benjamin, J., Krifcher, B., Moore, C., et al. (1992). Further evidence for family-genetic risk factors in attention deficit hyperactivity disorder: Patterns of comorbidity in probands and relatives in psychiatrically and pediatrically referred samples. *Archives of General Psychiatry, 49*, 728–738.

Biederman, J., Faraone, S. V., & Lapey, K. (1992). Comorbidity of diagnosis in attention-deficit hyperactivity disorder. *Child and Adolescent Psychiatry Clinics of North America, 1*, 335–360.

Biederman, J., Faraone, S. V., Mick, E., Spencer T., Wilens, T., Kiely, K., et al. (1995). High risk for attention deficit hyperactivity disorder among children of parents with childhood onset of the disorder: A pilot study. *American Journal of Psychiatry, 152*, 431–435.

Biederman, J., Faraone, S., & Monteaux, M. (2002). Impact of exposure to parental attention-deficit hyperactivity disorder on clinical features and dysfunction in the offspring. *Psychological Medicine, 32*, 817–827.

Biederman, J., Keenan, K., & Faraone, S. V. (1990). Parent-based diagnosis of attention deficit disorder predicts a diagnosis based on teacher report. *Journal of the American Academy of Child and Adolescent Psychiatry, 26*, 698–701.

Biederman, J., Kwon, A., Aleardi, M., Chouinard, V., Marino, T., Cole, H., et al. (2005). Absence of gender effects on attention deficit hyperactivity disorder: Findings in nonreferred subjects. *American Journal of Psychiatry, 162*, 1083–1089.

Biederman, J., Milberger, S., Faraone, S. V., Kiely, K., Guite, J., Mick, E., et al. (1995). Family–environment risk factors for attention-deficit hyperactivity disorder. A test of Rutter's indicators of adversity. *Archives of General Psychiatry, 52*, 464–470.

Biederman, J., Monuteaux, M. C., Doyle, A. E., Seidman, L. J., Wilens, T. E., Ferrero, F., et al. (2000). Strategy application disorder: The role of the frontal lobes in human multitasking. *Psychological Research, 63*, 279–288.

Biederman, J., Newcorn, J., & Sprich, S. (1991). Comorbidity of attention deficit hyperactivity disorder with conduct, depressive, anxiety and other disorders. *American Journal of Psychiatry, 148*, 564–577.

Biederman, J., Petty, C., Fried, R., Doyle, A., Spencer, T., Seidman, L., et al. (2007). Stability of executive function deficits into young adult years: A prospective longitudinal follow-up study of grown up males with ADHD. *Acta Psychiatrica Scandanavia, 116*, 129–136.

Blachman, D., & Hinshaw, S. (2002). Patterns of friendship among girls with and without attention deficit/hyperactivity disorder. *Journal of Abnormal Child Psychology, 30*, 625–640.

Blader, J. C., & Carlson, G. A. (2007). Increased rates of bi-polar disorder diagnoses among U.S. child, adolescent, and adult inpatients, 1996–2004. *Biological Psychiatry, 62*, 107–114.

Borrelli, B., Sepinwall, D., Ernst, D., Bellg, A. J., Czajkowski, S., Breger, R., et al. (2005). A new tool to assess treatment fidelity and evaluation of treatment fidelity across 10 years of health behavior research. *Journal of Consulting and Clinical Psychology, 73*, 852–860.

Bos, C., Nahmias, M., & Urban, M. (1999). Targeting home–school collaboration for students with ADHD. *Teaching Exceptional Children, 31*, 4–11.

Bradley, C. (1937). The behavior of children receiving benzendrine. *American Journal of Psychiatry, 94*, 577–585.

Braswell, L. (1998, February). Self-regulation training for children with ADHD: Response to Harris and Schmidt. *The ADHD Report, 6*, 1–3.

Breslau, J., Miller, E., Breslau, N., Bohnert, K., Lucia, V., & Schweitzer, J. (2009). The impact of early behavior disturbances on academic achievement in high school. *Pediatrics, 123,* 1472–1476.

Brock, S. W., & Knapp, P. K. (1996). Reading comprehension abilities of children with attention-deficit/hyperactivity disorder. *Journal of Attention Disorders, 1,* 173–186.

Broden, M., Hall, R. V., & Mitts, B. (1971). The effects of self-recording on the classroom behavior of two eighth-grade students. *Journal of Applied Behavior Analysis, 4,* 191–199.

Brook, U., & Boaz, M. (2005). Atttention deficit hyperactivity disorder (ADHD) and learning disabilities (LD): Adolescents perspective. *Parent Education and Counseling, 58,* 187–191.

Brophy, J. (1981). Teacher praise: A functional analysis. *Review of Educational Research, 51,* 5–32.

Brown, G. M., Kerr, M. M., Zigmond, N., & Harris, A. L. (1984). What's important for student success in high school?: "Successful" and "unsuccessful" students discuss school survival skills. *The High School Journal, 68,* 10–17.

Brown, T. E. (2000). Attention-deficit disorders with obsessive–compulsive disorder. In T. E. Brown (Ed.), *Attention-deficit disorders and comorbidities in children, adolescents, and adults* (pp. 209–230). Washington, DC: American Psychiatric Press.

Brown, T. E. (2005). *Attention deficit disorder: The unfocused mind in children and adults.* New Haven, CT: Yale University Press.

Bussing, R., & Gary, F. A. (2001). Practice guidelines and parental ADHD treatment evaluations: Friends or foes. *Harvard Review of Psychiatry, 9,* 223–233.

Bussing, R., Gary, F. A., Mills, T. L., & Garvan, C. W. (2003). Parental explanatory models of ADHD: Gender and cultural variations. *Social Psychiatry and Psychiatric Epidemiology, 38,* 563–575.

Bussing, R., Gary, F. A., Mills, T. L., & Garvan, C. W. (2007). Cultural variations in parental health beliefs, knowledge and information sources related to attention-deficit/hyperactivity disorder. *Journal of Family Issues, 28,* 291–318.

Bussing, R., Schoenberg, N., Rogers, K., Zima, B., & Angus, S. (1998). Explanatory models of ADHD: Do they differ by ethnicity, child gender, or treatment status? *Journal of Emotional and Behavioral Disorders, 6,* 233–242.

Bussing, R., Zima, B. T., Gary, F. A., & Garvan, C. W. (2002). Use of complimentary and alternative medicine for symptoms of attention-deficit hyperactivity disorder. *Psychiatric Services, 53,* 1096–1102.

Bussing, R., Zima, B. T., Gary, F., Mason, D., Leon, C., Sinha, K., & Garvan, C. W. (2003). Social networks, caregiver strain, and utilization of mental health services among elementary school students at high risk for ADHD. *Journal of the American Academy of Child and Adolescent Psychiatry, 42,* 842–850.

Bussing, R., Zima, B. T., Mason, D., Hou, W., Garvan, C. W., & Forness, S. (2005). Use and persistence of pharmacotherapy for elementary school students with attention-deficit/hyperactivity disorder. *Journal of Child and Adolescent Psychopharmacology, 15,* 78–87.

Cala, S., Crismon, M. L., & Baumgartner, J. (2003). A survey of herbal use in children with attention-deficit-hyperactivity disorder or depression. *Pharmacotherapy, 23,* 222–230.

Cantwell, D., & Baker, L. (1991). Association between attention deficit-hyperactivity disorder and learning disorders. *Journal of Learning Disabilities, 24,* 88–95.

Cantwell, D. P., & Satterfield, J. H. (1978). The prevalence of academic underachievement in hyperactive children. *Journal of Pediatric Psychology, 3,* 168–171.

Carey, W. (2002). Is ADHD a valid disorder? In P. S. Jensen & J. R. Cooper (Eds.), *Attention deficit hyperactivity disorder-state of the science-best practices* (pp. 3-13–3-19). Kingston, NJ: Civic Research Institute.

Carr, E., & Durand, M. (1985). Reducing behavior problems through functional communication training. *Journal of Applied Behavior Analysis, 18,* 111–126.

Casey, J. E., Rourke, B. P., & Del Otto, J. E. (1996). Learning disabilities in children with attention deficit disorder with and without hyperactivity. *Child Neuropsychology, 2,* 83–98.

Casey, K. J., Hagaman, J. L., Trout, A. L., Reid, R., Chmelka, M. B., Thompson, R., et al. (2008). Children with ADHD in residential care. *Journal of Child and Family Studies, 17,* 909–927.

Centers for Disease Control and Prevention. (2005, September 2). Mental health in the United States: Prevalence of diagnosis and medication treatment for attention-deficit/hyperactivity disorder—United States, 2003 [Electronic version]. *Morbidity and Mortality Weekly Report, 54,* 542–847.

Center for Health Care in Schools. (2007). State policies on the administration of medication in schools. Retrieved from *www.nasbe.org/index.php/file-repository?func=fileinfo&id=252.*

Chan, E., Rappaport, L. A., & Kemper, K. J. (2003). Complementary and alternative therapies in childhood attention and hyperactivity problems. *Journal of Developmental and Behavioral Pediatrics, 24,* 4–8.

Christakis, D. A., Zimmerman, F. J., DiGiuseppe, D. L., & McCarthy, C. A. (2004). Early television exposure and subsequent attentional problems in children. *Pediatrics, 113,* 708–713.

Chronis, A. M., Lahey, B. B., Pelham, W. E., Kipp, H. L., Baumann, B. L., & Lee, S. S. (2003). Psychopathology and substance abuse in parents of children with attention-deficit/hyperactivity disorder. *Journal of the American Academy of Child and Adolescent Psychiatry, 42,* 1424–1432.

Chronis-Tuscano, A., Raggi, V., Clarke, T., Rooney, M., Diaz, Y., & Pian, J. (2008). Associations between maternal attention-deficit/hyperactivity disorder symptoms and parenting. *Journal of Abnormal Child Psychology, 36,* 1237–1250.

Clark, C., Prior, M., & Kinsella, G. (2002). The relationship between executive function abilities, adaptive behaviour, and academic achievement in children with externalizing behaviour problems. *Journal of Child Psychology and Psychiatry, 43,* 785–796.

Clark, M., Cheyne, A., Cunningham, C., & Siegel, L. (1988). Dyadic peer interactions and task orientation in attention-deficit disordered children. *Journal of Abnormal Child Psychology, 16,* 1–15.

Cohen, N. J., Menna, R., Vallance, D. D., Barwick, M. A., Im, N., & Horodezky, N. (1998). Language, social cognitive processing, and behavioral characteristics of psychiatrically disturbed children with previously identified and unsuspected language impairments. *Journal of Child Psychology and Psychiatry, 39,* 853–864.

Cohen, P., Velez, C. N., Brook, J., & Smith, J. (1989). Mechanisms of the relation between perinatal problems, early childhood illness, and psychopathology in late childhood and adolescence. *Child Development, 60,* 701–709.

Cohen, S., & de Bettencourt, L. (1988). Teaching children to be independent learners: A step by step strategy. In E. L. Meyen, G. L. Vergason, & R. J. Whelan (Eds.), *Effective instructional strategies for exceptional children* (pp. 319–334). Denver, CO: Love.

Collipp, P. J., Chen, S. Y., & Maitinsky, S. (1983). Manganese in infant formulas and learning disability. *Annals of Nutrition and Metabolism, 27,* 488–494.

Conners, C. K. (1997). *Conners' Rating Scales—Revised: Technical manual.* Toronto, Canada: Multi-Health Systems.

Conners, C. K., Epstein, J. N., March, J. S., Angold, A., Wells, K. C., Klaric, J., et al. (2001). Multimodal treatment of ADHD in the MTA: An alternative outcome analysis. *Journal of the American Academy of Child and Adolescent Psychiatry, 40,* 159–167.

Connor, D., Glatt, S., Lopez, I., Jackson, D., & Melloni, R. (2002). Psychopharmacology and aggression: I. A meta-analysis of stimulant effects on overt/covert aggression-related behaviors in ADHD. *Journal of the American Academy of Child and Adolescent Psychiatry, 41,* 253–261.

Conway, A., Cowan, N., & Bunting, M. (2001). The cocktail party revisited: The importance of working memory capacity. *Psychonomic Bulletin and Review, 8,* 331–335.

Cooper, H. (2007). *The battle over homework.* Thousand Oaks, CA: Corwin.

Cooper, J., Heron, T., & Heward, W. (2007). *Applied behavior analysis* (2nd ed.). Upper Saddle River, NJ: Pearson.

Cooper, L., Wacker, D., Thursby, D., Plagmann, L., Harding, J., Millard, T., et al. (1992). Analysis of the effects of task preferences, task demands, and adult attention on child behavior in outpatient and classroom settings. *Journal of Applied Behavior Analysis, 25,* 823–840.

Copeland, E. D. (1995). *Medications for attention disorders (ADHD/ADD) and related medical problems.* Atlanta, GA: SPI Press.

Corbetta, M., & Shulman, G. L. (2002). Control of goal-directed and stimulus-driven attention in the brain. *Nature Reviews Neuroscience, 3,* 215–229.

Cornoldi, C., Barbieri, A., Gaiani, C., & Zocchi, S. (1999). Strategic memory deficits in attention deficit disorder with hyperactivity participants: The role of executive processes. *Developmental Neuropsychology, 15,* 53–71.

Council for Exceptional Children. (2009). *Best practices for administering medication in school.* Retrieved from *www.cec.sped.org/AM/Template.cfm?Section=Home&CONTENTID=11752&TEMPLATE=/CM/HTMLDisplay.cfm.*

Counts, C., Nigg, G., Stawicki, J., Rappley, M., & von Eye, A. (2005). Family adversity in DSM-IV ADHD combined and inattentive subtypes and associated disruptive behavior problems. *Journal of the American Academy of Child Adolescent Psychiatry, 44,* 690–698.

Coutinho, M. J., & Oswald, D. P. (2000). Disproportionate representation in special education: A synthesis and recommendations. *Journal of Child and Family Studies, 9,* 135–156.

Cox, D. (2005). Evidence-based interventions using home–school collaboration. *School Psychology Quarterly, 20,* 473–497.

Cunningham, C., & Cunningham, L. (2006). Student-mediated conflict resolution programs. In R. Barkley, *Attention-deficit hyperactivity disorder: A handbook for diagnosis and treatment* (3rd ed., pp. 590–607). New York: Guilford Press.

Cunningham, C., & Siegel, L. (1987). Peer interactions of normal and attention-deficit disordered boys during free-play, cooperative task, and simulated classroom situations. *Journal of Abnormal Child Psychology, 15,* 247–268.

Currie, J., & Stabile, M. (2006). Child mental health and human capital accumulation: The case of ADHD. *Journal of Health Economics, 25,* 1094–1118.

Davila, R., Williams, M. L., & MacDonald, J. T. (1991). *Clarification of policy to address the needs of children with attention deficit disorder within general and/or special education.* Washington, DC: U.S. Department of Education, Office of Special Education and Rehabilitative Services.

DeGrandepre, R. (2000). *Ritalin nation.* New York: Norton.

DePaepe, P., Shores, R. E., Jack, S. L., & Denny, R. K. (1996). Effects of task difficulty on the disruptive and on-task behavior of students with severe behavior disorders. *Behavioral Disorders, 21,* 216–225.

Diller, L. (1996). The run on Ritalin: Attention deficit disorder and stimulant treatment medication in the 1990's. *Hastings Center Report, 26*(2), 12–18.

Divoky, D. (1989). Ritalin: Education's fix-it-drug? *Phi Delta Kappan, 70,* 599–605.

dosReis, S., Zito, J., Safer, D., Soeken, K., Mitchell, J., & Ellwood, L. (2003). Parental perceptions and satisfaction with stimulant medication for attention deficit hyperactivity disorder. *Journal of Developmental and Behavioral Pediatrics, 24,* 155–162.

Douglas, V. I. (1983). Attention and cognitive problems. In M. Rutter (Ed.), *Developmental neuropsychiatry* (pp. 280–329). New York: Guilford Press.

Drabick, D. A. G., Gadow, K. D., & Sprafkin, J. (2006). Co-occurrence of conduct disorder and depression in a clinic-based sample of boys with ADHD. *Journal of Child Psychology and Psychiatry, 47,* 766–774.

Drasgow, E., & Yell, M. (2001). Functional behavioral assessments: Legal requirements and challenges. *School Psychology Review, 30,* 239–251.

Drasgow, E., Yell, M. L., Bradley, R., & Shriner, J. G. (1999). The IDEA Amendments of 1997: A school-wide model for conducting functional behavioral assessments and developing behavior intervention plans. *Education and Treatment of Children, 22,* 244–266.

Dulcan, M. K. (Ed.). (2007). *Helping parents, youth, and teachers understand medications for behavioral and emotional problems: A resource book of medication information handouts* (3rd ed.). Washington, DC: American Psychiatric Press.

Dunlap, G., dePerczel, M., Clarke, S., Wilson, D., Wright, S., White, R., et al. (1994). Choice making to promote adaptive behavior for students with emotional and behavioral challenges. *Journal of Applied Behavior Analysis, 27,* 505–518.

Dunlap, G., & Kern, L. (1993). Assessment and intervention for children within the instructional curriculum. In J. Reichle & D. Wacker (Eds.), *Communication alternatives to challenging behavior: Integrating functional assessment and intervention strategies* (pp. 177–203). Baltimore: Brookes.

Dunlap, G., Kern, L., dePerczel, M., Clarke, S., Wilson, D., Childs, K., et al. (1993). Functional analysis of classroom variables for students with emotional and behavioral disorders. *Behavioral Disorders, 18,* 275–291.

Dunlap, G., Kern-Dunlap, L., Clarke, S., & Robbins, F. R. (1991). Functional assessment, curricular revision, and severe behavior problems. *Journal of Applied Behavior Analysis, 24,* 387–397.

Dunlap, G., White, R., Vera, A., Wilson, D., & Panacek, L. (1996). The effects of multicomponent, assessment-based curricular modifications on the classroom behavior of children with emotional and behavioral disorders. *Journal of Behavioral Education, 6,* 481–500.

Dunn, L. M. (1968). Special education for the mildly retarded: Is much of it justifiable? *Exceptional Children, 35,* 5–22.

DuPaul, G. J., & Ervin, R. (1996). Functional assessment of behaviors related to attention-deficit/hyperactivity disorder: Linking assessment to intervention design. *Behavior Therapy, 27,* 601–622.

DuPaul, G. J., Ervin, R. A., Hook, C. L., & McGoey, K. E. (1998). Peer tutoring for children with attention deficit hyperactivity disorder: Effects on classroom behavior and academic performance. *Journal of Applied Behavior Analysis, 31,* 579–572.

DuPaul, G. J., & Henningson, P. A. (1993). Peer tutoring effects on the classroom performance of children with attention deficit hyperactivity disorder. *School Psychology Review, 22,* 134–143.

DuPaul, G. J., McGoey, K. E., Eckert, T. L., & VanBrakle, J. (2001). Preschool children with attention-deficit/hyperactivity disorder: Impairments in behavioral, social, and school functioning. *Journal of the American Academy of Child and Adolescent Psychiatry, 40,* 508–515.

DuPaul, G. J., Power, T. J., Anastopoulos, A. D., & Reid, R. (1998). *ADHD Rating Scale–IV: Checklists, norms and clinical interpretation*. New York: Guilford Press.

DuPaul, G. J., Rapport, M. D., & Perriello, L. M. (1991). Teacher ratings of academic skills: The development of the Academic Performance Rating Scale. *School Psychology Review, 20*, 284–300.

DuPaul, G. J., & Stoner, G. (2003). *ADHD in the schools: Assessment and intervention strategies* (2nd ed.). New York: Guilford Press.

DuPaul, G. J., & Weyandt, L. (2006). School-based intervention for children with attention deficit hyperactivity disorder: Effects on academic, social, and behavioural functioning. *International Journal of Disability, Development, and Education, 53*, 161–176.

DuPont, R., Bucher, R., Wilford, B., & Coleman, J. (2007). School-based administration of ADHD drugs decline along with diversion, theft, and misuse. *Journal of School Nursing, 23*, 349–352.

Durand, V. M., & Carr, E. G. (1991). Functional communication training to reduce challenging behavior: Maintenance and application in new settings. *Journal of Applied Behavior Analysis, 24*, 251–264.

Dyer, K., Dunlap, G., & Winterling, V. (1990). The effects of choice making on the serious problem behaviors of students with developmental disabilities. *Journal of Applied Behavior Analysis, 23*, 515–524.

Dykman, R. A., & Ackerman, P. T. (1992). Attention deficit disorder and specific reading disability: Separate but often overlapping disorders. In S. Shaywitz & B. A. Shaywitz (Eds.), *Attention deficit disorder comes of age: Toward the twenty-first century* (pp. 165–184). Austin, TX: PRO-ED.

Elliott, S. N., Gresham, F. M., & Heffer, R.W. (1987). Social-skills interventions: Research findings and training techniques. In C. A. Maher & J. E. Zins (Eds.), *Psychoeducational interventions in the schools* (pp. 141–159). New York: Pergamon Press.

Ellis, E. (1989). A metacognitive intervention for increasing class participation. *Learning Disabilities Focus, 5*(1), 36–46.

Engle, R. W. (2002). Working memory capacity as executive attention. *Current Directions in Psychological Science, 11*, 19–23.

Epstein, J. N., Willoughby, M., Valencia, E. Y., Tonev, S. T., Abikoff, H. B., Arnold, E. L., et al. (2005). The role of children's ethnicity in the relationship between teacher ratings of attention-deficit/hyperactivity disorder and observed classroom behavior. *Journal of Counseling and Clinical Psychology, 73*, 424–434.

Epstein, M. H., Polloway, E. A., Foley, R. M., & Patton, J. R. (1993). Homework: A comparison of teachers' and parents' perceptions of the problems experienced by students identified as having behavioral disorders, learning disabilities, or no disabilities. *Remedial and Special Education, 14*, 40–50.

Ernhardt, D., & Hinshaw, S. (1994). Initial sociometric impressions of attention-deficit hyperactivity disorder and comparison boys: Predictions from social behavior and from nonbehavioral variables. *Journal of Consulting and Clinical Psychology, 62*, 833–842.

Evangelista, N., Owens, J., Golden, C., & Pelham, W. E. Jr. (2008). The positive illusory bias: Do inflated self-perceptions in children with ADHD generalize to perceptions of others? *Journal of Abnormal Child Psychology, 36*, 779–791.

Exley, B. (2008). "Staying in class so no one can get to him": A case for the institutional reproduction of ADHD categories and behaviors. *International Journal of Inclusive Education, 12*, 65–80.

Fabiano, G. A., & Pelham, W. E. Jr. (2003). Improving the effectiveness of behavioral classroom interventions for attention-deficit/hyperactivity disorder: A case study. *Journal of Emotional and Behavioral Disorders, 11,* 122–128.

Fabiano, G. A., Pelham, W. E. Jr., Gnagy, E., Burrows-MacLean, L., Coles, E., Chacko, A., et al. (2007). The single and combined effects of multiple intensities of behavior modification and methylphenidate for children with attention deficit hyperactivity disorder in a classroom setting. *School Psychology Review, 36,* 195–216.

Fabiano, G. A., Pelham, W. E. Jr., Manos, M., Gnagy, E. M., Chronis, A. M., Onyango, A. N., et al. (2004). An evaluation of three time out procedures for children with attention-deficit hyperactivity disorder. *Behavior Therapy, 35,* 449–469.

Famularo, R., Kinscherff, R., & Fenton T. (1992). Psychiatric diagnoses of maltreated children: Preliminary findings. *Journal of the American Academy of Child and Adolescent Psychiatry, 31,* 863–867.

Fantuzzo, J., McWayne, C., Perry, M., & Childs, S. (2004). Multiple dimensions of family involvement and their relations to behavioral and learning competencies for urban, low-income children. *School Psychology Review, 33,* 467–480.

Fantuzzo, J., Tighe, E., & Childs, S. (1999). Relationships between family involvement in Head Start and children's interactive play. *NHSA Dialog, 3,* 60–67.

Faraone, S. V., & Biederman, J. (1997, October). *Familial transmission of attention-deficit/hyperactivity disorder and comorbid disorders.* Paper presented at the annual meeting of the American Academy of Child and Adolescent Psychiatry, Toronto, Canada.

Feindler, E. L., & Ecton, R. B. (1986). *Adolescent anger control: Cognitive-behavioral techniques.* New York: Pergamon Press.

Feingold, B. (1975). *Why your child is hyperactive.* New York: Random House.

Finn, J., & Cox, D. (1992). Participation and withdrawal among fourth-grade pupils. *American Educational Research Journal, 29,* 141–162.

Fischer, M., Barkley, R. A., Edelbrock, C. S., & Smallish, L. (1990). The adolescent outcome of hyperactive children diagnosed by research criteria: II. Academic, attentional, and neuropsychological status. *Journal of Consulting and Clinical Psychology, 58,* 580–588.

Fletcher, J. M., Lyon, G. R., Barnes, M. A., Stuebing, K. K., Francis, D. J., Olson, R., et al. (2002). Classification of learning disabilities: An evidence-based evaluation. In R. Bradley, L. Danielson, & D. P. Hallahan (Eds.), *Identification of learning disabilities: Research to practice* (pp. 185–250). Mahwah, NJ: Erlbaum.

Fletcher, J. M., Morris, R. D., & Lyon, G. R. (2003). Classification and definition of learning disabilities: An integrative perspective. In H. L. Swanson, K. R. Harris, & S. Graham (Eds.), *Handbook of learning disabilities* (pp. 30–56). New York: Guilford Press.

Forness, S. R., & Kavale, K. A. (2002). Impact of ADHD on school systems. In P. Jensen & J. Cooper (Eds.), *Attention deficit hyperactivity disorder: State of the science, best practices* (pp. 24–1 to 24–20). Kingston, NJ: Civic Research Institute.

Forness, S. R., Kavale, K. A., & Davanzo, P. A. (2002). The new medical model: Interdisciplinary treatment and the limits of behaviorism. *Behavioral Disorders, 27,* 168–178.

Foster-Johnson, L., Ferro, J., & Dunlap, G. (1994). Preferred curricular activities and reduced problem behaviors in students with intellectual difficulties. *Journal of Applied Behavior Analysis, 27,* 493–504.

Frame, K., Kelly, L., & Bayley, E. (2003). Increasing perceptions of self-worth in preadolescents diagnosed with ADHD. *Journal of Nursing Scholarship, 35,* 225–229.

Fraser, C., Belzner, R., & Conte, R. (1992). Attention deficit hyperactivity disorder and self-control: A single case study of the use of a timing device in the development of self-monitoring. *School Psychology International, 13,* 339–345.

Frazier, T. W., Demaree, H. A., & Youngstrom, E. A. (2004). Meta-analysis of intellectual and neuropsychological test performance in attention-deficit/hyperactivity disorder. *Neuropsychology, 18*, 543–555.

Frazier, T. W., Youngstrom, E. A., Glutting, J. J., & Watkins, M. W. (2007). ADHD and achievement: Meta-analysis of the child, adolescent, and adult literatures and a concomitant study with college students. *Journal of Learning Disabilities, 40*, 49–65.

Frick, P. J., Lahey, B. B., Applegate, B., Kerdyck, L., Ollendick, T., Hynd, G. W., et al. (1994). DSM-IV field trials for the disruptive behavior disorders: Symptom utility estimates. *Journal of the American Academy of Child and Adolescent Psychiatry, 33*, 529–539.

Galéra, C., Melchior, M., Chastang, J., Bouvard, M., & Fombonne, E. (2009). Childhood and adolescent hyperactivity-inattention symptoms and academic achievement 8 years later: The GAZEL youth study. *Psychological Medicine, 39*, 1895–1906.

Gathercole, S. E., Lamont, E., & Alloway, T. P. (2006). Working memory in the classroom. In S. Pickering (Ed.), *Working memory and education* (pp. 219–240). Oxford, UK: Elsevier Press.

Gaub, M., & Carlson, C. (1997). Gender differences in ADHD: A meta-analysis and critical review. *Journal of the American Academy of Child and Adolescent Psychiatry, 36*, 1036–1045.

Geist, E. A., & Gibson, M. (2000). The effect of network and public television programs on four and five year olds ability to attend to educational tasks. *Journal of Instructional Psychology, 27*, 250–262.

Gerber, M. M., & Semmel, M. I. (1984). Teacher as imperfect test: Reconceptualizing the referral process. *Educational Psychologist, 19*, 137–138.

Gershon, J. (2002). A meta-analytic review of gender differences in ADHD. *Journal of Attention Disorders, 5*, 143–154.

Gilchrist, R., & Arnold, E. (2005). Long term efficacy of ADHD pharmacotherapy in children. *Psychiatric Annals, 38*, 52–57.

Gladman, M., & Lancaster, S. (2003). A review of the Behavior Assessment System for Children. *School Psychology International, 24*, 276–291.

Glasser, W. (1992). *The quality school*. New York: HarperCollins.

Glomb, N., & West, R. P. (1990). Teaching behaviorally disordered adolescents to use self-management skills for improving the completeness, accuracy, and neatness for creative writing homework assignments. *Behavioral Disorders, 15*, 233–242.

Goldman-Rakic, P. S. (1987). Development of cortical circuitry and cognitive function. *Child Development, 58*, 601–622.

Graham, S., Harris, K. R., & Reid, R. (1992). Developing self-regulated learners. *Focus on Exceptional Children, 24*, 1–16.

Graham-Day, K., Gardner, R., & Hsin, Y. (2010). Increasing on-task behaviors of high school students with attention deficit hyperactivity disorder: Is it enough? *Education and Treatment of Children, 33*, 205–221.

Gresham, F., & Elliot, S. (2007). *Social Skills Improvement System Rating Scales*. San Antonio, TX: Pearson Assessments.

Gresham, F., Sugai, G., & Horner, R. (2001). Interpreting outcomes of social skills training for students with high-incidence disabilities. *Exceptional Children, 67*, 331–344.

Grice, K. (2002). Eligibility under IDEA for other health impaired children. *School Law Bulletin, 33*(3), 7–12.

Guilford, J. P. (1954). *Psychometric methods* (2nd ed.). New York: McGraw-Hill.

Gureasko-Moore, S., DuPaul, G. J., & White, G. (2006). The effects of self-management in general education classrooms on the organizational skills of adolescents with ADHD. *Behavior Modification, 30,* 159–183.

Gureasko-Moore, S., DuPaul, G. J., & White, G. (2007). Self-management of classroom preparedness and homework: Effects on school functioning of adolescents with attention deficit hyperactivity disorder. *School Psychology Review, 36,* 647–664.

Haenlein, M., & Caul, W. F. (1987). Attention deficit disorder with hyperactivity: A specific hypothesis of reward dysfunction. *Journal of the American Academy of Child and Adolescent Psychiatry, 26,* 356–362.

Hagaman, J., Luschen, K., & Reid, R. (2010). The "RAP" on reading comprehension. *Teaching Exceptional Children, 43*(1), 22–29.

Hale, G. A., & Lewis, M. (1979). *Attention and cognitive development.* New York: Plenum Press.

Hamlett, K. W., Pellegrini, D. S., & Conners, C. K. (1987). An investigation of executive processes in the problem-solving of attention deficit disorder-hyperactive children. *Journal of Pediatric Psychology, 12,* 227–240.

Handler, M. W., & DuPaul, G. J. (2005). Assessment of ADHD: Differences across psychology specialty areas. *Journal of Attention Disorders, 9,* 402–412.

Harborne, A., Wolpert, M., & Clarke, L. (2004). Making sense of ADHD: A battle for understanding?: Parents' views of their child being diagnosed with ADHD. *Clinical Child Psychology and Psychiatry, 9,* 327–339.

Harris, K. R. (1986). Self-monitoring of attentional behavior versus self-monitoring of productivity: Effects on on-task behavior and academic response rate among learning disabled children. *Journal of Applied Behavior Analysis, 19,* 417–423.

Harris, K. R. (1990). Developing self-regulated learners: The role of private speech and self-instructions. *Educational Psychologist, 25,* 35–49.

Harris, K. R., Friedlander, B. D., Saddler, B., Frizelle, R., & Graham, S. (2005). Self-monitoring of attention versus self-monitoring of academic performance: Effects among students with ADHD in the general education classroom. *Journal of Special Education, 39,* 145–156.

Harris, K. R., & Pressley, M. (1991). The nature of cognitive strategy instruction: Interactive strategy construction. *Exceptional Children, 57,* 392–404.

Harris, K. R., Reid, R., & Graham, S. (2004). Self-regulation among children with LD and ADHD. In B. Wong (Ed.), *Learning about learning disabilities* (pp. 167–195). San Diego, CA: Elsevier.

Harris, M., Milich, R., & McAninch, C. (1998). When stigma becomes self-fulfilling prophesy: Expectancy effects and the causes, consequences, and treatment of peer rejection. In J. Brophy (Ed.), *Advances in research on teaching* (pp. 243–272). Greenwich, CT: JAI Press.

Hartsough, C. S., & Lambert, N. M. (1985). Medical factors in hyperactive and normal children: Prenatal, developmental, and health history findings. *American Journal of Orthopsychiatry, 55,* 190–210.

Hechtman, L. (1996). Families of children with attention deficit hyperactivity disorder: A review. *Canadian Journal of Psychiatry, 41,* 350–360.

Hertzig, M. E. (1983). Temperament and neurological status. In M. Rutter (Ed.), *Developmental neuropsychiatry* (pp. 164–180). New York: Guilford Press.

Heward, W. L., Gardner, R., Cavanaugh, R., Courson, F. H., Grossi, T. A., & Barbetta, P. M. (1996). Everyone participates in this class. *Focus on Exceptional Children, 28,* 4–10.

Hinshaw, S. P. (2002). Is ADHD an impairing condition in childhood and adolescence? In

P. S. Jensen & J. R. Cooper (Eds.), *Attention deficit hyperactivity disorder-state of the science-best practices* (pp. 5.2–5.21). Kingston, NJ: Civic Research Institute.

Hinshaw, S. P. (2002). Preadolescent girls with attention deficit/hyperactivity disorder: I. Background characteristics, comorbidity, cognitive and social functioning, and parenting practices. *Journal of Consulting and Clinical Psychology, 70,* 1086–1098.

Hoban, T. (2008). Sleep disturbances and attention deficit hyperactivity disorder. *Sleep Medicine Clinics, 3,* 469–478.

Hogan, S., & Prater, M. (1993). The effects of peer tutoring and self-management on on-task, academic and disruptive behaviors. *Behavioral Disorders, 18,* 118–128.

Hoover-Dempsey, K., Walker, J., Sandler, H., Whetsel, D., Green, C., Wilkins, A., et al. (2005). Why do parents become involved?: Research findings and implications. *The Elementary School Journal, 106,* 105–130.

Hosterman, S. J., DuPaul, G. J., & Jitendra, A. K. (2008). Teacher ratings of ADHD symptoms in ethnic minority students: Bias or behavioral difference? *School Psychology Quarterly, 23,* 418–435.

Hoza, B., Gerdes, A. C., Hinshaw, S. P., Arnold, L. E., Pelham, W. E. Jr., Molina, B. S. G., et al. (2004). Self-perceptions of competence in children with ADHD and comparison children. *Journal of Consulting and Clinical Psychology, 72,* 382–391.

Hoza, B., Pelham, W. E. Jr., Waschbusch, D. A., Kipp, H., & Owens, J. S. (2001). Academic task performance of normally achieving ADHD and control boys: Performance, self-evaluations, and attributions. *Journal of Abnormal Child Psychology, 17,* 271–283.

Huizink, A. C., & Mulder, E. J. (2006). Maternal smoking, drinking or cannabis use during pregnancy and neurobehavioral and cognitive functioning in human offspring. *Neuroscience and Behavioral Reviews, 30,* 24–41.

Isaacs, D. (2006). Attention-deficit hyperactivity disorder: Are we medicating for social disadvantage? *Journal of Paediatrics and Child Health, 42,* 548–551.

Jackson, D., & Peters, K. (2008). Use of drug therapy in children with attention deficit hyperactivity disorder (ADHD): Maternal views and experiences. *Journal of Clinical Nursing, 17,* 2725–2732.

Jackson, D. A., & King, A. R. (2004). Gender differences in the effects of oppositional behavior on teacher ratings of ADHD symptoms. *Journal of Abnormal Child Psychology, 32,* 215–224.

Jacobs, J., Williams, A. L., Girard, C., Njike, V. Y., & Katz, D. (2005). Homeopathy for attention-deficit/hyperactivity disorder: A pilot randomized-controlled trial. *Journal of Alternative and Complementary Medicine, 11,* 799–806.

Jacobson, L., & Reid, R. (2010). Improving the persuasive essay writing of high school students with ADHD. *Exceptional Children, 76,* 157–174.

John, K., Gammon, D., Prusoff, B., & Warner, V. (1987). The Social Adjustment Inventory for Children and Adolescents (SAICA): Testing of a new semistructured interview. *Journal of the American Academy of Child and Adolescent Psychiatry, 26,* 898–911.

Johnson, J., Reid, R., & Mason, L. (in press). Improving the reading recall of high school students with ADHD. *Remedial and Special Education.*

Johnson, L., & Graham, S. (1990). Goal setting and its application with exceptional learners. *Preventing School Failure, 34,* 4–8.

Johnston, C. (1996). Parent characteristics and parent–child interactions in families of non-problem children and ADHD children with higher and lower levels of oppositional defiant behavior. *Journal of Abnormal Child Psychology, 24,* 85–104.

Johnston, C., & Mash, E. (2001). Families of children with attention-deficit/hyperactivity disorder: Review and recommendations for future research. *Clinical Child and Family Psychology Review, 4,* 183–207.

Kapalka, G. (2005). Avoiding repetitions reduces ADHD children's management problems in the classroom. *Emotional and Behavioural Difficulties, 10,* 269–279.

Kaplan, B. J., Crawford, S. G., Fisher, G. C., & Dewey, D. M. (1998). Family dysfunction is more strongly associated with ADHD than with general school problems. *Journal of Attention Disorders, 2,* 209–216.

Kaplan, J. S. (1995). *Beyond behavior modification: A cognitive-behavioral approach to behavior management in the school* (3rd ed.). Austin, TX: PRO-ED.

Karsh, K., Repp, A., Dahlquist, C., & Munk, D. (1995). In vivo functional assessment and multi-element interventions for problem behaviors of students with disabilities in classroom settings. *Journal of Behavioral Education, 5,* 189–210.

Kasten, E. F., Coury, D. L., & Heron, T. E. (1992). Educators' knowledge and attitudes regarding stimulants in the treatment of attention deficit hyperactivity disorder. *Journal of Developmental and Behavioral Pediatrics, 13,* 215–219.

Kats-Gold, I., Besser, A., & Priel, B. (2007). The role of simple emotion recognition skills among school aged boys at risk of ADHD. *Journal of Abnormal Child Psychology, 35,* 363–378.

Kats-Gold, I., & Priel, B. (2009). Emotion, understanding, and social skills among boys at risk of attention deficit hyperactivity disorder. *Psychology in the Schools, 46,* 658–678.

Kennedy, E. (2008). Media representations of attention deficit disorder: Portrayals of cultural skepticism in popular media. *Journal of Popular Culture, 41,* 91–117.

Kern, L., Childs, K., Dunlap, G., Clarke, S., & Falk, G. (1994). Using assessment-based curricular intervention to improve the classroom behavior of a student with emotional and behavioral challenges. *Journal of Applied Behavior Analysis, 27,* 7–19.

Kern, L., Dunlap, G., Clarke, S., & Childs, K. (1994). Student-Assisted Functional Assessment Interview. *Diagnostique, 19,* 29–39.

Kern-Dunlap, L., Clarke, S., & Dunlap, G. (1990). *Increasing the "meaningfulness" in curriculum content to reduce problem behaviors in a severely emotionally disturbed student.* Paper presented at the 10th annual convention of the Florida Association of Behavior Analysis, Orlando.

Klein, R., Abikoff, H., Klass, H., Ganeles, D., Seese, L., & Pollack, S. (1997). Clinical efficacy of methylphenidate in conduct disorder with and without attention deficit hyperactivity disorder. *Archives of General Psychiatry, 54,* 1073–1080.

Kliegel, M., Ropeter, A., & Mackinlay, R. (2006). Complex prospective memory in children with ADHD. *Child Neuropsychology, 12,* 407–419.

Knopf, H., & Swick, K. (2008). Using our understanding of families to strengthen family involvement. *Early Childhood Education, 35,* 419–427.

Kofler, M., Rapport, M., Bolden, J., Sarver, D., & Raiker, J. (2009). ADHD and working memory: The impact of central executive deficits and exceeding storage/rehearsal capacity on observed inattentive behavior. *Journal of Abnormal Child Psychology, 38,* 149–161.

Kofman, O., Larson, J. G., & Mostofsky, S. H. (2008). A novel task for examining strategic planning: Evidence for impairment in children with ADHD. *Journal of Clinical and Experimental Neuropsychology, 30,* 261–271.

Kollins, S. (2007). Abuse liability of medications used to treat attention-deficit/hyperactivity disorder (ADHD). *American Journal of Addiction, 16,* 35–44.

Kollins, S. (2008). ADHD, substance use disorders, and psychostimulant treatment: Current literature and treatment guidelines. *Journal of Attention Disorders, 12,* 115–125.

Konrad, M., Fowler, C. H., Walker, A. R., Test, D. W., & Wood, W. M. (2007). Effects of self-determination interventions on the academic skills of students with learning disabilities. *Learning Disabilities Quarterly, 30,* 89–113.

Krishnan, K., Feller, M., & Orkin, M. (2010). Goal setting, planning, and prioritizing. In L. Meltzer (Ed.), *Promoting executive function in the classroom* (pp. 57–85). New York: Guilford Press.

Kroth, R. L., & Edge, D. (2007). *Communicating with parents and families of exceptional children.* Denver, CO: Love.

Lahey, B. B., Applegate, B., McBurnett, K., Biederman, J., Greenhill, L., Hynd, G. W., et al. (1994). DSM-IV field trials for attention deficit hyperactivity disorder in children and adolescents. *American Journal of Psychiatry, 151,* 1673–1685.

Lalli, J., Browder, D., Mace, F., & Brown, D. (1993). Teacher use of descriptive analysis data to implement interventions to decrease students' problem behaviors. *Journal of Applied Behavior Analysis, 26,* 227–238.

Lambert, M. C., Puig, M., Lyubansky, M., Rowan, G. T., & Winfrey, T. (2001). Adult perspectives on behavioral and emotional problems in African American children. *Journal of Black Psychology, 27,* 64–85.

Larson, P. J., & Maag, J. W. (1998). Applying functional assessment in the general education classroom. *Remedial and Special Education, 19,* 338–349.

Lazarus, B. D. (1996). Flexible skeletons: Guided notes for adolescents. *Teaching Exceptional Children, 28*(3), 36–40.

Lehigh University Project Outreach. (n.d.). *Strategies for teachers.* Retrieved from *www.lehigh.edu/projectreach/teachers/peer_tutoring/peer_tutoring_step_1.htm.*

Leo, R., Khin, N., & Cohen, G. (1996). ADHD and thyroid dysfunction. *Journal of the American Academy of Child and Adolescent Psychiatry, 35,* 1572–1573.

Leslie, L., Plemmons, D., Monn, A., & Palinkas, L. (2007). Investigating ADHD treatment trajectories: Listening to families' stories about medication use. *Journal of Developmental and Behavioral Pediatrics, 28,* 179–188.

Levine, L. E., & Waite, B. M. (2000). Television viewing and attentional abilities in fourth and fifth grade children. *Journal of Applied Developmental Psychology, 21,* 667–679.

Levy, F., & Hay, D. A. (2001). *Attention, genes, and attention-deficit hyperactivity disorder.* Philadelphia: Psychology Press.

Lewis, T. J., & Sugai, G. (1996). Functional assessment of problem behavior: A pilot investigation of the comparative and interactive effects of teacher and peer social attention on students in general education settings. *School Psychology Quarterly, 11,* 1–19.

Lienemann, T. O., & Reid, R. (2008). Using self-regulated strategy development to improve expository writing with students with attention deficit hyperactivity disorder. *Exceptional Children, 74,* 471–486.

Locke, W. R., & Fuchs, L. S. (1995). Effects of peer-mediated reading instruction on the on-task behavior and social interaction of children with behavioral disorders. *Journal of Emotional and Behavioral Disorders, 3,* 92–99.

Loe, I., & Feldman, H. (2007). Academic and educational outcomes of children with ADHD. *Journal of Pediatric Psychology, 32,* 643–654.

Loo, S. K., & Barkley, R. A. (2005). Clinical utility of EEG in attention deficit hyperactivity disorder. *Applied Neuropsychology, 12,* 64–76.

Lorch, E. P., Berthiaume, K. S., Milich, R., & van den Broek, P. (2007). Story comprehension impairments in children with attention-deficit/hyperactivity disorder. In K. Cain & J. Oakhill (Eds.), *Children's comprehension problems in oral and written language: A cognitive perspective* (pp. 128–156). New York: Guilford Press.

Lynskey, M., & Hall, W. (2001). Attention deficit hyperactivity disorder and substance use disorders: Is there a causal link? *Addiction, 96,* 815–822.

Lyon, G. R., Fletcher, J. M., & Barnes, M. A. (2003). Learning disabilities. In E. J. Mash & R. Barkley (Eds.), *Child psychopathology* (pp. 520–588). New York: Guilford Press.

Maag, J. W. (2001). Rewarded by punishment: Reflections on the disuse of positive reinforcement in education. *Exceptional Children, 67,* 173–186.

Maag, J. W. (2004). *Behavior management: From theoretical implications to practical applications* (2nd ed.). Belmont, CA: Wadsworth/Thomson Learning.

Maag, J. W., Reid, R., & DiGangi, S. A. (1993). Differential effects of self-monitoring attention, accuracy, and productivity. *Journal of Applied Behavior Analysis, 26,* 329–344.

Mace, F. C., Belfiore, P. J., & Hutchinson, J. M. (2001). Operant theory and research on self-regulation. In B. Zimmerman & D. Schunk (Eds.), *Self-regulated learning and academic achievement* (pp. 39–65). Mahwah, NJ: Erlbaum.

Mace, F. C., & Kratochwill, T. R. (1988). Self-monitoring. In J. C. Witt, S. N. Elliott, & F. M. Gresham (Eds.), *Handbook of behavior therapy in education* (pp. 489–522). New York: Plenum Press.

Madan-Swain, A., & Zentall, S. (1990). Behavioral comparisons of liked and disliked hyperactive children in play contexts and the behavioral accommodations by their classmates. *Journal of Consulting and Clinical Psychology, 58,* 197–209.

Maheady, L., Mallette, B., & Harper, G. (2006). Four classwide peer tutoring models: Similarities, differences, and implications for research and practice. *Reading and Writing Quarterly, 22,* 65–89.

Mannuzza, S., & Klein, R. G. (2000). Long-term prognosis in attention-deficit/hyperactivity disorder. *Child and Adolescent Psychiatric Clinics of North America, 9,* 711–726.

Mannuzza, S., Klein, R. G., Bessler, A., Malloy, P., & Hynes, M. E. (1997). Educational and occupational outcome of hyperactive boys grown up. *Journal of the American Academy of Child and Adolescent Psychiatry, 36,* 1222–1227.

Margolis, H., & McCabe, P. (1997). Homework challenges for students with reading and writing problems: Suggestions for effective practice. *Journal of Educational and Psychological Consultation, 8,* 41–74.

Marsh, E. J., & Johnston, C. (1990). Determinants of parenting stress: Illustrations from families of hyperactive children and families of physically abused children. *Journal of Clinical Child Psychology, 19,* 313–328.

Martinussen, R., Hayden, J., Hogg-Johnson, S., & Tannock, R. (2005). A meta-analysis of working memory impairments in children with attention-deficit/hyperactivity disorder. *Journal of the American Academy of Child and Adolescent Psychiatry, 44,* 377–384.

Martinussen, R., & Tannock, R. (2006). Working memory impairments in children with attention-deficit hyperactivity disorder with and without comorbid language learning disorders. *Journal of Clinical and Experimental Neuropsychology, 28,* 1073–1094.

Mason, L. H., Kubina, R., & Taft, R. (2009). Developing quick writing skills of middle school students with disabilities. *Journal of Special Education, 44,* 205–222.

Mastropieri, M. A., & Scruggs, T. E. (2005). *Effective instruction for special education* (3rd ed.). Austin, TX: PRO-ED.

Mathes, M. Y., & Bender, W. N. (1997). The effects of self-monitoring on children with attention-deficit/hyperactivity disorder who are receiving pharmacological interventions. *Remedial and Special Education, 18,* 121–128.

Matson, J. L., Rotatori, A. F., & Helsel, W. J. (1983). Development of a rating scale to measure social skills in children: The Matson Evaluation of Social Skills with Youngsters (MESSY). *Behaviour Research and Therapy, 21,* 335–340.

Mautone, J., DuPaul, G., & Jitendra, A. (2005). The effects of computer-assisted instruction on the mathematics performance and classroom behavior of children with ADHD. *Journal of Attention Disorders, 9,* 301–312.

Mayes, R., Bagwell, C., & Erkulwater, J. (2008). ADHD and the rise in use of stimulant use among children. *Harvard Review of Psychiatry, 16,* 151–166.

Mayes, S. D., Calhoun, S. L., & Crowell, E. W. (2000). Learning disabilities and ADHD: Overlapping spectrum disorders. *Journal of Learning Disabilities, 33,* 417–424.

McAfee, J. (1987). Classroom density and the aggressive behavior of handicapped children. *Education and Treatment of Children, 10,* 134–145.

McCarney, S. B. (1995). *The Attention Deficit Disorders Evaluation Scale* (2nd ed.). Columbia, MO: Hawthorne Educational Services.

McConaughy, S. H., & Achenbach, T. M. (2004). *Manual for the Test Observation Form for ages 2–18.* Burlington: University of Vermont, Research Center for Children, Youth, and Families.

McIntosh, K., Herman, K., Sanford, A., McGraw, K., & Florence, K. (2004). Teaching transitions: Techniques for promoting success between lessons. *Teaching Exceptional Children, 37,* 32–38.

McLeer, S. V., Callaghan, M., Henry, D., & Wallen, J. (1994). Psychiatric disorders in sexually abused children. *Journal of the American Academy of Child and Adolescent Psychiatry, 33,* 313–319.

McLeod, J., Fettes, D., Jensen, P., Pescosolido, B., & Martin, J. (2007). Public knowledge, beliefs, and treatment preferences concerning attention-deficit hyperactivity disorder. *Psychiatric Services, 58,* 626–631.

Meltzer, L. (2007). Executive function difficulties and learning disabilities: Understandings and misunderstandings. In L. Meltzer (Ed.), *Executive function in education: From theory to practice* (pp. 77–105). New York: Guilford Press.

Mercer, J. (1973). *Labeling the mentally retarded.* Berkley and Los Angeles: University of California Press.

Merrell, K. (2001). Assessment of children's social skills: Recent developments, best practices, and new directions. *Exceptionality, 9,* 3–18.

Merrell, K. (2002). *School Social Behavior Scales* (2nd ed.). Baltimore: Brookes.

Meyer, K., & Kelley, M. (2007). Improving homework in adolescents with attention-deficit/hyperactivity disorder: Self vs. parent monitoring of homework behavior and study skills. *Child and Family Behavior Therapy, 29,* 25–42.

Mikami, A., Jack, A., & Lerner, M. (2010). Attention-deficit/hyperactivity disorder. In J. Matson (Ed.), *Social behavior and skills in children* (pp. 159–185). New York: Springer.

Milberger, S., Biederman, J., Faraone, S. V., Murphy, J., & Tsuang, M. T. (1995). Attention deficit hyperactivity disorder and comorbid disorders: Issues of overlapping symptoms. *American Journal of Psychiatry, 152,* 1783–1800.

Milich, R., & Greenwell, L. (1991, December). An examination of learned helplessness among attention-deficit hyperactivity disordered boys. In B. Hoza & W. E. Pelham (Chairs), *Cognitive biases as mediators of childhood disorders: What do we know?* Symposium presented at the annual meeting of the Association for the Advancement of Behavior Therapy, New York, NY.

Milich, R., & Okazaki, M. (1991). An examination of learned helplessness among attention-deficit hyperactivity disordered boys. *Journal of Abnormal Child Psychology, 19,* 607–623.

Miller, M. A. (2005). Using peer tutoring in the classroom: Applications for students with emotional/behavioral disorders. *Beyond Behavior, 15*(1) 25–30.

Miller, T., Nigg, J., & Miller, R. (2009). Attention deficit hyperactivity disorder in African American children: What can be concluded from the past ten years? *Clinical Psychology Review, 29,* 77–86.

Mirsky, A. F. (1996). Disorders of attention: A neuropsychological perspective. In R. G. Lyon & N. A. Krasnegor (Eds.), *Attention, memory, and executive function* (pp. 71–96). Baltimore: Brookes.

Monastra, V. (2008). Medical conditions that mimic ADHD. In V. J. Monastra (Ed.), *Unlocking the potential of patients with ADHD: A model for clinical practice* (pp. 49–66). Washington, DC: American Psychological Association.

Moore Partin, T., Robertson, R., Maggin, D., Oliver, R., & Wehby, J. (2010). Using teacher praise and opportunities to respond to promote appropriate student behavior. *Preventing School Failure, 54,* 172–178.

MTA Cooperative Group. (2004). National Institute of Mental Health Multimodal Treatment Study of ADHD follow-up: Changes in effectiveness and growth after the end of treatment. *Pediatrics, 113,* 762–769.

Munir, K., Biederman, J., & Knee, D. (1987). Psychiatric comorbidity in patients with attention deficit disorder: A controlled study. *Journal of the American Academy of Child and Adolescent Psychiatry, 26,* 844–848.

Murray, D., Rabiner, D., Schulte, A., & Newitt, K. (2008). Feasibility and integrity of a parent–teacher consultation intervention for ADHD students. *Child Youth Care Forum, 37,* 111–126.

National Association of School Psychologist. (2002). Social skills: Promoting positive behavior, academic success, and school safety. Retrieved from *www.nasponline.org/resources/factsheets/socialskills_fs.aspx.*

Needleman, H. L. (1982). Lead and impaired abilities. *Developing Medicine and Child Neurology, 24,* 196–198.

Neel, R. S., & Cessna, K. K. (1993). Replacement behaviors: A strategy for teaching social skills to children with behavior problems. *Rural Special Education Quarterly, 12*(1), 30–35.

Nelson, C., & Rutherford, R. (1983). Time out revisited: Guidelines for its use in special education. *Exceptional Education Quarterly, 3,* 56–67.

Nelson, R. O., & Hayes, S. C. (1981). Theoretical explanations for reactivity in self-monitoring. *Behavior Modification, 5,* 3–14.

Neufeld, P., & Foy, M. (2006). Historical reflections on the ascendancy of ADHD in North America, c. 1980–c. 2005. *British Journal of Educational Studies, 54,* 449–470.

Northup, J., Broussard, C., Jones, K., George, T., Vollmer, T. R., & Herring, M. (1995). The differential effects of teacher and peer attention on the disruptive classroom behavior of three children with a diagnosis of attention deficit hyperactivity disorder. *Journal of Applied Behavior Analysis, 28,* 227–228.

Olfson, M., Marcus, S., Weissman, M., & Jensen, P. (2002). National trends in the use of psychotropic medications by children. *Journal of the American Academy of Child and Adolescent Psychiatry, 41,* 514–521.

O'Neill, M. E., & Douglas, V. I. (1991). Study strategies and story recall in attention-deficit disorder and reading disability. *Journal of Abnormal Child Psychology, 19,* 671–692.

O'Neill, M. E., & Douglas, V. I. (1996). Rehearsal strategies and recall performance in boys with and without attention deficit hyperactivity disorder. *Journal of Pediatric Psychology, 21,* 73–88.

O'Neill, R., Horner, R., Albin, R., Sprague, J., Storey, K., & Newton, I. (1997). *Functional assessment and program development for problem behavior: A practical handbook* (2nd ed.). Pacific Grove, CA: Brooks/Cole.

O'Regan, F., & Cooper, P. (2001). Ruby Tuesday: A student with ADHD and learning difficulties. *Emotional and Behavioural Difficulties, 6,* 265–269.

Oswald, D. P., Coutinho, M. J., Best, A. M., & Singh, N. N. (1999). Ethnic representation in special education: The influence of school-related economic and demographic variables. *Journal of Special Education, 32,* 194–206.

Ota, K. R., & DuPaul, G. J. (2002). Task engagement and mathematics performance in children with attention deficit hyperactivity disorder: Effects of supplemental computer instruction. *School Psychology Quarterly, 17,* 242–257.

Owens, M., Stevenson, J., Norgate, R., & Hadwin, J. (2008). Processing efficiency theory in children: Working memory as a mediator between trait anxiety and academic performance. *Anxiety, Stress, and Coping, 21,* 417–430.

Packenham, M., Shute, R., & Reid, R. (2004). A truncated functional behavioral assessment procedure for children with disruptive classroom behaviors. *Education and Treatment of Children, 27,* 9–25.

Paine, S. C., Radicchi, J., Rosellini, L. C., Deutchman, L., & Darch, C. (1983). *Structure your classroom for success.* Champaign, IL: Research Press.

Park, R. (2003). *Seven signs of bogus science.* Retrieved from *www.quackwatch.com/01Quackery RelatedTopics/signs.html.*

Partin, T., Robertson, R., Maggin, D., Oliver, R., & Wehby, J. (2010). Using teacher praise and opportunities to respond to promote appropriate student behavior. *Preventing School Failure, 54,* 172–178.

Pelham, W. E., Foster, M., & Robb, J. A. (2007). The economic impact of attention-deficit/hyperactivity disorder in children and adolescents. *Journal of Pediatric Psychology, 32,* 711–727.

Pelham, W. E. Jr. (1993). Pharmacotherapy for children with attention-deficit hyperactivity disorder. *School Psychology Review, 22,* 199–227.

Pelham, W. E. Jr. (2002). How to establish a school–home daily report card. Retrieved from *www.utmem.edu/pediatrics/general/clinical/behavior.*

Pelham, W. E. Jr., & Fabiano, G. A. (2008). Evidence based psychosocial treatments for attention-deficit/hyperactivity disorder. *Journal of Clinical Child and Adolescent Psychology, 37,* 184–214.

Pelham, W. E. Jr., Fabiano, G. A., & Massetti, G. M. (2005). Evidence-based assessment of attention deficit hyperactivity disorder in children and adolescents. *Journal of Clinical Child and Adolescent Psychology, 34,* 449–476.

Pelham, W. E. Jr., & Hoza, B. (1996). Intensive treatment: A summer treatment program for children with ADHD. In E. D. Hibbs & P. S. Jensen (Eds.), *Psychosocial treatments for child and adolescent disorders: Empirically based strategies for clinical practice* (pp. 311–340). Washington, DC: American Psychological Association.

Pelham, W. E. Jr., Massetti, G. M., Wilson, T., Kipp, H., Myers, D., Standley, B. E. N., et al.

(2005). Implementation of a comprehensive schoolwide behavioral intervention: The ABC program. *Journal of Attention Disorders, 9*, 248–260.

Pelham, W. E. Jr., Wheeler, T., & Chronis, A. (1998). Empirically supported psychosocial treatments for attention deficit hyperactivity disorder. *Journal of Clinical Child and Adolescent Psychology, 27*, 190–205.

Perdue, N., Manzeske, D., & Estell, D. (2009). Early predictors of school engagement: Exploring the role of peer relationships. *Psychology in the Schools, 46*, 1084–1097.

Peterson, B. S. (1995). Neuroimaging in child and adolescent neuropsychiatric disorders. *Journal of the American Academy of Child and Adolescent Psychiatry, 34*, 1560–1576.

Pfiffner, L. J., & Barkley, R. A. (1998). Treatment of ADHD in school settings. In R. A. Barkley (Ed.), *Attention deficit hyperactivity disorder: A handbook for diagnosis and treatment* (2nd ed., pp. 458–490). New York: Guilford Press.

Pfiffner, L. J., Barkley, R. A., & DuPaul, G. J. (2006). Treatment of ADHD in school settings. In R. A. Barkley (Ed.), *Attention deficit hyperactivity disorder: A handbook for diagnosis and treatment* (3rd ed., pp. 547–589). New York: Guilford Press.

Pfiffner, L. J., McBurnett, K., Lahey, B. B., Loeber, R., Green, S., Frick, P. J., et al. (1999). Association of parental psychopathology to the comorbid disorders of boys with attention-deficit hyperactivity disorder. *Consulting and Clinical Psychology, 67*, 881–893.

Pfiffner, L. J., & O'Leary, S. G. (1987). The efficacy of all-positive management as a function of the prior use of negative consequences. *Journal of Applied Behavior Analysis, 20*, 265–271.

Pfiffner, L. J., Rosen, L., & O'Leary, S. G. (1985). The efficacy of an all-positive approach to classroom management. *Journal of Applied Behavior Analysis, 18*, 257–261.

Pisecco, S., Huzinec, C., & Curtis, D. (2001). The effect of child characteristics on teachers' acceptability of classroom-based behavioral strategies and psychostimulant medication for the treatment of ADHD. *Journal of Clinical Child Psychology, 30*, 413–421.

Podolski, C., & Nigg, J. (2001). Parent stress and coping in relation to child ADHD severity and associated child disruptive behavior problems. *Journal of Clinical Child Psychology, 30*, 503–513.

Powell, S., & Nelson, B. (1997). Effects of choosing academic assignments on a student with attention deficit hyperactivity disorder. *Journal of Applied Behavior Analysis, 30*, 181–183.

Power, T., Hess, L., & Bennett, D. (1995). The acceptability of interventions for attention-deficit hyperactivity disorder among elementary and middle school teachers. *Journal of Developmental and Behavioral Pediatrics, 16*, 238–243.

Power, T., & Mautone, J. (2008). Best practice in linking families and schools to educate children with attention problems. In A. Thomas & J. Grimes (Eds.), *Best practices in school psychology* (Vol. 5, pp. 839–850). Bethesda, MD: National Association of School Psychologists.

Psychogiou, L., Daley, D., Thompson, M., & Sonuga-Barke, E. (2008). Do maternal attention-deficit/hyperactivity disorder symptoms exacerbate or ameliorate the negative effect of child attention-deficit/hyperactivity disorder symptoms on parenting? *Development and Psychopathology, 2*, 121–137.

Puig, M., Lambert, M. C., Rowan, G. T., Winfrey, T., Lyubansky, M., Hannah, S. D., et al. (1999). Behavioral and emotional problems among Jamaican and African American children, ages 6 to 11: Teacher reports versus direct observations. *Journal of Emotional and Behavioral Disorders, 7*, 240–250.

Purvis, K. L., & Tannock, R. (1997). Language abilities in children with attention deficit hyperactivity disorder, reading disabilities, and normal controls. *Journal of Abnormal Child Psychology, 25*, 133–144.

Quay, H. C. (1988a). The behavioral reward and inhibition systems in childhood behavior disorder. In L. M. Bloomingdale (Ed.), *Attention deficit disorder: Vol. 3. New research in treatment, psychopharmacology, and attention* (pp. 176–186). New York: Pergamon Press.

Quay, H. C. (1988b). Attention deficit disorder and the behavioral inhibition system: The relevance of the neuropsychological theory of Jeffrey A. Gray. In L. M. Bloomingdale & J. Sergeant (Eds.), *Attention deficit disorder: Criteria, cognition, intervention* (pp. 117–126). New York: Pergamon Press.

Rapport, M. D., Denney, C., DuPaul, G. J., & Gardner, M. J. (1994). Attention deficit disorder and methyphenidate: Normalization rates, clinical effectiveness, and response prediction in 76 children. *Journal of the American Academy of Child and Adolescent Psychiatry, 33,* 882–839.

Reid, R. (1993). Implementing self-monitoring interventions in the classroom: Lessons from research. *Monograph in Behavior Disorders: Severe Behavior Disorders in Youth, 16,* 43–54.

Reid, R. (1996). Self-monitoring for students with learning disabilities: The present, the prospects, the pitfalls. *Journal of Learning Disabilities, 29,* 317–331.

Reid, R. (1999). Attention deficit hyperactivity disorder: Effective methods for the classroom. *Focus on Exceptional Children, 32,* 1–20.

Reid, R., DuPaul, G. J., Power, T. J., Anastopoulos, A. D., Rogers-Adkinson, D., Noll, M.-B., et al. (1998). Assessing culturally different students for attention deficit hyperactivity disorder using behavior rating scales. *Journal of Abnormal Child Psychology, 26,* 187–198.

Reid, R., Hakendorf, P., & Prosser, B. (2002). Use of psychostimulant medication for ADHD in South Australia. *Journal of the American Academy of Child and Adolescent Psychiatry, 41,* 906–913.

Reid, R., & Harris, K. R. (1993). Self-monitoring of attention versus self-monitoring of performance: Effects on attention and academic performance. *Exceptional Children, 60,* 29–40.

Reid, R., Hertzog, M., & Snyder, M. (1996). Educating every teacher every year: The public schools and parents of children with ADHD. *Seminars in Speech and Language, 17,* 73–90.

Reid, R., & Katsiyannis, A. (1995). Attention-deficit/hyperactivity disorder and section 504. *Remedial and Special Education, 16,* 44–52.

Reid, R., & Lienemann, T. O. (2006a). *Strategy instruction for students with learning disabilities.* New York: Guilford Press.

Reid, R., & Lienemann, T. O. (2006b). Self-regulated strategy development for written expression with students with attention deficit hyperactivity disorder. *Exceptional Children, 73,* 53–68.

Reid, R., & Maag, J. W. (1994). How many "fidgets" in a "pretty much": A critique of behavior rating scales for identifying students with ADHD. *Journal of School Psychology, 32,* 339–354.

Reid, R., & Maag, J. W. (1998). Functional assessment: A method for developing classroom-based accommodations for children with ADHD. *Reading and Writing Quarterly, 14,* 9–42.

Reid, R., Maag, J. W., & Vasa, S. F. (1994). Attention deficit hyperactivity disorder as a disability category: A critique. *Exceptional Children, 60,* 198–214.

Reid, R., & Nelson, J. R. (2002). The utility, acceptability, and practicality of functional behavioral assessment for students with high-incidence problem behaviors. *Remedial and Special Education, 23,* 15–23.

Reid, R., Riccio, C. A., Kessler, R. H., DuPaul, G. J., Power, T. J., Anastopoulos, A. D., et al.

(2000). Gender and ethnic differences in ADHD as assessed by behavior ratings. *Journal of Emotional and Behavioral Disorders, 8,* 38–49.

Reid, R., Trout, A. L., & Schartz, M. (2005). Self-regulation interventions for children with attention-deficit/hyperactivity disorder. *Exceptional Children, 71,* 361–377.

Reid, R., Vasa, S. F., Maag, J. W., & Wright, G. (1994). An analysis of teachers' perceptions of ADHD. *Journal of Research and Development in Education, 27,* 195–202.

Reynolds, C. R., & Kamphaus, R. W. (1992). *BASC: Behavior Assessment System for Children manual.* Circle Pines, MN: American Guidance.

Robin, A. (2006). Training families with adolescents with ADHD. In R. A. Barkley (Ed.), *Attention-deficit hyperactivity disorder: A handbook for diagnosis and treatment* (3rd ed., pp. 499–546). New York: Guilford Press.

Robinson, T. R., Smith, S. W., Miller, M. D., & Brownell, M. T. (1999). Cognitive behavior modification of hyperactivity–impulsivity and aggression: A meta-analysis of school-based studies. *Journal of Educational Psychology, 91,* 195–203.

Rock, M. (2005). Using strategic self-monitoring to enhance the academic engagement, productivity, and accuracy of students with and without exceptionalities. *Journal of Positive Behavior Interventions, 7,* 3–17.

Rogers, M., Wiener, J., Marton, I., & Tannock, R. (2009). Parental involvement in children's learning: Comparing parents of children with and without attention-deficit/hyperactivity disorder. *Journal of School Psychology, 47,* 167–185.

Rogevich, M. E., & Perin, D. (2008). Effects on science summarization of a reading comprehension intervention for adolescents with behavior and attention disorders. *Exceptional Children, 74*(2), 135–154.

Rojas, N. L., & Chan, E. (2005). Old and new controversies in the alternative treatment of attention-deficit hyperactivity disorder. *Mental Retardation and Developmental Disabilities Research Reviews, 11,* 116–130.

Rowland, A., Umbach, D., Stallone, L., Naftel, A., Bohlig, E., & Sandler, D. (2002). Prevalence of medication treatment for attention deficit-hyperactivity disorder among elementary school children in Johnston county, North Carolina. *American Journal of Public Health, 92,* 231–234.

Rutter, M. L. (1983). Issues and prospects in developmental neuropsychiatry. In M. L. Rutter (Ed.), *Developmental neuropsychiatry* (pp. 577–593). New York: Guilford Press.

Ryan, J. B., & Katsiyannis, A. (2009). The importance of teacher involvement in medication therapy. *Teaching Exceptional Children Plus, 6* Article 1. Retrieved from *escholarship.bc.edu/education/tecplus/vol6/iss2/art1.*

Ryan, J. B., Reid, R., & Ellis, C. (2008). A survey of special educator knowledge regarding psychotropic interventions for students with emotional and behavioral disorders. *Remedial and Special Education, 29,* 269–279.

Ryan, J. B., Reid, R., Gallagher, K., & Ellis, C. (2008). Prevalence rates of psychotropic medications for students placed in residential care. *Behavioral Disorders, 33,* 99–107.

Safer, D. J., & Krager, J. M. (1988). A survey of medication treatment for hyperactive/inattentive students. *Journal of the American Medical Association, 260,* 2256–2258.

Safer, D. J., & Malever, M. (2000). Stimulant treatment in Maryland public schools. *Pediatrics, 106,* 533–539.

Salend, S., & Schliff, J. (1989). An examination of homework practices of teachers of students with learning disabilities. *Journal of Learning Disabilities, 22,* 621–623.

Satterfield, J. H., Satterfield, B. T., & Cantwell, D. P. (1980). Multimodality treatment: A two-year evaluation of 61 hyperactive boys. *Archives of General Psychiatry, 37,* 915–919.

Satterfield, J. H., Satterfield, B. T., & Cantwell, D. P. (1981). Three-year multimodality treatment study of 100 hyperactive boys. *Journal of Pediatrics, 98*, 650–655.

Sawyer, A. M., Taylor, E., & Chadwick, O. (2001). The effect of off-task behaviors on the task performance of hyperkinetic children. *Journal of Attention Disorders, 5*, 1–10.

Sax, L., & Kautz, K. J. (2003). Who first suggests the diagnosis of attention-deficit/hyperactivity disorder? *Annals of Family Medicine, 1*, 171–174.

Schab, D. W., & Trinh, N.-H. T. (2004). Do artificial food colors promote hyperactivity in children with hyperactive syndromes?: A meta-analysis of double-blind placebo-controlled trials. *Journal of Developmental and Behavioral Pediatrics, 25*, 423–434.

Schachar, R. J., Tannock, R., & Logan, G. (1993). Inhibitory control, impulsiveness, and attention deficit hyperactivity disorder. *Clinical Psychology Review, 13*, 721–739.

Scheres, A., Oosterlaan, J., Geurts, H., Morein-Zamir, S., Meiran, N., Schut, H., et al. (2004). Executive functioning in boys with ADHD: Primarily an inhibition deficit? *Archives of Clinical Neuropsychology, 19*, 569–594.

Schlachter, S. (2008). Diagnosis, treatment, and educational implications for students with attention-deficit/hyperactivity disorder in the United States, Australia and the United Kingdom. *Peabody Journal of Education, 83*, 154–169.

Schnoes, C., Reid, R., Wagner, M., & Marder, C. (2006). ADHD among students receiving special education services: A national survey. *Exceptional Children, 72*(4), 483–496.

Schumaker, J. B., Denton, P. H., & Deshler, D. D. (1984). *The paraphrasing strategy.* Lawrence: University of Kansas.

Schunk, D. (1990). Goal setting and self-efficacy during self-regulated learning. *Educational Psychologist, 25*, 71–86.

Schunk, D. (2001). Social cognitive theory and self-regulated learning. In B. Zimmerman & D. Schunk (Eds.), *Self-regulated learning and academic achievement* (pp. 125–151). Mahwah, NJ: Erlbaum.

Scime, M., & Norvilitis, J. M. (2006). Task performance and response to frustration in children with attention deficit hyperactivity disorder. *Psychology in the Schools, 43*, 377–386.

Semrud-Clikeman, M., Biederman, J., Sprich-Buckminster, S., Lehman, B. K., Faraone, S. V., & Norman, D. (1992). Comorbidity between ADDH and learning disability: A review and report in a clinically referred sample. *Journal of the American Academy of Child and Adolescent Psychiatry, 31*, 439–448.

Semrud-Clikeman, M., & Pliszka, S. R. (2005). Neuroimaging and psychopharmacology. *School Psychology Quarterly, 20*, 172–186.

Seplocha, H. (2004). Partnerships for learning: Conferencing with families. *Beyond the Journal—Young Children on the Web.* Retrieved from *www.journal.naeyc.org.*

Shapiro, E. S., & Cole, C. L. (1994). *Behavior change in the classroom: Self-management interventions.* New York: Guilford Press.

Shapiro, E. S., DuPaul, G. J., Bradley, K. L., & Bailey, L. T. (1996). A school-based consultation program for a service delivery to middle school students with attention deficit hyperactivity disorder. *Journal of Emotional and Behavioral Disorders, 4*, 73–81.

Shapiro, E. S., DuPaul, G. J., & Bradley-Klug, K. L. (1998). Self-management as a strategy to improve the classroom behavior of adolescents with ADHD. *Journal of Learning Disabilities, 31*, 545–555.

Shaw, P., Eckstrand, K., Sharp, W., Blumenthal, J., Lerch, J. P., Greenstein, D., et al. (2007). Attention deficit/hyperactivity disorder is characterized by a delay in cortical maturation. *Proceedings of the National Academy of Sciences of the United States of America, 104*, 19649–19654.

Sherman, D. K., Iacono, W. G., & McGee, M. K. (1997). Attention-deficit hyperactivity disorder dimensions: A twin study of inattention and impulsivity and hyperactivity. *Journal of the American Academy of Child and Adolescent Psychiatry, 36,* 745–753.

Shimabukuro, S. M., Prater, M. A., Jenkins, A., & Edelen-Smith, P. (1999). The effects of self-monitoring of academic performance on students with learning disabilities and ADD/ADHD. *Education and Treatment of Children, 22,* 397–415.

Shin, M.-S., Kim, Y.-H., Cho, S.-C., & Kim, B.-N. (2003). Neurologic characteristics of children with attention deficit hyperactivity disorder (ADHD), learning disorder, and tic disorder on the Rey–Osterreith complex figure. *Journal of Child Neurology, 18,* 835–844.

Shinn, M. R. (Ed.). (1998). *Advanced applications of curriculum-based measurement.* New York: Guilford Press.

Silver, L. B. (1987). A review of the current controversial approaches for treating learning disabilities. *Journal of Learning Disabilities, 20,* 498–504.

Silver, L. B. (1990). Attention-deficit-hyperactivity disorder: Is it a learning disability or a related disorder? *Journal of Learning Disabilities, 23,* 394–397.

Silver, L. B. (1999). *Attention-deficit/hyperactivity disorder: A clinical guide to diagnosis and treatment for health and mental health professionals* (2nd ed.). Washington, DC: American Psychiatric Press.

Silverthorn, P., Frick, P. J., Kuper, K., & Ott, J. (1996). Attention deficit hyperactivity disorder and sex: A test of two etiological models to explain the male predominance. *Journal of Clinical Child Psychology, 25,* 52–59.

Singer, G., Singer, J., & Horner, R. (1987). Using pretask requests to increase the probability of compliance for students with severe disabilities. *Journal of the Association for Persons with Severe Handicaps, 12,* 287–291.

Singh, I. (2004). Doing their jobs: Mothering with Ritalin in a culture of mother blame. *Social Science and Medicine, 59,* 1193–1205.

Singh, I. (2007). Clinical implications of ethical concepts: The case of children taking stimulants for ADHD. *Journal of Child Psychology and Psychiatry, 12,* 167–182.

Singh, N., Curtis, W., Ellis, C., Wechsler, H., Best, A., & Cohen, R. (1997). Empowerment status of families whose children have serious emotional disturbance and attention-deficit/hyperactivity disorder. *Journal of Emotional and Behavioral Disorders, 5,* 223–229.

Smith, T. E. C., & Patton, J. R. (1998). *Section 504 and public schools: A practical guide for determining eligibility, developing accommodation plans, and documenting compliance.* Austin, TX: PRO-ED.

Snider, V. E., Busch, T., & Arrowood, L. (2003). Teacher knowledge of stimulant medication and ADHD. *Remedial and Special Education, 24,* 46–56.

Solanto, M., Marks, D., Wasserstein, J., Mitchell, K., Abikoff, H., Alvir, J., & Kofman, M. (2010). Efficacy of meta-cognitive therapy for adult ADHD. *American Journal of Psychiatry, 167,* 958–968.

Sonuga-Barke, E. J. (2002). Psychological heterogeneity in AD/HD—a dual pathway model of behaviour and cognition. *Behavioural Brain Research, 130,* 29–36.

Sonuga-Barke, E. J. S., Taylor, E., & Hepinstall, E. (1992). Hyperactivity and delay aversion: II. The effect of self versus externally imposed stimulus presentation periods on memory. *Journal of Child Psychology and Psychiatry, 33,* 399–409.

Spence, S. (2003). Social skill training with children and young people: Theory, evidence and practice. *Child and Adolescent Mental Health, 8,* 84–96.

Spencer, T., Biederman, J., Wilens, T., & Faraone, S. (2002). Novel treatments for attention-deficit/hyperactivity disorder in children. *Journal of Clinical Psychiatry, 63,* 16–22.

Sprague, R. L., & Ullman, R. K. (1981). Psychoactive drugs and child management. In J. M. Kaufman & D. P. Hallan (Eds.), *Handbook of special education* (pp. 749–766). New York: Prentice-Hall.

Stahr, B., Cushing, D., Lane, K., & Fox, J. (2006). Efficacy of a function-based intervention in decreasing off-task behavior exhibited by a student with ADHD. *Journal of Positive Behavior Interventions, 8,* 201–211.

Stenhoff, D., & Lignugaris-Kraft, B. (2007). A review of the effects of peer tutoring on students with mild disabilities in secondary settings. *Exceptional Children, 74,* 8–30.

Stevens, G. (1980). Bias in attributions of positive and negative behavior in children by school psychologists, parents, and teachers. *Perceptual and Motor Skills, 50,* 1283–1290.

Stevens, J., Harman, J., & Kelleher, K. (2005). Race/ethnicity and insurance status as factors associated with ADHD treatment patterns. *Journal of Child and Adolescent Psychopharmacology, 15,* 88–96.

Stevens, J., Quittner, A. L., & Abikoff, H. (1998). Factors influencing elementary school teachers' ratings of ADHD and ODD behaviors. *Journal of Clinical Child and Adolescent Psychology, 27,* 406–414.

Stewart, M. A., Pitts, F. N., Craig, A. G., & Dieruf, W. (1966). The hyperactive child syndrome. *American Journal of Orthopsychiatry, 36,* 861–867.

Still, G. F. (1902). Some abnormal psychical conditions in children. *Lancet, 1,* 1008–1012, 1077–1082, 1163–1168.

Stolzer, J. (2007). The ADHD epidemic in America. *Ethical Human Psychology and Psychiatry, 9,* 109–116.

Stormont, M. (2001). Social outcomes of children with AD/HD: Contributing factors and implications for practice. *Psychology in the Schools, 38,* 521–531.

Strauss, A. A., & Lehtinen, L. E. (1947). *Psychopathology and education of the brain-injured child: Vol. 2. Progress in theory and clinic.* New York: Grune & Stratton.

Strauss, M. E., Thompson, P., Adams, N. L., Redline, S., & Burant, C. (2000). Evaluation of a model of attention with confirmatory factor analysis. *Neuropsychology, 14,* 201–208.

Strayhorn, J. (2002). Self-control: Toward systematic training programs. *Journal of the American Academy of Child and Adolescent Psychiatry, 41,* 17–27.

Swanson, H. L., & Sachse-Lee, C. (2000). A meta-analysis of single-subject-design intervention research for students with LD. *Journal of Learning Disabilities, 33,* 114–136.

Swanson, J. M. (1992). *School-based assessments and interventions for ADD students.* Irvine, CA: K. C. Publishing.

Swanson, J. M., Kraemer, H. C., Hinshaw, S. P., Arnold, L. E., Conners, C. K., & Abikoff, H. B. (2001). Clinical relevance of the primary findings of the MTA: Success rates based on severity of ADHD and ODD symptoms at the end of treatment. *Journal of the American Academy of Child and Adolescent Psychiatry, 40,* 168–179.

Swanson, J. M., McBurnett, K., Wigal, T., Pfiffner, L. J., Lerner, M. A., Williams, L., et al. (1993). Effect of stimulant medication on children with attention deficit disorder: A "review of reviews." *Exceptional Children, 60,* 154–162.

Szatmari, P., Offord, D. R., & Boyle, M. H. (1989). Ontario Child Health Study: Prevalence of attention deficit disorder with hyperactivity. *Journal of Child Psychology and Psychiatry, 30,* 219–230.

Tannock, R. (2000). Attention-deficit/hyperactivity disorders with anxiety disorders. In T. E. Brown (Ed.), *Attention-deficit disorders and comorbidities in children, adolescents, and adults* (pp. 125–170). Washington, DC: American Psychiatric Press.

Taylor, M., O'Donoghue, T., & Houghton, S. (2006). To medicate or not to medicate?: The decision-making process of Western Australian parents following their child's diagnosis with attention deficit hyperactivity disorder. *International Journal of Disability and Education, 53*, 111–128.

Thomas, J. M., & Guskin, K. A. (2001). Disruptive behavior in young children: What does it mean? *Journal of the American Academy of Child and Adolescent Psychiatry, 40*, 44–51.

Timimi, S., & Radcliffe, N. (2005). The rise and rise of ADHD. In C. Newnes & N. Radcliffe (Eds.), *Making and breaking children's lives* (pp. 63–70). Ross-on-Wye, UK: PCCS Books.

Tingley, S. (2009). Eight great teacher habits parents love. *Instructor, 111*(5), 30–35.

Todd, R., Huang, H., & Henderson, C. (2008). Poor utility of the age of onset criterion for DSM-IV attention deficit/hyperactivity disorder: Recommendations for DSM-V and ICD-11. *Journal of Child Psychology and Psychiatry, 49*, 942–949.

Touchette, P., MacDonald, R., & Langer, S. (1985). A scatter plot for identifying stimulus control of problem behavior. *Journal of Applied Behavior Analysis, 18*, 343–351.

Trammel, D., Schloss, P., & Alper, S. (1994). Using self-recording, evaluation, and graphing to increase completion of homework assignments. *Journal of Learning Disabilities, 27*, 75–81.

Treacy, L., Tripp, G., & Bird, A. (2005). Parent stress management training for attention-deficit/hyperactivity disorder. *Behavior Therapy, 36*, 223–233.

Trout, A., Lienemann, T., Reid, R., & Epstein, M. (2007). A review of non-medication interventions to improve academic performance of children and youth with ADHD. *Remedial and Special Education, 28*, 207–226.

Umbreit, J. (1995). Functional assessment and intervention in a regular classroom setting for the disruptive behavior of a student with attention deficit hyperactivity disorder. *Behavioral Disorders, 20*, 267–278.

U.S. Department of Education. (2005). *National Assessment of Educational Progress (NAEP).* Washington DC: Author.

U. S. Department of Education. (2006a). *Building the legacy: IDEA 2004, October 2006.* Retrieved from *idea.ed.gov/explore/view/p/,root,regs,300,A.*

U. S. Department of Education. (2006b). *PART 104—Nondiscrimination on the basis of handicap in programs or activities receiving federal financial assistance, October 2006.* Retrieved from *www2.ed.gov/policy/rights/reg/ocr/edlite-34cfr104.html.*

U.S. Department of Education, Office of Intergovernmental and Interagency Affairs, Educational Partnerships and Family Involvement Unit. (2003). *Homework tips for parents.* Washington, DC: Author.

U. S. Department of Justice. (2000). Coordination and review section. Retrieved from *www.usdoj.gov/crt/cor/byagency/usda504.php.*

van Zomeren, A. H., & Brouwer, W. H. (1994). *Clinical neuropsychology of attention.* London: Oxford University Press.

Wakefield, J. C. (1992). The concept of mental disorder: On the boundary between biological facts and social values. *American Psychologist, 47*, 373–388.

Walcott, C. M., & Landau, S. (2004). The relation between disinhibition and emotion regulation in boys with attention deficit hyperactivity disorder. *Journal of Clinical Child and Adolescent Psychology, 33*, 772–782.

Walker, H. M., Block-Pedego, A., Todis, B., & Severson, H. (1998). *School archival records search (SARS): User's guide and technical manual.* Longmont, CO: Sopris-West.

Walker, J., Shea, T., & Bauer, A. (2004). *Behavior management: A practical approach for educators.* Columbus, OH: Pearson.

Walker, S. (1999). *The hyperactivity hoax.* New York: St. Martin's Press.

Waschbusch, D. A., Craig, R., Pelham, W. E. Jr., & King, S. (2007). Self-handicapping prior to academic-oriented tasks in children with attention deficit/hyperactivity disorder (ADHD): Medication effects and comparisons with controls. *Journal of Abnormal Child Psychology, 35,* 275–286.

Waschbusch, D. A., & King, S. (2006). Should sex-specific norms be used to assess attention-deficit/hyperactivity disorder or oppositional defiant disorder? *Journal of Consulting and Clinical Psychology, 74,* 179–185.

Waschbusch, D. A., Pelham, W. E. Jr., & Massetti, G. (2005). The Behavior Education Support and Treatment (BEST) school intervention program: Pilot project data examining schoolwide, targeted-school, and targeted-home approaches. *Journal of Attention Disorders, 9,* 313–322.

Waschbusch, D. A., Pelham, W. E. Jr., Waxmonsky, J., & Johnson, C. (2009). Are there placebo effects in the medication treatment of children with attention-deficit hyperactivity disorder? *Journal of Developmental and Behavioral Pediatrics, 30,* 158–168.

Wasserman, R. C., Kelleher, K. J., Bocian, A., Baker, A., Childs, G. E., Indacochea, F., et al. (1999). Identification of attentional and hyperactivity problems in primary care: A report from pediatric research in office settings and the Ambulatory Sentinel Practice Network. *Pediatrics, 103,* E38.

Weber, W., Vander Stoep, A., McCarty, R. L., Weiss, N. S., Biederman, J., & McClellan, J. (2008). Hypericum perforatum (St. John's Wort) for attention-deficit/hyperactivity disorder in children and adolescents: A randomized controlled trial. *Journal of the American Medical Association, 299,* 2633–2641.

Weiss, M., Hechtman, L., & Weiss, G. (2000). ADHD in parents. *Journal of the American Academy of Child and Adolescent Psychiatry, 39,* 1059–1061.

Welner, Z., Welner, A., Stewart, M., Palkes, H., & Wish, E. (1977). A controlled study of siblings of hyperactive children. *Journal of Nervous and Mental Disease, 165,* 110–117.

Weyandt, L. L. (2001). *An ADHD primer.* Boston: Allyn & Bacon.

Weyandt, L. L. (2005). Executive function in children, adolescents and adults with attention deficit hyperactivity disorder: Introduction to the special issue. *Developmental Neuropsychology, 27,* 1–10.

Whalen, C., Henker, B., Collins, B., Finck, D., & Dotemoto, S. (1979). A social ecology of hyperactive boys: Medication effects in structured classroom environments. *Journal of Applied Behavior Analysis, 12,* 65–81.

Whalen, C., Henker, B., Ishikawa, S., Jamner, L., Floro, J., Johnston, J., et al. (2006). An electronic diary study of contextual triggers and ADHD: Get ready, get set, get mad. *Journal of the American Academy of Child and Adolescent Psychiatry, 45,* 166–174.

Wilens, T. E., Adler, L., Adams, J., Sgambati, S., Rotrosen, J., Sawtelle, R., et al. (2008). Misuse and diversion of stimulants prescribed for ADHD: A systematic review of the literature. *Journal of the American Academy of Child and Adolescent Psychiatry, 47,* 21–31.

Wilens, T. E., Biederman, J., Brown, S., Tanguay, S., Monuteaux, M. C., Blake, C., & Spencer, T. J. (2002). Psychiatric comorbidity and functioning in clinically-referred preschool children and school-age youth with ADHD. *Journal of the American Academy of Child and Adolescent Psychiatry, 41,* 262–268.

Wilson, J. (2007). ADHD and substance use disorders: Developmental aspects and the impact of stimulant treatment. *American Journal on Addiction, 16,* 5–13.

Wolraich, M. L., Wilson, D. B., & White, J. W. (1995). The effect of sugar on behavior or cognition in children: A meta-analysis. *Journal of the American Medical Association, 274,* 1617–1621.

Wymbs, B., Pelham, W., Molina, B., Gnagy, E., Wilson, T., & Greenhouse, J. (2008). Rate and predictors of divorce among parents of youths with ADHD. *Journal of Consulting and Clinical Psychology, 76,* 735–744.

Xu, C., Reid, R., & Steckelberg, A. (2002). Technology applications for children with ADHD: Assessing the empirical support. *Education and Treatment of Children, 25,* 224–248.

Zachor, D., Roberts, A., Hodgens, J., Isaacs, J., & Merrick, J. (2006). Effects of long-term psychostimulant medication on growth of children with ADHD. *Research in Developmental Disabilities, 27,* 162–174.

Zametkin, A. J., Ernst, M., & Silver, R. (1998). Laboratory and diagnostic testing in child and adolescent psychiatry: A review of the past 10 years. *Journal of the American Academy of Child and Adolescent Psychiatry, 37,* 464–472.

Zentall, S. S. (1985). A context for hyperactivity. In K. D. Gadow & I. Bialer (Eds.), *Advances in learning and behavioral disabilities* (Vol. 4, pp. 273–343). Greenwich, CT: JAI Press.

Zentall, S. S. (1993). Research on the educational implications of attention deficit hyperactivity disorder. *Exceptional Children, 60,* 143–153.

Zentall, S. S. (2006). *ADHD and education.* Columbus, OH: Pearson.

Zentall, S. S., Harper, G., & Stormont-Spurgin, M. (1993). Children with hyperactivity and their organizational abilities. *Journal of Educational Research, 87,* 112–117.

Zentall, S. S., & Meyer, M. J. (1987). Self-regulation of stimulation for ADD-M children during reading and vigilance task performance. *Journal of Abnormal Child Psychology, 15,* 519–536.

Zentall, S. S., & Stormont-Spurgin, M. (1995). Educator preferences of accommodations for students with attention deficit hyperactivity disorder. *Teacher Education and Special Education, 18,* 115–123.

Zigmond, N., Kerr, M., & Schaeffer, A. (1988). Behavior patterns of learning disabled and non-learning disabled adolescents in high school academic classes. *Remedial and Special Education, 9,* 6–11.

Zimmerman, B. J., & Schunk, D. (1989). *Self-regulated learning and academic achievement: Theory, research, and practice.* New York: Springer Verlag.

Index

f following a page number indicates a figure; *t* following a page number indicates a table.